SOCIAL ANXIETY

EMOTIONS AND SOCIAL BEHAVIOR

Series Editor
Peter Salovey, *Yale University*

Social Anxiety
Mark R. Leary and Robin M. Kowalski

Breaking Hearts: The Two Sides of Unrequited Love
Roy F. Baumeister and Sara R. Wotman

Jealousy: Theory, Research, and Clinical Strategies
Gregory L. White and Paul E. Mullen

Social Anxiety

Mark R. Leary
Wake Forest University

Robin M. Kowalski
Western Carolina University

THE GUILFORD PRESS
New York   London

© 1995 The Guilford Press
A Division of Guilford Publications, Inc.
72 Spring Street, New York, NY 10012

Printed in the United States of America
This book is printed on acid-free paper.
Last digit is print number: 9 8 7 6 5 4 3 2 1

Library of Congress Cataloging-in-Publication Data

Leary, Mark R.
    Social anxiety / Mark R. Leary and Robin M. Kowalski.
        p.   cm.—(Emotions and social behavior)
    Includes bibliographical references and indexes.
    ISBN 1-57230-007-8
    1. Anxiety.   2. Self-presentation.   3. Interpersonal relations.
I. Kowalski, Robin M.   II. Title.   III. Series.
BF575.A6L387   1995
152.4'6—dc20   95-32612
                                                                    CIP

To Kevin and Collin
—M.R.L.

To Dad, Mom, Kelly, Jeff, Sarah, and Serena
—R.M.K.

Preface

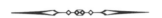

For centuries, people have been fascinated by horror stories. From ancient myths and legends, to early novels such as *Dracula* and *Frankenstein*, to recent books by Stephen King, stories and movies that play upon deep human fears have always been popular. Although we know that the horrible things in the book or movie are not real, we are frightened by imagining what it might be like to be awakened some night by cold skeletal fingers or pursued by a decaying corpse brandishing an ax.

In everyday life, the things that cause us anxiety are much more mundane. We occasionally worry about the safety of ourselves and our loved ones (but more often at the hands of a drunk driver or gun-wielding criminal than a flesh-eating alien), and we sometimes worry about our financial situation or job stability. But our most common fears center around our interactions and relationships with other people. If movies were made about our most common anxieties, they would have titles such as *Stage Fright, Journey to the Center of Attention, Bill and Ted's Blind Dates, Faces of Disapproval, The Fugitive: Running from Social Encounters*, and *Attack of the Butterflies*. Although people rarely give much thought to the possibility of encountering a nightmarish creature from a horror film, they do worry about their dealings with other people.

We wrote the present volume to review the research literatures dealing with anxiety and discomfort in social encounters that have emerged in the past several years. We use the plural, *literatures*, because theory and research on social anxiety appear in the journals of virtually every area of human behavioral science, including social psychology, personality psychology, developmental psychology, psychophysiology, clinical psychology, counseling psychology, health psychology, industrial–organizational psychology, sport psychology, communication, management, psychiatry, sociology, and education. Our goal was to review and integrate the theory and research in these areas.

Readers who are familiar with *Understanding Social Anxiety: Social, Personality, and Clinical Perspectives* (Leary, 1983d) will see some similarities between this and the earlier book; indeed, given that both books deal with the same topic, some points of overlap are unavoidable. But the present volume is much more than an update of *Understanding Social Anxiety*. In the past 15 years, hundreds of studies have been published that deal with social anxiety and related constructs, and several scholarly books on social anxiety and shyness have been published, not to mention books intended primarily for nonprofessional audiences.

For example, research on social phobia, which became a separate diagnostic category only in 1980, has greatly informed us regarding the antecedents and treatment of excessively high trait social anxiety. Similarly, the explosion of work on embarrassment during the 1980s led us to include an entire chapter on this interesting variant of social anxiety. New theoretical perspectives have been offered, refined, and tested, and some degree of consensus reached about the most useful paradigms for thinking about social anxiety. Evolutionary analyses have furthered our understanding of possible adaptive functions of social anxiety for human beings, and research in developmental psychology and behavioral genetics has advanced our knowledge of why some people are so much more socially anxious than others. In addition, much research has focused on specific manifestations of social anxiety that were not recognized or that were rarely studied just a few years ago, such as sport performance anxiety and physique anxiety. Physiological aspects of social anxiety, including blushing, have also received increased attention.

In addition to work on social anxiety specifically, recent theory and research on other topics in psychology have advanced our understanding of social anxiety. Notably, work on self-processes (such as self-awareness, self-esteem, and self-referenced thought), emotion, impression management, relationships, interpersonal interaction, and nonconscious processing has provided insight into the processes involved in social anxiety and interpersonal behavior.

This book was written for three primary audiences. First, it is intended as a review of the social anxiety literature for researchers, therapists, and others with a professional interest in the topic. The approach of the book is quite eclectic, and the material should be as palatable to social and personality psychologists as it is to practitioners.

Second, undergraduate and graduate students in psychology and other behavioral sciences will benefit from the book, and we hope it finds its way onto the reading lists of courses in social, personality, clinical, and counseling psychology. One of the book's underlying themes is that a full understanding of psychological phenomena can be attained only by integrating work across diverse areas of basic and applied behavioral research. Among other things, we hope the book will show students that psychology and the other behavioral sciences are not as fragmented or as conflicted as they often appear once one makes the effort to integrate what the various areas have to contribute to our understanding of a particular phenomenon.

Finally, people who have a personal interest in social anxiety arising out of curiosity or because they are troubled by excessive social anxiety or know someone for whom social anxiety is a problem should find the book useful. We have kept technical discussions to a minimum and explained all specialized terms, and the book is certainly accessible to the educated layperson.

For those who decide not to read further, we hope you are not waiting for the book to be made into a movie . . . although we do think *Fatal Embarrassment* might make a heck of a thriller.

MARK R. LEARY
ROBIN M. KOWALSKI

Contents

------⟨⟩◇⊗◇⟨⟩------

CHAPTER 1

The Stage Fright
of Everyday Life

All the world's a stage, and all the men and
women merely players. They have their exits
and their entrances; And one man in his
time plays many parts. . . .
—SHAKESPEARE, *As You Like It*

ALTHOUGH HIS ANALOGY of the world as a stage is among his best-
known lines, Shakespeare was neither the first nor the last writer to
draw a parallel between the theatre and everyday life. One hundred
years earlier, for example, Erasmus asked, "What after all is human
life if not a continuous performance in which all go about wearing
different masks, in which everyone acts a part assigned to him until
the stage director removes him from the boards?" Later, Goldberg
talked about "that smaller world which is the stage, and that larger
stage which is the world." Sociologist Erving Goffman analyzed
daily life using theatrical metaphors, complete with performers,
audiences, sets, roles, props, and backstage areas.

Although few people would agree that the world is really a
stage or that life is nothing more than a rather long play, the
dramaturgical metaphor contains a grain of truth. Human beings
do, in fact, resemble actors in many ways, and our daily lives share
many features with the theatre. Like an actor, each of us plays many
roles. In one situation, we find ourselves in the role of a friend, in
another we play the role of a student, in yet others we enact the role

of a parent, partygoer, customer, employee, or citizen. As we change roles, we not only play different parts and speak different lines, but we may even change costumes (e.g., wearing different clothes as we play the role of "employee" vs. "tourist"). Like actors, we sometimes arrange the "sets" on which we play out our roles and even use "props" to help us play our parts more effectively.

Furthermore, like an actor, we feel ourselves to be "onstage" in the presence of certain audiences, but "offstage" when alone or in the company of those with whom we can forgo our lines and completely be ourselves. And, just as actors in the theatre sometimes experience stage fright before or during their performances, we, too, sometimes get the jitters as we grace the stage of everyday life.

This book is about the "stage fright" of everyday life—those feelings of nervousness, self-consciousness, uncertainty, and dread that we sometimes experience before and during encounters with other people. People experience anxiety in a variety of social situations, ranging from important, meaningful encounters to mundane, seemingly trivial ones. People may feel nervous in job interviews, on dates, in interactions with their superiors, while speaking or performing in public, when leading a meeting, or in casual conversations with strangers. Sometimes their unease is only a minor annoyance, merely detracting from their enjoyment of a social encounter; at other times, people may be so anxious that they are unable to function normally and may even flee the stressful situation.

These feelings of anxiety in social settings are quite common. Virtually everybody experiences social anxiety at least occasionally, and some people experience such feelings frequently. Who has never experienced "butterflies" before addressing a large audience, blushed after commiting a *faux pas*, or felt bashful while trying to carry on a stilted conversation with new acquaintances?

Between 11% and 37% (depending on the study) of college students report feeling nervous while interacting with people of the other sex (Arkowitz, Hinton, Perl, & Himadi, 1978; Borkovec, Stone, O'Brien, & Kaloupek, 1974; Glass, Gottman, & Shmurak, 1976). At least 20% report an excessively high degree of apprehension about public speaking (McCroskey, 1970, 1977; Pollard & Henderson, 1988), and this does not include people who feel only mildly anxious when speaking in public. Similarly, musicians and other performers commonly experience stage fright; even among relatively elite symphony and opera musicians, 24% reported that stage fright was a problem (Fishbein, Middlestadt, Ottati, Strauss, & Ellis, 1988). All told, over 90% of Americans indicate that they sometimes feel shy (Zimbardo, 1977). At least 2% are so distressed in social encounters that their reactions can be characterized as social phobic (Pollard & Henderson, 1988).

Although most research on social anxiety has been conducted in North America, Europe, and Australia, social anxiety is by no means a uniquely Western phenomenon. Cross-cultural research shows that social anxiety occurs in all cultures that have been studied, and that the prevalence of social phobia is at least as high in other cultures (including non-Western countries such as India, Japan, and Saudi Arabia) as it is in the United States (Chaleby, 1987; Hansford & Hattie, 1982; Ishiyama, 1984; Karno et al., 1989; Takahashi, 1989).

Feelings of discomfort in social encounters are so common that we typically don't even stop to ask ourselves the most basic question about them: What is so scary about certain social situations that people often feel uncomfortable when in them? We can easily understand why people are sometimes afraid of threats to their physical well-being—afraid, for example, when they come upon a poisonous snake in the woods or witness an approaching tornado. We can also see why people are sometimes afraid of other individuals who have some potential to hurt them—the ex-convict who lives next door or the disagreeable boss who's trimming the size of the company staff. But why are we afraid of perfectly ordinary people in otherwise normal interactions? Where do such feelings come from and what purpose, if any, do they serve? Why are such feelings associated with awkward and disrupted behavior, and what can be done to reduce exceptionally high levels of social anxiety?

This book attempts to answer such questions, drawing upon theory and research from many domains of behavioral science. We will draw upon social psychology as we examine the situational factors that cause feelings of social anxiety, personality psychology to inform us about individual differences in social anxiety, and developmental psychology to address the question of why some people grow up to be socially anxious. We will turn to psycho-physiological research to explore the physiological underpinnings of social anxiety, and to evolutionary psychology for insight into why human beings developed the capacity to feel socially anxious. We consult communication research to understand communication apprehension, sport psychology to examine sport performance and physique anxiety, and educational psychology to elucidate the causes of test anxiety. We will also explore the work of researchers in clinical psychology, counseling psychology, and psychiatry who have studied various treatments for excessively high social anxiety. Only by drawing upon the work of behavioral researchers from these varied domains can we fully understand the complex and multifaceted phenomenon known as social anxiety.

A DEFINITION

People become anxious about many things, only some of which involve social situations or other people. Numerous studies have attempted to identify basic types of fear-producing situations, trying to reduce a nearly infinite number of frightening stimuli to a few basic categories. Although the particular dimensions differ slightly from study to study, at least one category of "social" or "inter-personal" anxieties has been obtained in each study (H. D. Bates, 1971; Bernstein & Allen, 1969; Braun & Reynolds, 1969; Endler, Hunt, & Rosenstein, 1962; Landy & Gaupp, 1971; L. C. Miller, Barrett, Hampe, & Noble, 1972; Neiger, Atkinson, & Quarrington, 1981; Strahan, 1974).

Given that people feel anxious for a variety of reasons, we must distinguish social anxiety from anxieties arising from nonsocial sources. It is not accurate to conclude that all instances of anxiety that occur in interactions with others or that are caused by other people reflect social anxiety. If you are anxious because you are being followed by a street gang or because you think the pilot of your flight is intoxicated, other people are causing your anxiety, but we would not characterize your feelings as *social* anxiety.

A great deal can be learned about the nature of social anxiety by examining the kinds of interpersonal situations that are most likely to cause people to feel anxious. D. Russell, Cutrona, and

Jones (1986) asked university students to describe the situations that caused them to feel shy. Strangers and authority figures were most likely to cause such feelings, reported by nearly 80% of the respondents. Other common anxiety-eliciting situations included public performances (such as giving speeches), meeting new people, embarrassing situations, heterosexual risks (such as asking for a date), social functions, evaluations (oral exams, interviews), and impressive people (high status, attractive others). What such situations seem to have in common is that they make the prospect of evaluation by other people salient.

Holt, Heimberg, Hope, and Liebowitz (1992) suggested that the situations that precipitate social anxiety can be classified into four primary categories (see Table 1.1). The most anxiety-producing are situations involving formal speaking and interaction: giving a talk in front of an audience, performing on stage, giving a report to a group, speaking up at a meeting, and the like. A second category of situations that induce social anxiety involves informal speaking and interaction. This category includes situations such as going to a party, meeting strangers, and trying to pick up someone (e.g., at a bar). Third, interactions requiring assertive behavior (expressing disagreement, returning goods to a store, or resisting a high-pressure salesperson) also precipitate social anxiety. Fourth, people sometimes feel socially anxious when they are simply observed by others while working, writing, or eating, for example. What all of these situations have in common is that they tend to evoke concerns with other people's evaluations of oneself.

TABLE 1.1. Situational Domains of Social Anxiety

Formal speaking and interaction
 Examples: participating in small groups, acting

Informal speaking and interaction
 Examples: giving a party, calling someone you don't know very well

Assertive interaction
 Examples: talking to authority figures, expressing disapproval of someone

Observation of behavior
 Examples: eating while others are watching, modeling clothes

---

Note. Data from Holt, Heimberg, Hope, and Liebowitz (1992).

Specifically, the defining characteristic of social anxiety is that, unlike other anxieties, social anxiety arises from *the prospect or presence of interpersonal evaluation in real or imagined social settings* (Schlenker & Leary, 1982, p. 642). In fact, social anxiety could just as easily be called "evaluation anxiety" (A. T. Beck & Emery, 1985), but social anxiety is by far the more common term. As we will see throughout the book, people have many good reasons to be concerned with how others perceive them, and it is not unreasonable that they sometimes become worried about others' reactions. Social anxiety occurs when people become concerned about how they are being perceived and evaluated by others.

As the preceding definition notes, people become socially anxious not only when they are currently being evaluated, but also when the possibility or *prospect* of interpersonal evaluation exists. In fact, people may worry as much, if not more, about how others are likely to regard them prior to a social encounter as they do during the interaction itself. Thus, people may experience social anxiety even when they are alone if they worry about how others may regard them in an upcoming interaction.

In fact, people may become anxious about social interactions that are entirely imagined rather than real. We may become as distressed about an encounter that we imagine *might* happen as a real social situation. For example, a spectator at a celebrity golf tournament may feel nervous when merely anticipating the possibility of meeting one of his or her favorite stars. Other people need not actually be present, except in the person's mind.

THE EXPERIENCE OF SOCIAL ANXIETY

Chances are you've had firsthand experience with what it's like to be socially anxious, although you may not have used that term to describe your feelings. If you think about it, you may see that anxiety generally entails four distinct, though obviously interrelated, experiences reflecting cognitive, somatic, behavioral, and affective aspects (e.g., Fremouw, Gross, Monroe, & Rapp, 1982; Lehrer & Woolfolk, 1982).

First, by definition, anxiety involves apprehensive thoughts or cognitions. When anxious, people dwell on the awful things they are currently experiencing or that they might experience in the future. For example, a socially anxious man interacting with a woman may think things such as "I bet she thinks I'm a geek" or "I wish I could get out of here." A person waiting to give a speech to a large audience may ruminate about how ill-prepared he or she is and worry about what others will think of his or her performance.

Second, anxiety is accompanied by somatic symptoms—physical reactions such as sweaty palms and increased heart rate. As we will explore in detail in Chapter 7, anxiety is mediated by the sympathetic nervous system, the portion of the nervous system that prepares us to deal with threats to our well-being. When the sympathetic nervous system is activated, heart rate, respiration, and muscular tension increase, digestion slows (sometimes producing a nauseated feeling), and sweat pores open. Together, these and other reactions prepare individuals to meet threats to their well-being.

Third, behaviorally, anxiety is typically accompanied by attempts to avoid or escape the anxiety-producing situation. The person may or may not act on the urge to flee, but the tendency certainly increases. In the case of social anxiety, people may withdraw either by participating less in ongoing interactions or by actually leaving the social situation altogether. We will deal with the behavioral concomitants of social anxiety in Chapter 8.

Although socially anxious people tend to withdraw, there is no necessary relationship between social anxiety and these behavioral reactions. To understand fully the experiences and behavior of socially anxious people, we must maintain the distinction between subjective feelings of anxiety and behavioral inhibition. People who feel socially anxious are often quiet, inhibited, and withdrawn, a finding we will explore in later chapters. Yet, some people may feel quite anxious without showing it, and other people may behave in an unsociable, withdrawn, or introverted manner, but not feel anxious. We shouldn't confuse a quiet nature or a desire for solitary activities with anxious avoidance of interpersonal situations (Leary, 1983b). Although social anxiety and inhibition often occur together, the distinction between them should be maintained.

Finally, anxiety is characterized by subjective feelings that are virtually always unpleasant (although they may be accompanied by other, pleasant reactions). When anxious, people report feeling nervous or tense. Often feelings of subjective anxiety or nervousness are accompanied by other negative emotions, such as anger, hope-lessness, or depression.

Taken all together, then, anxiety is an aversive emotional ex-perience involving apprehension regarding the possibility of phys-ical or psychological harm, increased physiological arousal, and the motive to avoid or escape the anxiety-producing situation. We dis-cuss the cognitive, physiological, behavioral, and affective compo-nents of social anxiety in detail throughout the book.

TYPES OF SOCIAL ANXIETY

We will examine not only research that has focused on social anxi-ety, broadly defined, but also research dealing with particular "types" of social anxiety. Some researchers, for example, have stud-ied what they call *heterosexual–social anxiety* (social anxiety expe-rienced in interactions with members of the other sex), and others have studied the related construct of *dating anxiety*. Researchers interested in public speaking have focused on constructs such as *public speaking anxiety, communication apprehension, stage fright* and *audi-ence anxiety*. Sport psychologists have used the terms *competition anxiety* and *sport performance anxiety* to refer to anxiety experienced while playing sports, and *physique anxiety* to refer to anxiety that arises from concerns with others' evaluations of one's body. *Test anxiety* is also sometimes considered a type of social anxiety. Fur-thermore, other research suggests subtypes of social anxiety involv-ing, for example, fears of revealing one's inferiority, being the center of attention, losing bodily control, and having to assert one-self (Dixon, de Monchaux, & Sandler, 1957).

Don't let the number and variety of these terms blind you to the fact that they all refer to essentially the same psychological reaction—social anxiety. In fact, referring to these experiences as different "types" of anxiety is a bit misleading. What differs among these constructs is not so much the experience of anxiety as the social context in which the anxiety occurs. If social anxiety is ex-perienced on a date, we might call it dating anxiety, whereas if social anxiety is experienced while speaking in public, we might call it speech anxiety or stage fright. But using different terms obscures the fact that each refers to essentially the same experience.

If carried to an extreme, we could identify a virtually endless number of types of social anxiety, leading to a proliferation of terms such as "attractive people anxiety," "talking-to-the-boss-before-raises-are-announced anxiety," "being-naked-in-the-locker-room anxiety," and "having-Happy-Birthday-sung-to-you anxiety." Although an endless list of types of social anxiety is unneccessary, we find it useful to make two distinctions among the conditions that precipitate social anxiety.

First, some instances of social anxiety are anticipatory, whereas others are reactive. That is, people may be anxious either because of a situation that might arise (anticipatory) or because of an event that has already occurred (reactive). We may be distressed either because we might forget our lines in a play or because we've already flubbed our part. Most writers have used the term social anxiety to refer to the anticipatory variety only, but the reactive form (which we popularly call embarrassment) involves social anxiety as well. We will return to the anticipatory–reactive distinction and to the topic of embarrassment at various points (particularly Chapter 5).

A second distinction involves whether social anxiety is experienced in a contingent or a noncontingent encounter (cf. E. E. Jones & Gerard, 1967). As we will see in later chapters, whether an encounter is contingent or noncontingent has implications for both the factors that precipitate social anxiety and for the anxious person's response in such situations. In a contingent encounter, people's behaviors are highly dependent, or contingent, on the behavior of others. In an ordinary conversation, for example, people are expected to tailor their behavior to the responses of other interactants.

In noncontingent encounters, by contrast, people's behaviors are based less on the reactions of others who are present and more on their own script or agenda. A person giving a prepared speech, performing a piano recital, or acting in a play is in a noncontingent encounter. The person's behavior in the situation is more or less predetermined and, assuming everything goes as planned (the audience does not begin to boo or throw things), only minimally responsive to the behavior of others who are present.

A construct that is closely related to and often confused with social anxiety is shyness. As we use the term, shyness is an "affec-

tive-behavioral syndrome characterized by social anxiety and interpersonal inhibition that results from the prospect or presence of
interpersonal evaluation" (Leary, 1986a, p. 30). That is, if a person
is both socially anxious *and* inhibited (withdrawn, reticent, unsociable) in a particular situation, we characterize his or her behavior
as "shy." Thus, we do not regard shyness as a type of social anxiety
per se (Buss, 1980; Leary & Schlenker, 1981), but rather as subjective social anxiety paired with behavioral avoidance or inhibition.

Although social anxiety and shyness are not identical, research
on shyness sheds a great deal of light on social anxiety, particularly
if researchers measure how shy subjects *feel* (see W. H. Jones,
Cheek, & Briggs, 1986). We caution, however, that although the
most commonly used definitions of shyness are consistent with
ours (that is, a combination of subjective anxiety and behavioral
inhibition; e.g., Cheek & Buss, 1981; Crozier, 1979; W. H. Jones,
Briggs, & Smith, 1986), not all researchers have defined shyness in
this way. Some researchers define shyness solely in terms of behavioral inhibition or timidity, irrespective of whether evidence of
subjective anxiety is present (Pilkonis, 1977b; Reznick, Gibbons,
Johnson, & McDonough, 1989). Shyness research that deals only
with inhibited behavior is less relevant to understanding social
anxiety than shyness research that also examines anxious feelings.

INDIVIDUAL DIFFERENCES

Although virtually everyone occasionally experiences social anxiety,
people differ widely in how often they feel socially anxious. Some
people feel socially anxious only rarely (if at all), whereas others feel
nervous in a great many of their dealings with others.

Given that some people are characteristically more socially
anxious than others, we can regard the tendency to experience social
anxiety as a personality trait or disposition (Crozier, 1979). Several
measures of trait social anxiety (sometimes called dispositional social anxiety or social anxiousness) have been developed to assess
differences among individuals along this dimension, and a great
deal of research has examined how people scoring low versus high
in trait anxiety differ from one another (see Leary, 1991, for a
review of these measures). We will deal with individual differences

in trait social anxiety throughout the book and devote all of Chapter 6 to this topic.

At the extreme, some people are so troubled by feelings of anxiety in interpersonal situations that they can be diagnosed as social phobic according to psychiatric criteria. The difference between a normal degree of anxiety and a *clinical fear* or *phobia* rests on several criteria. If a person is phobic, his or her level of anxiety is out of proportion to the degree of threat that is really present, yet, though the person may realize this, the intense feelings of anxiety cannot be reasoned away. Phobias lead the person to avoid the feared situation (and, thus, are typically maladaptive), and they persist over an extended period of time, usually for many years (see Marks, 1969; L. C. Miller, Barrett, & Hampe, 1974).

According to the fourth edition of the *Diagnostic and Statistical Manual of Mental Disorders* (DSM-IV), people are labeled social phobic when they manifest

> a marked and persistent fear of one or more social or performance situations in which the person is exposed to unfamiliar people or to possible scrutiny by others. The individual fears that he or she will act in a way (or show anxiety symptoms) that will be humiliating or embarrassing. . . . (American Psychiatric Association, 1994, p. 411)

When people who are social phobic are exposed to the feared social situations, they almost invariably experience anxiety, often anxiety that is intense enough to be characterized as a panic attack. For a person to receive a diagnosis of social phobia (also called *social anxiety disorder*), the person's anxiety must be so extreme that it interferes markedly with the person's daily life, occupational or academic functioning, social life, or relationships, or otherwise becomes very troubling to the person.

One interesting feature of social phobia that distinguishes it from other clinical anxiety syndromes is that social fears are, in one sense, more reasonable than many of the other things about which people are commonly phobic (Beck & Emery, 1985). A person who panics when thunderstorms approach, who is afraid of heights, or who refuses to ride in elevators is, in reality, in very little danger of being hit by lightning, falling from a high place, or being in an elevator crash. In contrast, a social phobic person may reasonably be concerned about being evaluated in undesired ways; the probability of experiencing distressing interpersonal difficulties is much greater than becoming a human lightning rod, plummeting to one's death, or being maimed in an elevator accident. Social phobics certainly overestimate the frequency and severity of experiencing interpersonal difficulties, but their worries are, in many ways, more realistic than those of many other phobics.

Studies show that approximately 2% of the adult population of the United States are so chronically nervous in social situations that they can be characterized as social phobic, but some experts suggest that the actual incidence may be higher (Heimberg, Dodge, & Becker, 1987). The lifetime prevalence (the percentage of people who experience symptoms of social phobia during their lives) is between 3% and 13% (American Psychiatric Association, 1994).

In brief, like most personality characteristics, trait social anxiety is normally distributed, with most people experiencing moderate levels of anxiety in particular social situations only occasionally. Relatively few people fall at the extremes, either experiencing no anxiety at all or experiencing intense anxiety so frequently that they may be classified as social phobic.

BEHAVIORAL SCIENCE AND SOCIAL ANXIETY

Given the pervasiveness of social anxiety and the degree to which it constitutes a significant problem for many people, you might imagine that behavioral researchers, particularly psychologists, would have attacked the topic long ago. On the contrary, scientific research into social anxiety is relatively recent.

Darwin was among the first to systematically address topics such as shyness, embarrassment, and blushing. In writing about social anxiety in *The Expression of the Emotions in Man and Animals*, Darwin (1872/1955) noted that "shyness . . . is closely related to fear; yet it is distinct from fear in the ordinary sense. A shy man no doubt dreads the notice of strangers, but can hardly be said to be afraid of them; he may be as bold as a hero in battle, yet have no self-confidence about trifles in the presence of strangers" (p. 330).

The Japanese philosopher Yoritomo-Tashi (1915) also dealt extensively with social anxiety and embarrassment. In his teachings,

Yoritomo not only presaged contemporary perspectives on social anxiety, but offered what was essentially a cognitive-behavioral model for overcoming excessive anxiety and timidity in social situations.

The earliest empirical research on social anxiety emerged in the context of developing and validating early inventories to measure the basic dimensions of personality (e.g., Cattell, 1946; Comrey, 1965; Guilford & Guilford, 1936; see Crozier, 1979, for a review). Many investigators independently found that distress and inhibition in social situations constituted one of the basic dimensions of personality, but, with a few exceptions, these researchers did not study social anxiety per se.

The systematic study of social anxiety was fueled by the publication of two measures of trait social anxiety—one in psychology and the other in communication. The Social Avoidance and Distress Scale (Watson & Friend, 1969) provided researchers in psychology with the first freestanding, well-validated measure of social anxiety and stimulated a wave of social anxiety studies during the 1970s. At about the same time, McCroskey's (1970) Personal Report of Communication Apprehension gave researchers in speech communication a measure of communication apprehension that improved on earlier scales (e.g., Paul, 1966), likewise stimulating a flurry of interest in the topic.

Most early work on social anxiety focused on individual differences in trait social anxiety, but dealt little with the situational factors that cause people to feel anxious. During the 1970s, Zimbardo and his students adopted a social psychological approach to shyness that delved into both the dispositional and situational antecedents of social anxiety and inhibition (e.g., Pilkonis, 1977a, 1977b; Zimbardo, 1977). Later, Schlenker and Leary (1982, 1985; Leary, 1983d; Leary & Schlenker, 1981) offered integrative reviews of the social anxiety literature, as well as a social psychological theory of social anxiety.

If one looks at the literature on social anxiety as a whole, four themes can be discerned. One cluster of studies has examined the situational antecedents of social anxiety, trying to address the question: What are the characteristics of social situations that cause people to feel nervous? A second group of studies has examined individual differences in social anxiety and how trait social anxiety is related to people's affective, cognitive, physiological, and behavioral reactions to social encounters. A third collection of studies adopted a developmental perspective to examine the sources of these individual differences in trait social anxiety, answering the question of why some people are more socially anxious than others. A fourth set of studies involves investigations of treatment approaches designed to reduce high levels of social anxiety.

This book examines all four of these categories of research. In Chapter 2, we discuss a theory of social anxiety that provides a framework for the rest of the book, followed by an examination of the primary situational and dispositional antecedents of social anxiety in Chapters 3 and 4. Chapter 5 then focuses specifically on the reactive variety of social anxiety (i.e., embarrassment). Individual differences in trait social anxiety and social phobia are the topic of Chapter 6. Chapter 7 examines the physiological, cognitive, and emotional aspects of social anxiety, and Chapter 8 deals with its behavioral manifestations. The book concludes with a look at the treatment of excessively high social anxiety and social phobia in Chapter 9.

CHAPTER 2

The Interpersonal Basis
of Social Anxiety

———◇◦⊗◦◇———

FEELINGS OF SOCIAL anxiety are precipitated by a large variety of situations. People sometimes feel socially anxious when they meet new people, talk to their teachers or bosses, have memory lapses during interactions, or perceive that others are uninterested or rejecting. They also feel distressed when they do stupid or foolish things, find themselves in novel situations, can't think of anything to say during conversations, or are closely scrutinized by others. Meeting celebrities makes some people nervous, as does being interviewed on television or radio. People sometimes experience anxiety when they speak or perform in front of groups, are called on in class, take examinations, have sex, compete in sports, or have their pictures taken. The number and variety of situations that cause social anxiety seem nearly endless. The key to understanding social anxiety is identifying the least common denominator of these diverse situations. What do all of these situations share that causes people to feel nervous and to behave in uncertain, awkward ways?

For many years, researchers interested in social anxiety focused primarily on factors that lead some people to be more socially anxious than others. For example, theorists traced high social anxiety to poor social skills (Curran, 1977), negative self-thoughts (Ellis, 1962), or conditioned responses (Wolpe, 1958). Although these interpretations provided viable explanations of trait social anxiety and phobia, they did not address the broader question of why people feel more socially anxious in some situations than in others.

Schlenker and Leary (1982) offered a social psychological explanation of social anxiety that accounts for both the social situations that cause state social anxiety as well as individual differences in trait social anxiety. Because this theory not only helps us to understand the antecedents of social anxiety but also provides a framework for reviewing the diverse literatures that deal with social distress, we examine this model in detail in this chapter.

SELF-PRESENTATION AND INTERPERSONAL BEHAVIOR

Most of social life involves influencing other people and being influenced by them. Although many of us do not like to see ourselves as engaged in a continual struggle for social influence, we spend a great deal of our time trying to lead other people to respond as we would like. We try to get others to treat us well, to reward and affirm our efforts, to do the things we would like, to consent to our requests, and so on.

There is nothing Machiavellian or manipulative in our pervasive emphasis on influencing other people. On the contrary, social influence is an essential and valuable aspect of social life. We simply cannot achieve many of our goals without influencing other people's behavior. Most of what people want can be obtained only by influencing others. Whether people need material goods (such as food, clothing, or personal belongings), social commodities (such as friendship, love, or companionship), or psychological rewards (such as self-esteem, positive feelings, or security), they usually must influence others to respond in certain desired ways. Similarly, most negative events in life—such as rejection, a denied promotion, physical punishment, and public humiliation—occur because of the actions of other people. And, just as we try to induce other people to treat us in desired ways, we also try to influence them not to treat us in undesired ways.

People try to influence others through a variety of means. They may try to persuade them through reason or appeals to emotion, play upon their sympathy, provide incentives for desired behavior, shame them into compliance, or threaten them into submission. One important set of tactics for influencing other people involves self-presentational behaviors. Self presentation (which is also called impression management) involves the processes by which people attempt to control the impressions others form of them (Leary & Kowalski, 1990; Schlenker, 1980).

Self-presentation is an important mode of social influence because other people's reactions depend greatly on their impressions of us. Think for a moment about the potent effect that others' impressions of us have on our daily lives. The impressions we make on others affect the development and dissolution of our personal relationships, including friendships and romantic involvements. In fact, whether we have a supportive social network of friends and acquaintances or are a social isolate depends, in part, on the impressions others have of us. Our public image also affects our job success because the kinds of impressions we make affect the likelihood that we will be hired, promoted, or terminated. Our personal effectiveness depends on being perceived in particular ways (such as credible or honest) and on not being perceived in other ways (such as selfish or untrustworthy). It is not an overstatement to suggest that one's happiness and success in life depend to a large degree on the kinds of impressions one makes on other people.

In light of the importance of their public impressions, people are understandably motivated to control how others perceive them. Such efforts to control others' impressions are not necessarily deceitful or manipulative; quite often people convey impressions of themselves that are entirely accurate. For example, the highly qualified job applicant will make every effort to bring his or her abilities to the attention of the job interviewer. Although obviously designed to influence the impressions the interviewer forms, the applicant's self-presentations are truthful. Of course, people sometimes do lie about themselves, presenting public images that they know are contrary to the truth, but, as often as not, their self-presentations are neither deceitful nor manipulative (Leary, 1993, 1994; Schlenker, 1980).

In most instances, the impressions people desire to create are positive, socially desirable ones. This is because, under most circumstances, people are more likely to achieve their goals when others hold favorable impressions of them. For example, people typically find it more advantageous to be perceived as friendly, competent, and ethical than as cold, incompetent, and dishonest.

Even so, on some occasions, people believe that their goals can be met best if they influence others to perceive them in socially un-desirable ways. For example, being perceived as threatening or in-timidating can be an effective means of getting one's way, and con-veying impressions of weakness and dependence may influence others to be supportive (E. E. Jones & Pittman, 1982; Leary & Mil-ler, 1986).

A great deal of human behavior is affected by the desire to convey certain impressions to other people. Much of our behavior is an explicit attempt to convey impressions that will influence other people to react in desired ways. In addition, no matter what else they do, people generally try not to jeopardize their social images in others' eyes. This is not to say that everything people do is done only for the impressions their behavior creates. However, as we will see, there are few social contexts in which people are entirely free of the constraints imposed by their desire to be re-garded in certain ways and not to be regarded in other ways.

Many studies have documented the ubiquity of self-presenta-tion and its pervasive influence on interpersonal behavior. People manage others' impressions of them not only through what they say (and don't say) about themselves, but through the attitudes they express, the explanations they give others for their behavior, their nonverbal behaviors (including their physical appearance, gestures, and expressions), the connections they draw between themselves and other people, their use of physical "props" (for example, the possessions they display), and the sports they play. People even do things that are hazardous to their personal well-being if they think doing so will make desired impressions. For example, health risks such as excessive suntanning, eating disorders, failure to practice safe sex, and unwillingness to receive cervical cancer screening are partly affected by people's concerns with how other people perceive and evaluate them. Wanting to be perceived as attractive leads many people to maintain a tan or to diet excessively, worrying about being perceived as promiscuous may inhibit people from carrying con-doms, and concerns with personal appearance or cleanliness may deter some women from receiving gynecological examinations (Kowalski & Brown, 1994; Leary, Tchvidjian, & Kraxberger, 1994). (For reviews of research on tactics of self-presentation, see Baumeister, 1982; Leary, 1995; Leary & Kowalski, 1990; Schlenker, 1980; Tedeschi, 1981).

THE SELF-PRESENTATIONAL BASIS
OF SOCIAL ANXIETY

Think for a moment about those social situations that you find most relaxing and enjoyable. Such situations are typically ones in which you have few pressing self-presentational concerns. As long as people believe they are projecting the kinds of impressions they desire to convey in a particular interpersonal encounter, they typically feel confident and relaxed. However, when people begin to think they are not conveying the impressions they desire, they feel tense, flustered, and awkward—in other words, socially anxious.

The self-presentational theory of social anxiety posits that social anxiety arises when people are motivated to make a desired impression on others but are not certain they will do so (Schlenker & Leary, 1982). According to this view, then, social anxiety is a function of two factors: the motivation to make a desired impression and the subjective probability of doing so.

People are not always motivated to manage the impressions others form of them. In some social settings, people are relatively unconcerned with the impressions others are forming. For example, when few outcomes are contingent upon the impressions they make, people are unlikely to feel socially anxious because little is to be gained by self-presentational success or lost by self-presentational failure. When the stakes are higher, however, people are more motivated to impression-manage. Overall, the higher the individual's motivation to convey certain desired impressions, the more likely he or she is to experience social anxiety.

Although necessary, self-presentational motivation alone is not sufficient to cause social anxiety. People will not feel socially anxious if they believe they will successfully convey the impressions they desire to make (and, thus, expect to influence others to react as they desire). Given that people have the goal of making certain impressions, they will feel socially anxious to the degree they doubt they will make those impressions.

The two factors that together precipitate social anxiety are multiplicatively related (Leary, 1983d). Expressed symbolically,

$$SA = f[M \times (1 - p)],$$

where *SA* is the level of social anxiety, *M* is the level of motivation to make a desired impression, and *p* is the the subjective probability of making the impressions the individual desires.

As can be seen from this formula, if either $M = 0$ (self-presentational motivation is zero) or $p = 1$ (the person's subjective probability of making the desired impression is certainty, or 1.00), social anxiety should not occur. However, when *M* is greater than zero and *p* is less than 1.00, social anxiety increases with increases in *M* and decreases in *p*. In other words, as the motivation to make a desired impression increases and the subjective probability of making that impression decreases, social anxiety should increase.

The worst possible situation, from a self-presentational perspective, is one in which the individual's motivation to make a desired impression is sky-high, but events have occurred that lead the person to believe the probability of making the impression is zero. Imagine being interviewed for one's "dream job" and suddenly realizing that one's imprudent response has led the interviewer to regard one as an incompetent, insensitive idiot.

A Point of Clarification

Some researchers have misinterpreted the self-presentational theory to say that people experience social anxiety when they do not think they will make desirable or positive impressions on others. This interpretation is incorrect on two counts.

The theory refers not to making a favorable impression, but to making a *particular* or a *desired* impression (Leary, 1983d; Schlenker & Leary, 1982). In every situation in which impression motivation is greater than zero, there are impressions the person desires to make, those he or she does not want to make, as well as potential impressions that the person does not care about one way or another. In most instances, the impressions people want others to form involve socially desirable characteristics, and the ones they do not want to convey involve socially undesirable attributes. For example, respondents indicated in one study that the impressions they most desired to make on others were likeable, happy, interesting, humorous, confident, and attractive (Trower, in press, reported in Trower, Gilbert, & Sherling, 1990). As this list shows, desired impressions also tend to be desirable.

However, as we noted earlier, people sometimes want to convey images of themselves that most would regard as socially *undesirable*. Perhaps they wish to be seen as intimidating or prone to violence to threaten others to behave in certain ways. Or they may wish to appear unfriendly, aloof, or even antagonistic to discourage another person from interacting with them. They may want to appear incompetent to avoid being asked to perform a particular onerous task, or to convey impressions of weakness to obtain nurturance and support (Kowalski & Leary, 1990; Leary & Miller, 1986). In cases such as these, the desired impressions are undesirable. Once we recognize that people are sometimes motivated to convey impressions of themselves that are socially undesirable, we can see that they should experience social anxiety to the extent that they doubt they will make these undesirable (but desired) impressions.

Second, even when people are motivated to make positive, desirable impressions, they do not have to think they will make a negative impression to feel socially anxious. People who want to make a good impression (whatever that may be in a particular situation) will feel anxious even when they think they are making a positive impression if they think the impression they are making is not *adequate* (i.e., good or bad enough) to achieve their goals in the situation. For example, a job applicant may expect to make a good impression on the interviewer, yet feel socially anxious because she is not certain she will make a good enough impression to get the job. Similarly, an adolescent boy may feel nervous not because he thinks his date will dislike him, but because he doubts he can make a good enough impression to really pique her interest.

From the standpoint of the self-presentational theory, social anxiety depends on people's own judgments of their self-presentational success relative to their interpersonal goals. Whether the desired impression is socially desirable or undesirable, and whether the person is, in fact, making a good or bad impression is irrelevant to the theory.

The Reasonableness of Social Anxiety

Viewed from a self-presentational perspective, social anxiety is a reasonable response to many social situations. Given that other interactants' perceptions often have important consequences, it makes some degree of sense that people will become apprehensive at the prospect of failing to make desired impressions on those whom they are, for whatever reason, motivated to impress. The notion that social anxiety is a reasonable response to certain situations runs counter to some views of social anxiety. Social anxiety is often discussed as if it were always indicative of a psychological or interpersonal problem, or at least that it is somehow irrational or maladaptive to experience anxiety in social encounters. In fact, for many, the word anxiety itself has connotations of personal weakness and maladjustment.

There is nothing inherent in the concept of anxiety in general or social anxiety in particular to warrant such a view. In fact, the case can be made that *failing* to feel socially anxious in certain social situations indicates that the individual is maladjusted. A person who is never concerned with others' perceptions nor apprehensive at the prospect of making undesired impressions would likely be a selfish, egocentric, brazen, and highly unlikeable individual. This is not to say that social anxiety never reflects social or psychological difficulties or never creates problems for people. We simply note that there is nothing inherently unreasonable about social anxiety, and in fact, social anxiety may have positive features (see following box).

The Two Sides of Social Anxiety

Given their propensity for focusing on the maladaptive aspects of human behavior, it is not surprising that psychologists and other behavioral researchers have emphasized the negative, dysfunctional features of social anxiety. Social anxiety typically has been discussed as an unpleasant experience that interferes with people's interpersonal effectiveness and that constitutes a personal problem for many people. Socially anxious people themselves are usually described as inhibited, withdrawn, and meek, and as having negative self-images.

(continued)

(continued from p. 22)

Although this view of social anxiety is accurate as far as it goes, the emphasis on the negative aspects should not blind us to the fact that social anxiety has positive features as well. Viewed from another angle, the behaviors of socially anxious people have decidedly positive connotations. People who feel socially anxious are modest, self-controlled, serious, and tactful. They are rarely obnoxious, overbearing, argumentative, bossy, or boastful (Gough & Thorne, 1986). In fact, in the right combinations, the characteristics of socially anxious people may actually be endearing. This can be seen by considering fictional characters such as Bashful (from *Snow White and the Seven Dwarfs*), the cowardly lion (from *The Wizard of Oz*), and Piglet (from *Winnie-the-Pooh*), each of whom is socially anxious, yet quite likeable.

We are not suggesting that social anxiety is a positive experience or that practitioners should try to help their clients become more socially anxious. However, it is not the uniformly negative phenomenon that much of the literature seems to indicate.

THE EVOLUTIONARY BASIS OF SOCIAL ANXIETY

Many psychologists assume that human beings developed the capacity for emotional experience because emotions possess survival value. According to this view, emotions evolved because individuals who had a capacity to experience anger, fear, love, anxiety, and other emotions were more likely to survive and reproduce than individuals who lacked the capacity for these feelings. Among other things, emotions mobilize psychobiological responses that prepare individuals to avoid, escape from, or defend against threats to their well-being.

If emotions conferred an adaptive advantage, prehominids who experienced emotions were more likely to pass their genes on to future generations—genes that carried the blueprints for nervous systems that were capable of emotional experience (Hatfield & Rapson, 1990; Izard, 1977; Plutchik, 1980). If this is so, we may ask what function *social anxiety* in particular might have served our evolutionary ancestors and, indeed, what function it may serve us today. Two evolutionary explanations of social anxiety have been offered that differ regarding whether social anxiety evolved as a mechanism for promoting the individual's integration into the group or as a system for negotiating issues of dominance and submission.

The Need to Belong

Human beings appear innately predisposed to develop and sustain relationships with other people (Ainsworth, 1989; Barash, 1977; Baumeister & Tice, 1990). The most basic and notable psychological fact about human beings is that they are a highly gregarious species. They spend a great deal of time in the company of other people, even when doing so has no immediate benefits and may even be aversive. Furthermore, they develop various kinds of relationships quickly, and they resist the dissolution of existing relationships, both casual and intimate (Baumeister & Leary, 1995).

This strong and pervasive motivation to develop connections with other people undoubtedly had immense survival value for prehistoric people, as it does in some places today. Solitary humans are quite vulnerable. Not only are they ill prepared to defend themselves against nonhuman predators and human enemies, but they find it difficult to meet single-handedly all of their survival needs (such as food and shelter). A prehistoric inhabitant of the African savanna who was not inclined to stay with the clan would have been unlikely to survive for long by him- or herself and, thus, unlikely to produce many, if any, offspring. As a result, evolutionary processes selected humans who preferred to associate with other people and to live in groups. Because we are the descendents of the most gregarious individuals among our ancestors, modern humans possess a strong "need to belong." This fundamental motive toward sociality undoubtedly continues to promote the survival of people who live in inhospitable environments and may even serve those of us living in developed societies.

To function optimally, a psychological system for promoting social inclusion must not only provide an impetus or motivation for the person to be sociable, but it must deter people from behaving in ways that would jeopardize their acceptance by other members of their social groups. After all, it would do people little good to want to be with others if their own behavior was so aversive to other group members that they were rejected, ostracized, or even killed (Gilbert & Trower, 1990).

Social anxiety in particular may be the emotion primarily involved in the avoidance of social rejection. Specifically, the emotional distress that people feel when they think they have made undesired impressions may serve to (1) deter them from making undesired impressions in the first place, (2) interrupt whatever they are doing when anxiety occurs (thereby stopping socially offensive actions in progress), and (3) motivate remedial behaviors that repair their damaged images, restore their relations with others, and, thereby, reduce their anxiety (Baumeister & Leary, 1995; Baumeister & Tice, 1990; Miller & Leary, 1992).

An analogy between social anxiety and physical pain demonstrates the point. We would be unable to survive without physical pain to deter us from seriously hurting ourselves, stopping injurious behaviors, and motivating us to attend to injuries once they occur. Similarly, we would have difficulty surviving socially without social anxiety to deter us from conveying images that would damage our interpersonal relationships, to stop behaviors that threaten our images in others' eyes, and to repair damage to our identities that may occur (R. S. Miller & Leary, 1992).

In addition to its effects on inclusion and, thus, survival, the capacity to experience social anxiety may have a *direct* effect on reproductive fitness. To the extent that social anxiety prompts people to behave in ways that enhance their social desirability, the capacity for social concern may promote socially adaptive behavior and increase one's breeding potential.

Dominance Relations

Gilbert and Trower (1990; Trower et al., 1990) proposed a slightly different evolutionary analysis that emphasizes the role of social anxiety in negotiating dominance. They suggested that, like other animals, humans exhibit intrasexual and intersexual "display behaviors" that affect their control over breeding resources and op-

portunities. Intrasexual displays are relevant to conveying dominance and status (thereby laying claim to resources), whereas intersexual displays are relevant to appearing attractive to others,
particularly those of the other sex. They suggested that social anxiety may have evolved as part of a system for promoting successful
displays of these types.

Trower and colleagues (1990) distinguished between two different systems that facilitate group living among the primates, including humans. The *agonic* system involves a dominance hierarchy
sustained by behavioral displays relevant to dominance and submissiveness. Through a system of facial, postural, and vocal cues,
animals negotiate their places in the social hierarchy, thereby allowing them to live in groups without having to continually resort
to physical aggression to resolve disputes regarding territory, mates,
and other resources. Without an agonic system, members of the
same species would have difficulty living together.

The *hedonic* system, in contrast, is involved in fostering cooperation among members of the same species. When in the hedonic mode, social encounters are based on sending and receiving
reassurance signals between mutually dependent individuals (rather
than on threat and submission displays). In apes, these signals
involve a wide array of kisses, hugs, grooming behaviors, grins, and
vocal signals. The analogous signals in humans may involve behaviors such as greetings and signs of affection.

According to Trower and colleagues (1990), social anxiety
evolved primarily as part of the agonic system. A heightened state
of anxious arousal alerted individuals to threats by more dominant
members of the group, put them in a state of "braced readiness" to
respond to these threats, and motivated submissive behaviors to
diminish the threat. Extending this perspective to an analysis of trait
social anxiety, Trower and colleagues suggested that

> socially anxious people are locked into an "agonic mentality"
> which precludes them from processing information or recruit-
> ing response repertoires in any other than a defensive way. This
> leads them to perceive themselves as subordinates in hostile
> hierarchies and to utilize submissiveness and other "reverted
> escape" behaviors to minimize loss of status and rejection. (p.
> 39)

An Integration

These two evolutionary perspectives share many fundamental assumptions regarding the evolutionary significance of social anxiety in making it possible for humans to live together. However, they differ in emphasis. Although no data exist to support one approach over the other, we favor the idea that social anxiety evolved as a mechanism for fostering social inclusion and minimizing the possibility of rejection and exclusion. Put differently, social anxiety appears to be more clearly involved in the hedonic system than the agonic system described by Trower and colleagues (1990).

Although encounters involving dominant people often arouse anxiety (D. Russell et al., 1986), social anxiety is also quite common in situations in which issues of dominance and submissiveness do not appear relevant. Furthermore, although displays of dominance can trigger anxiety, so can the failure to obtain "reassurance signals" from those with whom we are interdependent. Thus, it seems unlikely that social anxiety evolved only in the service of the agonic system.

One resolution would be to conclude that social anxiety is involved in both the agonic and hedonic systems, helping us to negotiate status and to promote our inclusion into cooperative social groups. It would not be unreasonable to conclude that a single affective–motivational system could be involved in responses to two different kinds of intraspecies encounters.

Alternatively, one could argue that social anxiety evolved primarily as a hedonic mechanism for fostering social inclusion. The fact that social anxiety sometimes occurs in response to dominance displays and similar social threats may be explained by the fact that many agonistic encounters involve the threat of social exclusion. More dominant people often have the power of social exclusion: for example, to fire us from our jobs, to deny our membership in an organization, to impede our entry into certain social circles, or to banish us from the clan.

In our (admittedly unsubstantiated) view, the most parsimonious evolutionary explanation of social anxiety is that it evolved as a mechanism for fostering and maintaining one's membership in supportive (i.e., mutually interdependent) groups and relationships. Thus, it is involved not only in encounters where dominance is relevant, but in interactions with peers, real and potential romantic partners, and even strangers.

Many people may object to this evolutionary analysis of social anxiety, arguing that it seems ludicrous to suggest that a capacity for experiencing anxiety over a perceived failure to make desired impressions enhances survival and reproductive success. However, one must remember that our evolutionary ancestors spent most of the last several million years as foragers or hunter-gatherers, and that whatever psychological mechanisms evolved did so because of the evolutionary pressures under which these prehistoric beings lived (Cosmides, Tooby, & Barkow, 1992). In the time before modern cultural constructions (such as formal government, education, transportation, and agriculture), solitary individuals were unlikely to survive and reproduce. Thus, evolution selected persons who behaved in ways that attracted mates and facilitated their inclusion in social groups. Because of these evolutionary processes, modern humans have innate tendencies to foster connections with others, pay attention to others' reactions to them, and experience anxiety when self-presentational difficulties are detected (Gilbert & Trower, 1990).

Researchers have found it nearly impossible to garner direct research support for evolutionary theories of emotion and behavior that will satisfy critics of sociobiological perspectives. Even so, an evolutionary analysis provides plausible explanations regarding why people have a universal capacity for social anxiety, and why the experience of social anxiety centers on self-presentational concerns.

IMPLICATIONS OF THE SELF-PRESENTATIONAL APPROACH

If social anxiety stems from the motivation to make desired impressions and uncertainty that one will successfully do so, then any situational or dispositional factor that affects one or both of these components should precipitate or heighten the experience of social anxiety. In other words, factors that affect the experience of social anxiety do so by either increasing the degree to which people are motivated to make an impression on others or by decreasing the subjective probability that the individual will convey the desired impression.

Thus, the self-presentational theory provides us with a framework for organizing and understanding the diverse literatures on antecedents and correlates of social anxiety. In the next three chapters, we use this framework to examine the primary causes of social anxiety.

CHAPTER 3

Self-Presentational Motivation

---◇◈◇---

SOCIAL ANXIETY IS essentially a reaction to real or imagined self-presentational difficulties. An individual in a social encounter is not likely to experience social anxiety unless self-presentational concerns arise. According to the self-presentational theory, such worries cause social anxiety when people are motivated to make a desired impression, but are not certain they will do so. As we will discuss, people who are either unmotivated to manage their impressions or who feel certain that they will do so will not experience social anxiety even if the social encounter is disrupted.

The degree to which people are motivated to manage their impressions differs across situations, people, and time. In some encounters and with some people, a person may have no interest whatsoever in how he or she is perceived by others—that is, his or her impression motivation is zero. As we saw in Chapter 2, when impression motivation is zero (indicating no interest whatsoever in making a particular impression), people will not feel socially anxious. In other situations, people are motivated to have others form certain impressions of them (or not form certain undesired impressions). As impression motivation increases beyond zero, the probability of social anxiety increases.

A variety of factors precipitate or heighten social anxiety by increasing people's motivation to make impressions on others. In this chapter, we examine factors that affect social anxiety via their effects on self-presentational motivation. In Chapter 4, we turn to the second component of the self-presentational theory to look at factors that influence social anxiety by affecting people's beliefs that they can or cannot make the impressions they desire.

IMPRESSION MONITORING

Impression monitoring refers to the amount of thought and effort that a person devotes to the impressions others are forming. In order for people to be motivated to manage their impressions, they must monitor, on one level or another, how they are being perceived by others. People who are not monitoring how they are being perceived and evaluated will not be motivated to control their impressions, and social anxiety should not occur (Asendorpf, 1994). Although impression monitoring is, in reality, a continuum running from no monitoring whatsoever to monitoring that requires all of the person's attentional capacity and cognitive resources, it is useful to distinguish four levels of impression monitoring (Leary, 1995).

Levels of Impression Monitoring

At one extreme is the state of *impression oblivion* in which people are oblivious to others' reactions. When in this state, people are unaware at any level of how others are perceiving them or even of the possibility that others are forming impressions (Leary, 1995; see following box). For example, many of us have become so immersed in a movie or play that we were totally unaware not only of the impressions others might form of us but also of the fact that other people were, in fact, around at all. Only when the movie or play ends do we "snap back" into reality and become cognizant of the presence of other people and the evaluative implications of our behavior.

Although impression oblivion sometimes occurs, people more often monitor others' reactions to them at a *nonconscious or pre-attentive level* (Leary, 1995; Leary & Kowalski, 1990). While devoting their conscious attention to other things, people scan the social environment for cues relevant to how others perceive them. Even when people do not appear to be monitoring or controlling how they are regarded by others (and, thus, might claim that they don't

Are People Ever Free of Self-Presentational Concerns?

We've all met people who say they don't care what others think of them—in essence, that their self-presentational motivation is zero all or most of the time. Given the importance of the impressions people make on others to the quality of their lives, situations in which people are absolutely free of self-presentational concerns are probably rare. In fact, we believe that self-presentational motivation is truly zero in only three kinds of situations.

First, when people are deindividuated, their ability to monitor and control their behavior is compromised (Lindskold & Propst, 1981). People who are caught up in very strong emotions (such as rage or ecstasy) or who are pulled into highly involving situations (such as finding themselves in the path of an approaching tornado or aboard an airplane that has lost its engines) are often in a state of impression oblivion in which they pay scant attention to how they are being perceived by other people. Still, unless the inner emotion or external threat is extremely strong, even people under extreme duress appear to behave in ways that don't convey highly undesirable impressions to others. Indeed, even in the face of potentially traumatizing events, such as the approaching tornado, many people attempt to give others the impression that they are "cool" and composed, even though internally they are experiencing intense anxiety. To the extent that the person is truly deindividuated, however, social anxiety should not occur.

Second, self-presentational motivation is lowered by internal conditions that interfere with self-relevant thought. Alcohol, for example, diminishes self-awareness (Hull, 1981), which may account for why people who are inebriated often seem unconcerned with others' impressions of them. People who are very drunk have diminished self-presentational motivation. Only in sober retrospect are they sometimes mortified by how they appeared while inebriated. Other conditions that compromise the effective operation of the nervous system, such as mental retardation and schizophrenia, can also lower or eliminate self-presentational motives.

Finally, situations sometimes arise in which people are neither deindividuated nor cognitively impaired yet are not the least bit concerned with others' impressions of them. These situations are quite rare, however. If a situation truly engenders no self-pre-

(continued)

(*continued from p. 32*)

sentational motivation, the person will suffer no distress whatsoever regardless of the damage that may occur to his or her social
image. The person will be unaffected no matter what impression
others may form of him or her—as being rude, dishonest, unattractive, boring, shallow, cowardly, simple-minded, stupid, or
whatever. In our view, situations in which otherwise non-
impaired people would not be bothered if others formed highly
undesirable impressions are extremely rare.

We've met a few people who claim that they are unconcerned with others' impressions of them. Yet, in every case, careful probing shows that they are motivated to be perceived in certain ways and not to be perceived in others. For example, imagine
a situation in which you honestly believe that you have no interest
in others' opinions of you. Now picture vomiting on yourself in
front of all of those people. How would you react? Most of us
would feel greatly embarrassed and would want to leave the situation as quickly as possible. The question is why do people feel so
terrible about committing a social infraction if they don't care in
the least how others regard them? The answer is, of course, that
most of us *are* motivated to convey particular impressions of ourselves to others, and the image of a "public vomiter" is not among
them. In many cases we are not consciously aware of the degree to
which we are monitoring and controlling our demeanor until we
find ourselves in an embarrassing incident such as this.

really care how others see them), they are, nonetheless, impression
monitoring. Just as people who are engrossed in conversation easily
detect their name against the backdrop of the hubbub of a lively
party (the cocktail party effect; Cherry, 1953; W. Schneider & Shiffrin, 1977), people who are engaged in other activities can detect
evaluative cues from other people.

In his discussion of the "looking-glass self," Charles Horton
Cooley (1902/1922) observed that

> many people of balanced mind and congenial activity scarcely
> know that they care what others think of them, and will deny,
> perhaps with indignation, that such care is an important factor
> in what they are or do. But this is illusion. If failure or disgrace

arrives, if one suddenly finds that the faces of men show cold-
ness or contempt instead of the kindliness and deference that he
is used to, he will perceive from the shock, fear, the sense of
being outcast and helpless, that he was living in the minds of
others without knowing it, just as we walk the solid ground
without thinking how it bears us up. (p. 208)

When people think *consciously* about others' reactions to them,
they are in a state of *impression awareness.* Sometimes we consciously
contemplate others' reactions to us: What do they think of me? Boy,
what a stupid thing for me to say! Do they notice my hands shaking? I'm really underdressed in this situation.

Occasionally, people are not only consciously aware of others'
impressions, but self-presentation completely dominates their
thoughts (a state called *impression focus*). People can become so
focused on their self-presentational worries that it interferes with
their behavior (Leary, 1995). For example, a public speaker may
become so concerned with the impressions that the audience is
forming that he or she becomes debilitated in his or her attempt to
deliver a smooth, coherent speech.

Public Self-Awareness

Any situational or dispositional factor that leads people to impression monitor should heighten their motivation to make impressions on those present and increase the chance they will become
socially anxious. Several writers have suggested that public self-
awareness—the state in which people are thinking about the public,
observable aspects of themselves—is necessary, though not sufficient for social anxiety to occur (Buss, 1980; Elliott, 1984; Fenigstein, Scheier, & Buss, 1975; Leary & Schlenker, 1981). Because
people who are publicly self-aware are conscious of how they might
be appearing to others, they are more concerned with how others
perceive and evaluate them than people who are not publicly self-
aware (Buss, 1980; Fenigstein, 1979). Conversely, when an individual is not publicly self-aware, he or she is not attending to
public dimensions of the self, nor contemplating others' reactions
to them. Some people become publicly self-aware more frequently
and easily than others. Consistent with Buss's (1980) use of the

terms, we use *public self-awareness* to refer to the state of focusing one's attention upon public aspects of the self, and *public self-con-sciousness* to refer to individual differences in the tendency to be publicly self-aware across situations and time.

The trait of public self-consciousness is typically measured by the public self-consciousness subscale of the Self-Consciousness Scale (Fenigstein et al., 1975; Scheier & Carver, 1985). This scale is a seven-item self-report measure of the degree to which people think about the public aspects of themselves and contemplate others' reactions to them. Representative items include: "I'm concerned about what other people think of me," "I'm usually aware of my appearance," and "One of the last things I do before I leave the house is look in the mirror."

People who score high in public self-consciousness think more about public aspects of themselves, are more attuned to others' evaluations of them, and are more concerned with managing their impressions than people who score low on the scale (Buss, 1980; Fenigstein, 1979; Fenigstein et al., 1975). As Fenigstein (1979) puts it, "A major consequence of self-consciousness is an increased concern with the presentation of self and the reactions of others to that presentation" (p. 75). Thus, public self-consciousness is associated with higher levels of social anxiety. Several studies report a significant correlation between public self-consciousness and trait social anxiety (Cheek & Buss, 1981; Fenigstein, 1979; Fenigstein et al., 1975; Hope & Heimberg, 1988; Leary & Kowalski, 1993; R. G. Turner, 1977). However, this should not lead us to conclude that public self-consciousness and social anxiety are the same thing. People who are publicly self-conscious and people who are socially anxious are both concerned with the public aspects of themselves. However, unlike individuals who are purely publicly self-conscious, socially anxious people become apprehensive at the prospect or presence of others' evaluations (Bylina, 1991).

Although public self-awareness and self-consciousness are associated with impression monitoring and with social anxiety, it is not true that public self-awareness is necessary for either impression motivation or social anxiety to occur, as many have suggested. When people impression-monitor, they often reflect on how others regard *unobservable, nonpublic* aspects of themselves. We sometimes want others to form certain impressions of our intentions, morals, attitudes, interests, or feelings, for example. In fact, we may wonder or worry about what someone who has never seen us thinks about us. In such cases, we are not monitoring or controlling the public, observable aspects of ourselves (i.e., we are not publicly self-aware), but we are monitoring our impressions nonetheless. Thus, although public self-awareness always involves impression monitoring, impression monitoring need not involve public self-awareness.

As we explore in Chapter 9, the literature on public self-awareness, self-consciousness, and social anxiety suggests that it may be possible to reduce social anxiety by helping people learn to focus their attention away from themselves. Although a certain level of awareness of how one is coming across to others is sometimes necessary for smooth and effective interactions, it is often neither necessary nor desirable. People who are unable to enjoy a party because they are constantly wondering about how they are coming across are inappropriately self- focused. It may be possible to help highly self-conscious individuals learn to focus their attention less on themselves and more upon others in social encounters, thereby reducing their social anxiety.

Scrutiny and Conspicuousness

The realization that others are attending to our physical appearance or public behavior can quickly induce impression monitoring, raise impression motivation, and trigger social anxiety. People begin to impression-monitor when others ask about, comment on, or are seen to be observing their features or behavior.

Simply being the center of attention often triggers impression monitoring because it alerts the individual to the fact that he or she is being observed and, possibly, evaluated. It is often difficult *not* to think about what others are thinking when one is the center of attention. (How do I look? Is my hair neat? Do I look relaxed? How am I coming across?) One situation that people indicate is likely to make them feel particularly shy is being the center of attention of a large group (Zimbardo, 1977).

Not only does being the center of attention induce public self-awareness, thereby increasing the person's motivation to make certain impressions, but many people doubt their ability to handle such situations adroitly. The demands of being the center of attention are somewhat different than those encountered in more common contingent interactions. As a result, many people expect to project a less-than-satisfactory image of themselves. Being the center of attention delivers a "double whammy" that sends social anxiety soaring in many people.

THE VALUE AND IMPORTANCE OF HOPED-FOR OUTCOMES

When people are motivated to convey images of themselves, they expect that the impressions others form will affect how others evaluate and treat them, how they see themselves, or how they feel. By monitoring and controlling their self-presentations, people actively try to maximize their social rewards and minimize their social costs (Schlenker, 1980). Thus, the degree to which people are motivated to convey impressions of themselves is affected by the perceived *value* of the outcomes they desire. The more valuable or important others' evaluations and reactions, the more concerned people will be with obtaining those outcomes, the more motivated they will be to impression-manage, and the more likely they will be to feel socially anxious.

At one extreme are situations in which people believe that they have nothing whatsoever to gain or lose as a result of a particular social encounter. Others' perceptions and evaluations of them are of absolutely no concern. In such situations, people should not be motivated to convey impressions of themselves and, according to the self-presentational theory, should not experience social anxiety.

At the other extreme are encounters in which the stakes are very high. In such situations, the consequences of projecting desired images to those who are in the position to reward and punish are substantial. When the value of hoped-for outcomes is very high, individuals are strongly motivated to come across in certain ways and, thus, are likely to feel socially anxious if they are not certain they will make the impressions they desire. Under these circumstances, people are likely to react to even minor flubs with discomfort and nervousness, whereas they would not give them a second thought under other circumstances.

People are more motivated to manage their impressions when they believe that how they are perceived by others has important consequences for them. As a result, people are likely to experience social anxiety and experience it more intensely as the potential positive and negative outcomes they may receive from others in the encounter become greater. For example, a person interviewing for a job that he or she wants badly will be very motivated to impression-manage, and, thus, likely to experience social anxiety. Nearly all of the other factors discussed in this chapter can be regarded as affecting social anxiety by increasing the value or importance of the outcomes people desire to obtain as a result of their participation in interpersonal encounters.

Initial Encounters

Most people are convinced of the importance of first impressions, as exemplified by adages such as "Put your best foot forward," and "You never get a second chance to make a first impression." Research shows that the layperson's intuitions are correct: First impressions are weighed more heavily in forming an impression of other people than information that is received later (E. E. Jones & Goethals, 1972). Thus, the emphasis that people put on making good first impressions is not misplaced.

One consequence of recognizing the importance of making good first impressions is that people are highly motivated to manage their impressions when they meet others for the first time, resulting in an increased likelihood of social anxiety. Meeting people for the first time, being introduced to new people, and interacting with strangers are highly anxiety-arousing situations for many people (Curran, 1977; W. H. Jones & Russell, 1982; D. Russell et al., 1986; Strahan, 1974; Zimbardo, 1977). For example, many college professors, even those with many years experience, report that they become socially anxious on the first day of each new class. Wanting to get the course off to a good start but not having the benefit of rapport with this group of students, many professors worry about making a good impression on the first day. Presumably, if, on the first day of class, the professor faced a group of students with whom he or she was already acquainted, his or her feelings of anxiety would be minimal.

Evaluative Salience

Social settings differ in the degree to which interpersonal evaluation is salient. In some encounters, evaluation is present but implicit, as when it is obvious to people that others are sizing them up for one reason or another. In other settings, the evaluation is explicit, such as when a person is being interviewed for a job or is participating in a public speaking contest. In such situations, everyone present, including the target of the evaluation, knows that an evaluation is occurring. In yet other cases, it appears that interactants are not evaluating one another at all.

Whether implicit or explicit, evaluative overtones increase the person's desire to project certain images to the evaluators. Because evaluation by others carries the potential for positive and negative outcomes, people should be concerned with the impressions others are forming and, thus, more likely to feel socially anxious. A woman who is normally quite comfortable chatting with her boss might become anxious and awkward during her annual evaluation interview with the supervisor. The immediacy of her boss's evaluation makes her more motivated to manage her impressions. Inasmuch as social anxiety arises from the prospect or presence of interpersonal evaluation, situational cues that make evaluation salient should increase the likelihood of social anxiety.

Characteristics of Others

People value the opinions, evaluations, and reactions of certain kinds of people more highly than they do those of others. Most people are more concerned with how they are perceived, evaluated, and treated by those whom they regard as attractive, competent, socially desirable, and powerful than by those with less desirable characteristics. The evaluations of those with desirable characteristics are often perceived as more diagnostic and valid than the reactions of undesirable others. Whose evaluation would you take more seriously—that of a talented, competent, and socially desirable individual, or that of an incompetent, inept, socially undesirable one? Clearly, people place more importance on the evaluations of socially desirable others. Because others' evaluations have effects upon people's self-esteem and feelings of worth, they are more motivated to obtain positive and avoid negative evaluations from desirable than from undesirable others. As a result, they should be more motivated to convey particular impressions of themselves and more likely to feel anxious when dealing with competent, high status, and attractive people.

Another reason why people value the evaluative reactions of competent, powerful, high-status others is that such individuals are often in a position to mediate valuable rewards as well as punishments. Employers, teachers, supervisors, and others in positions of authority are likely to bestow positive outcomes upon those who suitably impress them and negative outcomes upon those who do not. Thus, it is not surprising that people are often concerned about how they are being perceived and evaluated by authority figures.

One personal characteristic that commonly precipitates or exacerbates social anxiety in our culture is the gender of the other interactant. A high proportion of Americans report that they are often uncomfortable interacting with those of the other gender (Arkowitz et al., 1978; Glass et al., 1976; Zimbardo, 1977). Viewed from the self-presentational perspective, it is easy to see why cross-gender encounters are anxiety arousing (at least for heterosexuals). In a society that emphasizes male–female relationships, sex appeal, and heterosexuality, those of the other gender are in the position to mediate valued social rewards. When people make appropriate impressions upon those of the other gender, they are likely to receive self-affirming feedback indicating that they are socially and/or sexually desirable. In addition, success in one's heterosocial dealings demonstrates one's social worth to onlookers; in some circles, a major benefit of attracting members of the other gender is to impress one's own friends. And, of course, being perceived in favorable ways by the other gender has the potential to result in the acquisition of a dating, romantic, sexual, or marital partner, along with the attendant benefits of such a relationship. The emphasis that much of Western culture places on female–male relationships leads people to be highly motivated to make particular impressions upon the other gender.

Number of People Present

People are more likely to feel socially anxious as the number of people present increases. People generally indicate that they are more anxious at large parties than at small ones, and when speaking or performing before large than small audiences (Knight & Borden, 1978; Latané & Harkins, 1976; Zimbardo, 1977).

The self-presentational approach suggests two possibilities for why increases in audience size result in heightened social anxiety. First, larger groups increase people's motivation to make desired impressions upon those present. The interpersonal evaluations of many people have the potential for greater impact upon the individual than the evaluations of just a few. Put another way, it is better to make a good impression, but worse to make a bad impression, on 50 as opposed to 5 other people. Thus, we would expect to find that people are more motivated to manage their impressions as the number of observers increases.

A second reason why social anxiety increases with audience size might be that most people are less confident of their ability to project desired images of themselves as the size of the group increases. Speaking to larger groups, whether in public speaking or semiconversational settings such as parties, often requires the individual to be a bit of a storyteller or performer. The interpersonal skills required in such settings are somewhat different from those needed for more common contingent conversations. Individuals who are comfortable conversing with a handful of others may experience acute anxiety when they become the focus of attention of a large group and feel compelled to "perform" (i.e., tell a story, anecdote, or joke).

Although social anxiety increases with the number of interactants, the impact of each additional person added to the situation has less and less of an effect upon the individual's level of social anxiety. A person at a party with 25 other people might be more likely to feel nervous than if he or she were at a party with 5 others. However, those 20 additional partiers would have minimal, if any, impact upon the individual's anxiety if there were already 200 people at the party. Similarly, giving a speech in front of 20 people may be more anxiety producing than speaking for a group of 10, but the addition of those 10 to an audience of 800 is not likely to have any discernible effect upon the speaker. Research by Latané and his colleagues (see Latané, 1981, for a review) clearly demonstrates this effect. Within a number of quite disparate social contexts (e.g., conformity, prosocial behavior, crowding in rats, tipping in restaurants, stage fright), constant increases in the number of others present had less and less social impact upon the individual's responses. An early study of stuttering showed that speech dysfluencies—presumably indicative of subjective anxiety—increased with audience size (H. Porter, 1939). Reanalyzing Porter's data, Latané (1981) found that, like subjective tension, the stuttering of Porter's subjects fit a decelerating curve.

SELF-IMAGE AND SELF-ESTEEM

Even when people are not directly affected by others' evaluations of them, they are able to *imagine* the kinds of impressions others are forming. People are sometimes as distressed about these imagined reactions as they are about actual ones, even when there are no material or social outcomes at stake. There are at least two ways of interpreting this observation. First, because others' evaluations of us are often associated with real positive or negative consequences, others' real or imagined evaluations acquire secondary reinforcing and punishing properties. (A secondary or conditioned reinforcer is one that acquires its reinforcing qualities by having been associated with other reinforcers.) Thus, we take pride when others view our accomplishments and feel ashamed when others learn of our transgressions even though we may receive absolutely no direct or indirect feedback from them.

Second, people's views of themselves are affected by how they believe they are perceived and evaluated by others (Cooley, 1902/1922). Others' real or imagined perceptions and evaluations have implications for one's own self-concept and self-esteem. If we assume that people generally desire to enhance and maintain their self-esteem, it follows that they will be motivated to behave in ways that will result in real or imagined positive reactions from others. It deflates one's self-esteem to even *imagine* that one is being viewed in undesired ways.

The constructs that make up people's self-concepts may be arranged in a hierarchy according to how important or central they are to the person's identity; some self-constructs are more important to an individual than are others. For example, the construct that one is an "animal lover" may be more important to one's sense of self than the construct that one is "athletic." Although both constructs may be equally descriptive, the individual values one attribute more than the other and considers it more important to his or her self-concept. Although there is no empirical evidence to bear upon this hypothesis, it seems likely that people are more motivated to convey impressions of themselves that are more central to their self-concepts. Using the example above, a person might be more interested in being perceived by others as an animal lover than as an athlete.

Creating the desired impressions (e.g., of being an animal lover) would allow a person to receive the satisfaction of being regarded by others in ways that he or she considers personally important. In addition, successfully projecting a social identity that embodies constructs central to one's self-concept provides the individual with self-validating feedback. It is important for people to receive confirmation that they are the things they believe and desire themselves to be. One source of such confirmation is others' reactions to one's self-presentations. If other people accept at face value the images one projects, one obtains validation for one's self-constructs. Thus, people will be motivated to project images of themselves that will result in the confirmation of important self-constructs. If the self-construct "animal lover" is central to a woman's self-concept, she may wish to convey to others the image of a person who likes animals. When other people comment, "It sure seems you like animals" or "It's great that you give so much time to the humane society," she receives feedback indicating that others regard her as an animal lover as well. Such feedback regarding attributes that are central to one's self-concept is quite rewarding—more so than feedback regarding constructs that are peripheral to one's identity.

Social and Personal Identity

Personal aspects of identity reflect characteristics of an individual that exist independently of other people, such as one's personal goals, morals, and feelings of being a unique individual (Barnes et al., 1988; Brewer, 1991; Cheek, 1989b; J. C. Turner, 1984). Social aspects of identity, on the other hand, are based on a person's relationships with others. Although nearly everyone's identity is based on both personal and social aspects of identity, people differ in the value they place on these identity orientations (Cheek & Briggs, 1982; Deaux, 1992; Triandis, 1989).

Conceptualizing the self in terms of personal or social identity orientations has implications for a person's self-presentational behavior (Kowalski & Wolfe, 1994). Individuals whose identity is based heavily on personal aspects will be less concerned with the impressions and evaluations of others than people whose identities are more socially grounded. Thus, people with a predominantly social identity orientation will be more motivated to manage their impressions and, thus, have a heightened probability of experiencing social anxiety. Any foible by the individual may be perceived as threatening to valued social relationships, and, thus, trigger feelings of anxiety.

As we will see in Chapter 8, feelings of social anxiety may precipitate avoidant and withdrawn behavior. People who feel socially anxious may attempt to avoid social encounters, as a means of reducing the aversive experience of anxiety. For persons with a social identity orientation, this withdrawal may be particularly problematic. By cutting themselves off from social interactions, they distance themselves from the people and relationships on which their identity is based. For example, whereas people with a predominantly personal identity orientation prefer solitary jobs and individual sports, those with a social identity orientation seek jobs that involve interactions with others and team sports (Leary, Wheeler, & Jenkins, 1986). To the extent that impression management concerns (and thus social anxiety) are heightened in the presence of others, individuals with a social identity orientation may avoid interactive work and sport activities, thereby forgoing the very social relationships on which their identities are based.

APPROVAL SEEKING

Certain characteristics of social settings and of people's personalities heighten the degree to which they are motivated to seek others' approval or avoid their disapproval. Because people manage their impressions to a greater degree when their need for approval is high (Schlenker, 1980), factors that heighten people's motivation to seek approval or avoid disapproval should be associated with increased social anxiety.

Situational Determinants

Sometimes people seem not to care about others' evaluations of them, whereas at other times they seem starved for affection and acceptance. For example, recent failure experiences heighten people's attempts to gain approval from others, as does social disapproval and interpersonal rejection (D. Schneider, 1969; Walster, 1965). Presidential candidates are not the only ones to attempt to bolster their social images when they perceive that their "approval ratings" have dropped.

Failure heightens the desire for social approval for two reasons. First, if one's shortcomings are public knowledge, the individual will want to enhance his or her image in others' eyes to repair the damage caused by the failure. Because others' evaluations can have important consequences for the individual, people are motivated to forestall negative social repercussions of failure by improving their tarnished image.

Second, as we noted, people's feelings of self-worth partly depend on others' evaluations of them (Cooley, 1902/1922; Coopersmith, 1967; Mead, 1934). Others' appraisals are a major determinant of how people perceive and evaluate themselves (Backman, Secord, & Pierce, 1963; H. T. Haas & Maehr, 1965; Videbeck, 1960). Because people's feelings about themselves are partially based on how they believe others regard them, people can raise their self-esteem by obtaining positive evaluations from others. Following a failure in which one's self-perceptions of competence, control, and worth are called into question, successfully obtaining favorable reactions from others may lead the individual to feel better about him- or herself. As a result, after having failed, people are often motivated to make impressions that will elicit others' acceptance and approval.

Because people desire approval more after they have failed, they are more susceptible to feelings of social anxiety. Not only are they highly motivated to convey particular impressions, but the failure itself may lead them to doubt that they will make the impressions they desire.

Dispositional Factors

Although the degree to which people desire approval from others fluctuates over situations and time, some people are characteristically more interested in obtaining social approval or avoiding disapproval than are other people (S. E. Berger, Levin, Jacobsen, & Milham, 1977; Crowne & Marlowe, 1964). Because people who are highly apprehensive about being evaluated negatively are more concerned with making good impressions on others and try harder to do so, one would expect a strong relationship between measures of evaluation apprehension and social anxiety. Because people who are high in need for approval or in fear of negative evaluation are more motivated to make good impressions upon others, they experience social anxiety more frequently than people low in approval seeking.

In a study of social phobic individuals, Nichols (1974) observed that the most common characteristic of these subjects was sensitivity to and fearfulness of receiving disapproval and criticism. Similarly, Goldfried and Sobocinski (1975) found moderate correlations between subjects' endorsement of the belief that it is essential to be loved and approved of by others (presumably indicative of a concern for others' evaluations) and trait social anxiety.

People who are excessively concerned about being accepted and approved of by others tend to score higher in trait social anxiety than those who are lower in their need for acceptance (e.g., Ellis, 1962; Goldfried & Sobocinski, 1975). Research has shown that scores on the Fear of Negative Evaluation Scale (see box on page 48) are strongly related to the motivation to seek approval and avoid disapproval from others. Compared to subjects classified as low in fear of negative evaluation, high fear of negative evaluation individuals worked harder on a boring letter-substitution task when they believed that hard work would be acknowledged by their group leader (Watson & Friend, 1969). They also attempted to avoid potentially self-threatening social comparison information to a greater degree (Friend & Gilbert, 1973), indicated they felt worse about being evaluated negatively (R. E. Smith & Sarason, 1975), and were more concerned with making good impressions on others (Leary, 1980). Also, fear of negative evaluation correlates with social approval seeking (Watson & Friend, 1969). Taken together, these findings portray the person high in fear of negative evaluation as highly motivated both to gain approval and to avoid disapproval (Watson & Friend, 1969). Not surprisingly, then, fear of negative evaluation correlates moderately to highly with several measures of trait social anxiety (Goldfried & Sobocinski, 1975; Leary, 1983a; Leary & Kowalski, 1993; Montgomery & Haemmerlie, 1982; Watson & Friend, 1969). These correlations clearly implicate fear of negative evaluation as an important factor in social anxiety.

In an experimental study, participants high and low in fear of negative evaluation interacted with another subject under conditions in which the way to make a good impression on the other subject either was made explicit or was left ambiguous. Whereas subjects low in fear of negative evaluation reported being equally relaxed whether they knew what kind of image to project or not, participants high in fear of negative evaluation felt significantly less relaxed when they did not know how to make a good impression on the other subject than when they did know how to respond. People who are high in fear of negative evaluation appear to become more anxious when they do not know how to make a good impression on others (Leary, 1980).

From a logical standpoint, people's motivation to do well on a task (to obtain social approval) should depend, in part, on the performance of others on the task. When *everyone* performs poorly on a test, little diagnostic information is provided regarding your own abilities. As a result, knowing that others performed poorly should reduce people's concerns with the potentially negative evaluations of others following failure. However, Gregorich, Kemple, and Leary (1986) found that this effect occurs with people low but not high in fear of negative evaluation. When they knew that others

The Fear of Negative Evaluation Scale

Fear of negative evaluation is one of the strongest predictors of social anxiety (Leary & Kowalski, 1993; Watson & Friend, 1969). The original Fear of Negative Evaluation (FNE) Scale consisted of 28 items answered on a true–false response format. Leary (1983a) developed a shortened version of the scale—the Brief FNE Scale—that includes 12 items that are answered on a 5-point scale. The Brief FNE Scale is shown below.

Instructions: Read each of the following statements carefully and indicate how characteristic it is of you according to the following scale:

1 = Not at all characteristic of me
2 = Slightly characteristic of me
3 = Moderately characteristic of me
4 = Very characteristic of me
5 = Extremely characteristic of me

1. I worry about what other people will think of me even when I know it doesn't make any difference.
2. I am unconcerned even if I know people are forming an unfavorable impression of me. (R)
3. I am frequently afraid of other people noticing my shortcomings.
4. I rarely worry about what kind of impression I am making on someone. (R)
5. I am afraid others will not approve of me.
6. I am afraid that people will find fault with me.
7. Other people's opinions of me do not bother me. (R)
8. When I am talking to someone, I worry about what they may be thinking about me.
9. I am usually worried about what kind of impression I make.
10. If I know someone is judging me, it has little effect on me. (R)
11. Sometimes I think I am too concerned with what other people think of me.
12. I often worry that I will say or do the wrong things.

Note. (R) indicates item is reverse-scored before summing. From M. R. Leary, *Personality and Social Psychology Bulletin,* Vol. 9, p. 373. Copyright 1983 by the Society for Personality and Social Psychology. Reprinted by permission of Sage Publications, Inc.

had also performed poorly, subjects high in fear of negative evaluation were more concerned with an interviewer's impressions,
whereas people low in fear of negative evaluation were more preoccupied with self-presentational concerns when others had performed well. This suggests that people who are sensitive to the
disapproval of others are more threatened by the possibility of
negative evaluation regardless of how well others perform.

Given the large number of factors that enhance people's motivation to manage their impressions, it is little wonder that social
anxiety may rear its head at any time and in any place. The impressions that others form have important consequences for the
individual, leading to a nearly chronic concern with making the
sorts of impressions that help to achieve one's desired goals while
avoiding impressions that lead to undesired consequences. However, merely being motivated to impression-manage does not automatically lead to social anxiety. As we discuss in the next chapter,
self-presentational motivation must be accompanied by doubt regarding one's self-presentational effectiveness.

CHAPTER 4

Self-Presentational Expectancies

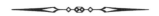

THE QUALITY OF most people's lives would undoubtedly improve if they could always make the kinds of impressions they desire. Wouldn't it be nice to always have others perceive us as we wish—to know that, no matter what, we would never convey images of ourselves that worked against our best interests?

Interpersonal life is not that easy, however. Although we sometimes believe we will make the impressions we desire, we often harbor some degree of doubt that everything will go as we hope. Sometimes we are convinced that we will be perceived in highly undesirable ways. At other times, we reasonably expect to come across well, yet realize that unforeseen events might trample on our social images at any time. Rarely are we absolutely certain that we will make the impressions on others we desire and that there is absolutely no possibility of events contradicting those impressions.

SELF-PRESENTATIONAL EFFICACY

Whenever people are motivated to manage their impressions, they hold an expectancy regarding the probability that they will convey the desired impression. This subjective expectancy is referred to as self-presentational efficacy. As a probability, self-presentational efficacy in a particular situation can range from zero to one.

When self-presentational efficacy is zero, the individual sees absolutely no possibility of making the impressions he or she is motivated to convey. In such instances, as when someone has clearly made a fool of him- or herself, the likelihood of experiencing social anxiety is quite high, given at least minimal motivation to make a particular impression. When self-presentational efficacy is 1.00, on the other hand, people are absolutely sure they will make the desired impressions, and thus do not experience social anxiety.

Of course, in most instances, self-presentational efficacy lies between these two extremes. Returning to the formula introduced in Chapter 2, we see that, holding constant the motivation to make a particular impression, decreases in self-presentational efficacy (which we earlier designated as *p*) are associated with increased social anxiety:

Social Anxiety =
f[Motivation × (1 − Self-Presentational Efficacy)]

Note that, if people are not at all motivated to make a particular impression (i.e., motivation is zero), they will not feel socially anxious no matter how low their self-presentational efficacy.

In this chapter, we examine variables that influence social anxiety by affecting self-presentational efficacy. For ease of presentation, we conceptualize self-presentational efficacy as a function of two types of cognitive appraisal. Specifically, self-presentational efficacy may be low because the person perceives (1) that the social situation imposes an excessively high interpersonal load (interpersonal load appraisal), or (2) that he or she does not possess the psychological or social resources to meet the interpersonal demand (resource appraisal). For example, interactions with strangers may decrease self-presentational efficacy for one of two reasons. On the one hand, because interactions with strangers are typically ambiguous, they are often self-presentationally problematic (i.e., the interpersonal load is high). On the other hand, people who feel they do not possess the social skills needed to successfully interact with strangers also have low self-presentational efficacy, not because the interpersonal load is unusually high but because they appraise their resources to be inadequate.

APPRAISAL OF INTERPERSONAL LOAD

Situations vary in the degree to which they create an interpersonal load on the interactants involved. From a self-presentational perspective, interpersonal load refers to the degree to which an interactant must invest attention, effort, and conscious thought to create desired impressions on others. Some situations are so familiar and scripted that they require little attention or effort. In such situations, interpersonal load is low and, consequently, self-presentational efficacy is generally high.

In other situations, however, interpersonal load is high. Such situations may be characterized by uncertainty, ambiguity, and novelty or by the presence of other people who are perceived as difficult to impress. Because such situations require considerable attention, effort, and conscious thought, interpersonal load is high, resulting in decreased self-presentational efficacy and increased social anxiety.

Uncertainty and Ambiguity

Factors that heighten uncertainty in a social encounter tend to increase interpersonal load and lead individuals to perceive the situation as self-presentationally demanding. When people want others to perceive and evaluate them in particular ways, they seek information regarding how to elicit the reactions they desire. People access such information from memory or glean it from cues in the current situation. Whatever its source, people use this information to modify their self-presentations in ways they expect will produce the desired reactions.

In many situations, people believe that they know how others are likely to react to various self-presentations. When dealing with those we know well, for instance, we generally have a good idea how other interactants will respond to particular behaviors and fostered impressions. A fraternity member may recognize that his brothers appreciate his capacity for consuming large quantities of beer, whereas his parents do not.

In other situations, cues regarding how to make the "right"

impressions are absent, ambiguous, or contradictory. When this is the case, the individual has few clues about how he or she should respond. This seems to be particularly true in interactions with strangers. Strangers have a special power to cause us to feel socially anxious; encounters with strangers cause feelings of shyness and anxiety in a high percentage of the population (D. Russell et al., 1986). Furthermore, people are more often embarrassed in front of those they do not know well and far more likely to blush in front of strangers than friends (Edelmann, 1987; Leary & Meadows, 1991).

When interacting with others for the first time, we typically know little if anything about their personalities, religious and political orientations, likes and dislikes, life-styles, occupations, interests, values, or the kinds of people they like or detest. Without such information, people may have difficulty deciding how to behave, leading to lowered self-presentational efficacy. This may be one reason why encounters with strangers focus initially on gathering information about one another (e.g., "Where did you go to school? What do you do? Married?"). Once the interactants acquire information about one another, uncertainty is reduced and each interactant is able to respond more confidently.

The effects of reducing uncertainty on social anxiety were demonstrated in a study by Leary, Kowalski, and Bergen (1988). Low and high socially anxious students who interacted with a stranger were given one of two sets of instructions. Half of the participants were told to "find out as much as you can about the other person." The other participants were not given any instructions regarding how they should behave. Subjects provided with information-seeking instructions reported feeling more confident and less awkward than subjects not provided with instructions. Interestingly, the effects of the information-seeking instructions were evident even prior to the interaction, suggesting that the mere provision of a script was sufficient to reduce anxiety and apprehension (see also Trentham, Searcy, Jeffcoat, Watters, & Carpenter, 1992).

Uncertainty is also high in interactions that are ambiguous or unstructured. In such situations, the "rules" regarding how to behave are not immediately obvious (Phillips, 1968; Pilkonis, 1977a;

Trentham et al., 1992). When people are sure how to act in a given social encounter, they should not worry that they might convey an undesired impression by behaving inappropriately. However, situational ambiguity increases interpersonal load and reduces self-presentational efficacy.

Uncertainty may occur when other interactants break implicit rules of social behavior, casting everyone present into the position of having to figure out how best to proceed. When others behave in an unexpected or socially inappropriate fashion, everyone in the encounter is spun into an ambiguous situation. When one participant says or does something inappropriate, such as unknowingly making a remark offensive to another interactant (e.g., telling a joke about homosexuals in the presence of a lesbian), others present may become uneasy because they do not know how to respond without complicating the situation (Goffman, 1967). Should they ignore the impropriety? Should they dismiss it with a laugh or lighthearted remark? Should they call the offending individual to account for his or her action? Uncertain about how to respond without conveying an undesired impression, people in such a situation may feel socially anxious (R. S. Miller, 1986). In fact, these kinds of awkward, stilted interactions are a primary cause of social discomfort (Parrott, Sabini, & Silver, 1988). One could imagine being seated near former President George Bush when, at a state dinner in Japan, Mr. Bush vomited. One's uncertainty about how to respond to the pale, faint President would likely cause awkwardness, concerns about doing the wrong thing, and social anxiety. A similar concern about the appropriateness of one's response leads to social anxiety in interactions with physically challenged people (see box on page 55).

Uncertainty is a much greater problem in contingent than noncontingent encounters. As we discussed in Chapter 1, contingent encounters are interactions in which a person modifies his or her behavior on the basis of what others say and do. In noncontingent encounters, on the other hand, what a person says and does is not contingent on others' actions but rather stems from a prepared plan or script. In most (but not all) noncontingent social settings—such as plays, speeches, concerts, and other public performances before audiences—people's actions are guided by explicit plans, whether they are speeches, scripts, or musical scores. These prepared scripts are generally not open to extensive revision during the course of the performance. As a result, people in noncontingent encounters are unlikely to have doubts about how they should behave during the encounter itself, and interpersonal load is low. (They may, however, doubt their ability to execute the script successfully, as we discuss below.) Uncertainty in a noncontingent encounter results only if the performer forgets part of a memorized script or attempts to ad-lib or improvise.

Stigma and Social Anxiety

Most people feel uncomfortable interacting with people who are physically challenged, disfigured, or possess other physical stigmas, such as an amputated limb, severe acne, chemotherapy-induced hair loss, or prominent scars. They not only show signs of being nervous, but often end encounters with stigmatized people sooner than they otherwise would (Comer & Piliavin, 1972; Kleck, Ono, & Hastorf, 1966). People will even avoid interacting with disabled people if they can do so without appearing to be rejecting (M. L. Snyder, Kleck, Strenta, & Mentzer, 1979).

In large part, the discomfort people feel in interactions with stigmatized others appears to be due to uncertainty about how to behave. Most people have limited experience with disabled people and with the norms regarding how to act around them. Should you openly acknowledge the stigma or pretend it's not there? Should you help the paralyzed person with his or her wheelchair, or offer the infirm companion your arm as you cross the street? How should you react to the individual's self-deprecating humor about his or her condition? Are you conveying your discomfort by obviously avoiding looking at the stigma? Without knowing how best to respond, people may worry about offending the stigmatized person and conveying an undesired impression to boot.

At the same time, the person with a physical stigma may experience social anxiety as well. Not only may the person worry about how his or her condition may affect others' impressions (Kowalski & Chapple, 1994), but he or she may also be uncertain about how to act so as to make encounters with others as normal and relaxed as possible.

In noncontingent encounters, uncertainty about how best to respond occurs *before* the encounter actually begins, while the plan is being devised. For example, a person preparing a speech may not be sure of the best way to influence his audience and may feel apprehensive while writing the text. Having written the speech, however, there should be no uncertainty about how to act, although, again, the speaker may doubt that the speech will be well-received. In contrast, because people in a contingent encounter modify their behavior on the basis of what other interactants say and do, uncertainty about how to respond at any given moment is more likely, interpersonal load is high, and the probability of social anxiety increases.

Situational and Role Novelty

Interpersonal load is also high in novel situations (Buss, 1980; W. H. Jones & Russell, 1982; G. M. Phillips, 1968; Pilkonis, 1977a; Trentham et al., 1992; Zimbardo, 1977). Unsure of how to respond in a new situation, an individual's self-presentational efficacy is likely to be low.

Typically, people report that new situations, such as a first date or the first day on a new job, are particularly anxiety arousing. Viewed in light of the self-presentational theory, this is not surprising. When in novel situations, people have few guidelines about how to respond. The vague prescription "When in Rome, do as the Romans do" is of some help, but the individual mimicking others is not likely to hold high expectations of creating a desired impression (see following box). Uncertainty about how to respond raises a person's doubts about his or her ability to make desired impressions on others, thus increasing the likelihood of social anxiety.

Role novelty is another source of self-presentational uncertainty. Social behavior is often guided by the roles people play within a given social context. Every person plays many different roles in the course of a typical day: employee, spouse, parent, teacher, club member, friend, supervisor, and so on. Associated with each role is a set of expectations regarding the appropriate behaviors for occupants of that role to perform and not perform. For example, teachers are supposed to attend to the needs of their students, and leaders to provide proper guidance to their followers.

Role novelty occurs when people find themselves in roles they have not previously occupied. When playing new roles, people may be unsure of the behaviors that are appropriate for the role or how to perform the behaviors they perceive to be appropriate. In addition, they may be concerned about their ability to *appear* to be playing the role appropriately. For example, ministers, particularly those who have recently been ordained, are frequently concerned that they will not convey the impressions expected of a person occupying a pastoral role. Many go to extremes to assure that they do not engage in out-of-role behavior that might jeopardize their image in the eyes of parishioners or members of the community. For example, however they might behave in the privacy of their own homes, ministers typically refrain from cursing, rudeness, boisterousness, and earthiness in public. People who do not conform to role demands risk being negatively evaluated and possibly losing the right to occupy a particular role. The uncertainty caused by role novelty may lead people in new roles to experience social anxiety.

Adolescence is a particularly insecure, awkward, and anxiety-ridden period in many people's lives. Studies of social anxiety across the lifespan suggest that junior high school students are more likely to label themselves "shy" than any other group in American society (Zimbardo, 1977). Part of the traumatic impact of adolescence may be traced to the fact that, during the teenage years, adolescents enter a large number of new, adult-oriented roles. For the first time in their lives, most young people get a job, have their first date, take on responsibilities in school and civic organizations and, in general, are forced to behave like adults rather than children. The occupation of new roles, often without sufficient training and preparation, results in uncertainty about how the roles should be performed. Role novelty is not limited to adolescence, however. Any time people take on new roles, they may experience increased social anxiety because their self-presentational efficacy is likely to be low.

Mind Your Manners

All societies have standards of conduct involving behaviors that, although having little or no functional value, are nonetheless expected of all "polite" people. These standards of etiquette specify, for example, forms of interpersonal address, the proper way to eat various foods, appropriate clothing for particular situations, and rules regarding courtesy. People who violate these standards—by belching at dinner or failing to respond to an RSVP— are sometimes perceived negatively.

As a result, people sometimes feel socially anxious because they worry that, out of their own ignorance, they may breach standards of etiquette, leading others to form undesired impressions. People unaccustomed to formal dinners are often uncertain, for example, about such things as which item of silverware to use, whether to eat chicken with their fingers or fork, how to appropriately summon a waiter, and whether to wait for others to receive their food before starting to eat. Similarly, a person who has been invited to dinner may wonder what sort of attire is appropriate, whether to bring a bottle of wine, or how fashionably late to arrive.

People who place a great deal of importance on manners might be expected to experience social anxiety more often when they are uncertain of the rules of proper etiquette. Some people appear unconcerned when they are unsure of the prevailing social norms. Others are mortified by the possibility that they may display "bad manners." The publishing industry has capitalized on people's insecurities regarding appropriate etiquette by publishing dozens of books that teach readers how to deal with situations as diverse as paying condolences, addressing invitations, and eating chicken.

Attributes of Others Present

People often feel socially anxious when interacting with those they perceive as competent, expert, or highly skilled (W. H. Jones & Russell, 1982; Zimbardo, 1977). As we discussed in Chapter 3, this is partly because people are more highly motivated to make an impression on those they hold in high esteem than those they do not.

In addition, highly esteemed audiences often increase the interpersonal load of a social situation because people who are seen as knowledgeable, competent, or skilled are regarded as harder to please. Thus, not only will people be more highly motivated to impress such audiences, but they may also be more likely to doubt they will do so.

Social impact theory deals with the effects of other people on emotion, motivation, and interpersonal behavior. According to the theory, social impact—the effect of others on an individual—is a function of the strength, immediacy, and number of others present. Strength refers to the power, salience, or importance of other people as reflected in attributes such as their status or age. Immediacy involves the physical closeness of others; people who are nearby exert a stronger influence on us than those who are distant. Number obviously indicates the number of people present (Latané, 1981).

Each of these three determinants of social impact can affect interpersonal load and, thus, social anxiety. Latané and Harkins (1976) had subjects imagine reciting a poem before an audience composed of either teenagers or middle-aged adults. To simulate an audience, from one to 16 pictures of audience members were placed in front of the subject. Participants indicated how nervous they felt by adjusting the brightness of a light. Subjects' feelings of nervousness increased with the perceived expertise (e.g., strength) and size (e.g., number) of the audience. Similarly, Jackson and Latané (1981) showed that subjects singing before an audience felt significantly more anxious when they thought the audience was composed of graduate students and faculty members from the music department than when the audience was composed of partially tone-deaf undergraduates.

Although interpersonal load and social anxiety increase with the number of people present, the relationship between number and social impact is what economists would call a marginally decreasing one. As discussed in Chapter 3, as the number of people increases, each additional person exerts less impact on the individual's behavior. Latané and Harkins (1976) found, for example, that subjects reported feeling about twice as tense performing in front of four people as in front of only two, but about three times as tense in front of eight than two. More precisely, social anxiety increased in proportion to the square root of the number of people present.

Coperformers

Although the prospect of speaking or performing in front of an audience is anxiety arousing for many people, the aversiveness of the experience is lowered when people perform as members of a group rather than alone. Among musicians, for example, solo performances engender greater social anxiety than ensemble performances (Cox & Kenardy, 1993). In a field study by Jackson and Latané (1981, Study 2), college students participated in a talent show in front of an audience of approximately 2,500. The number of performers in the various musical, dancing, and comedy acts ranged from 1 to 10, allowing the researchers to examine the relationship between the number of performers in an act and the individual's level of social anxiety. As expected, the greater the number of coperformers, the less nervous each performer felt. As with increases in the size of the audience discussed earlier, more coperformers had an increasingly smaller effect on performers' anxiety as the size of the group in the act increased; although performers felt much less nervous when they performed with four than two other people, there was not much difference in the nervousness of performers performing in groups of 10 versus 7, for example.

An earlier study also demonstrated the effects of the number of coperformers on overt manifestations of social anxiety. A common indication that a person is very anxious is an increase in speech dysfluencies, such as hesitating, stammering, stuttering, repeating oneself, and using an oversupply of "ahs" and "uhs." In a study of chronic stutters, Barber (1939) showed that people stuttered less when they read a passage in unison with others rather than alone. The difference in stuttering between the conditions was quite pronounced: Those reading alone stuttered on an average of 21% of the words, whereas those who read with three coperformers stuttered on only 1% of the words!

When people perform with others, the interpersonal load is diminished because they perceive that the audience's attention is divided among all performers. As a result, coperforming reduces people's concerns that they will personally make unfavorable impressions upon members of the audience. The solo speaker or performer stands or falls on the merits of his or her performance. By performing in a group, the self-presentational risks are generally lowered. Although one's sense of accomplishment for superior performances is diminished somewhat when the performance is a group endeavor, this is more than enough to offset the potential negative repercussions of inferior performances for many people. Not only are the individual performer's weaknesses less easily discernable and possibly compensated for by others in the group, but the blame for an unsatisfactory performance can be distributed among all participants.

An exception to this general principle arises when people believe they are potentially capable of a satisfactory performance, but think that their coperformers are not as skilled, talented, or prepared as themselves. In such cases, the individual may expect that coperformers' poor performances will make the entire group, including him- or herself, look bad. In this instance, social anxiety is not likely to be lowered by increasing numbers of incompetent coperformers.

APPRAISAL OF SELF-PRESENTATIONAL RESOURCES

Once people assess the demands of an interpersonal encounter, they engage in a process of self-evaluation in which they evaluate their probability of meeting the self-presentational demands of the situation. This appraisal involves an assessment of their self-presentational resources—factors that affect the extent to which people believe they can convey the impressions they are motivated to make. Some of these resources involve personal characteristics, whereas others involve features of the social situation.

Self-Evaluations

One's primary self-presentational resource is oneself. People who believe that they possess characteristics relevant to the impression they want to make should have relatively high self-presentational efficacy and, thus, should not feel socially anxious. On the other hand, people who think either that they don't possess characteristics relevant to the desired impression or who otherwise feel uncertain of their ability to convey the desired impressions will experience low self-presentational efficacy.

People become socially anxious when they evaluate themselves unfavorably on important social dimensions. When people regard themselves negatively or believe they will be unable to handle the social demands of an encounter, they are likely to experience social anxiety (Breck & Smith, 1983; Clark & Arkowitz, 1975; Meichenbaum, Gilmore, & Fedoravicius, 1971; O'Banion & Arkowitz, 1977; Rehm & Marston, 1968; Trentham et al., 1992). Whether their negative self-evaluations are warranted is beside the point. Imagined social deficiencies are as likely to trigger social anxiety as real ones.

Socially anxious people generate a greater number of negative self-statements before and during interpersonal encounters. When asked to report what they are thinking, socially anxious individuals say they are thinking about how poorly they expect to perform in the encounter, how negatively they are likely to be evaluated by other interactants, and that they are pondering their social deficiencies (Burgio, Glass, & Merluzzi, 1981; Cacioppo, Glass, & Merluzzi, 1979; Clark & Arkowitz, 1975; Glass, Merluzzi, Biever, & Larsen, 1982; Lucock & Salkovskis, 1988; Pozo, Carver, Wellens, & Scheier, 1991; Sutton-Simon & Goldfried, 1979). There is no way to show that these sorts of self-thoughts actually *cause* social anxiety, but an association between self-derogation and nervousness in social encounters is undisputed.

Several studies have obtained moderately strong negative correlations (in the vicinity of $-.50$ in most cases) between measures of self-evaluation, notably self-esteem, and self-report measures of trait social anxiety or shyness (Cheek, 1982; Cheek & Buss, 1981; Clark & Arkowitz, 1975; Leary, 1983a; Leary & Kowalski, 1993; McCroskey, 1975, 1977; Zimbardo, 1977). Thus, evaluating oneself unfavorably is associated with higher than average social anxiousness. Indeed, parallels can be drawn between the appraisals of individuals high in social anxiety and those low in self-esteem (Frey, Stahlberg, & Fries, 1986). For example, both socially anxious and low self-esteem people are particularly likely to derogate themselves following failure.

Low self-evaluation should result in social anxiety only to the degree that it leads people to anticipate that they are unable to project the social images they desire. In most instances, individuals who perceive some aspect of themselves negatively will assume that others will rate them unfavorably as well. However, *if* people do not think that their self-perceived deficiencies will be detected by others, social anxiety should not occur. It is possible to imagine a situation in which a person with low self-esteem believes that the other interactants in a particular encounter will, nonetheless, form desired impressions. Will the person feel socially anxious? The self-presentational model of social anxiety says "no," because the individual has a high sense of self-presentational efficacy in the encounter despite his or her negative self-evaluation. Thus, self-evaluation is related to social anxiety only indirectly via the individual's assumptions regarding how he or she is perceived and evaluated by others. Similarly, low self-evaluations are related to social anxiety only to the extent that the person's negative self-perceptions are relevant to his or her public image in a specific encounter (Sutton-Simon & Goldfried, 1979). Negative self-perceptions on attributes that are not detectable by others should not result in social anxiety.

The social difficulties of low self-esteem people are exacerbated by the fact that people remember information about themselves more easily when it is consistent with their self-schema (Breck & Smith, 1983; Markus, 1980). Research on memory for self-relevant information suggests that once people view themselves and their social performances negatively, they are more likely to recall incidents in which they performed poorly rather than skillfully and more likely to remember unfavorable than favorable reactions from others. As a result, these easily accessed negative memories serve to precipitate social anxiety in future encounters (Breck & Smith, 1983; O'Banion & Arkowitz, 1977).

Physical Appearance

Despite clichés such as "You can't judge a book by its cover," and "Beauty is only skin deep," people's impressions and evaluations of others *are* influenced by their level of physical attractiveness. Attractive persons are generally assumed to rank higher than less attractive persons on virtually every positive personality characteristic. They are perceived to be more warm, kind, responsive, interesting, poised, sociable, modest, strong, outgoing, socially adept, and humorous than less attractive persons (Berscheid & Walster, 1974; Feingold, 1992). Not only are attractive individuals liked better than less attractive ones, but people also respond more favorably to them. Physically attractive people report that their daily interactions, particularly those with persons of the other sex, are more intimate and satisfying than less attractive persons report their interactions to be (Garcia, Stinson, Ickes, Bissonnette, & Briggs, 1991; Reis, Nezlek, & Wheeler, 1980; Reis et al., 1982). In light of the emphasis placed on appearance in social encounters, it would be surprising if self-perceived attractiveness was not related to one's subjective probability of making a good overall impression on others. After all, why do we go to such lengths to make ourselves look better?

Given the emphasis placed on physical appearance, people who perceive themselves as relatively unattractive may hold a lower sense of self-presentational efficacy than people who see themselves as attractive. They are more likely to doubt that they will create sufficiently favorable impressions upon others and be evaluated and treated as they desire. Because their self-presentational efficacy is low, people who perceive themselves to be unattractive will be more likely to experience social anxiety when they are motivated to make a favorable impression. Self-presentational efficacy is further compromised by the fact that behavioral manifestations of social anxiety may decrease others' perceptions of an individual's physical attractiveness, thereby lowering self-presentational efficacy further (Funder & Colvin, 1988).

Empirical data bearing upon the link between physical attractiveness and social anxiety are scanty and equivocal. On one hand, experimenters, confederates, and trained observers rate shy subjects as significantly less physically attractive than nonshy subjects, and dating-anxious students as less attractive than students who are not date anxious (Arkowitz, 1977; Pilkonis, 1977a). However, Cheek and Buss (1981) found no differences in observers' attractiveness ratings for women classified as high versus low in shyness. Even so, it is clear that people who perceive themselves as less attractive— whether or not their self-perceptions are accurate—tend to be higher in social anxiety than people who view their appearance positively. At the extreme, individuals with body dysmorphic disorder—people who are preoccupied with an imagined defect in their physical appearance—are excessively concerned that others are forming negative impressions based on their physical defect. As a result, individuals suffering from body dysmorphism tend to be socially anxious and to avoid social encounters (K. A. Phillips, 1991).

In American culture, judgments of physical attractiveness are based, in part, on the form and structure of people's bodies. Several considerations go into such judgments, particularly the person's body weight, bodily proportions, and, often, level of physical conditioning (Hayes & Ross, 1987). In particular, being overweight or physically unfit is a stigma in many parts of our society; overweight people are often perceived not only as aesthetically displeasing, but as being lazy or lacking self-control (Brownell, 1991). The stigmatization of obesity is a relatively recent phenomenon in American society; contemporary Americans are far less accepting of those who are overweight than previous generations have been (Rodin, Silberstein, & Striegel-Moore, 1985).

In light of the emphasis placed on the physical body, many people work to maintain a minimally acceptable weight and degree of fitness through dieting and exercise. In addition, people often become distressed about being overweight or out of shape, which is essentially yet another manifestation of social anxiety. Although many people have occasional concerns with their physiques, some individuals are so preoccupied with how their bodies appear that they can be characterized as physique anxious.

Scores on the Physique Anxiety Scale correlate with objective measures of people's physiques, as well as their self-perceptions. (The Social Physique Anxiety Scale is shown in the following box.) For example, physique anxiety correlates moderately to strongly with negative evaluations of one's body, particularly evaluations of one's weight and physical condition (Hart, Leary, & Rejeski, 1989). The negative self-perceptions that promote physique anxiety may be partly accurate. Compared to women low in physique anxiety, highly physique anxious women have a higher percent body fat and are rated as larger by others. Apparently, concerns involving others' evaluations of one's physique may predispose people to be generally socially anxious as well; physique anxiety correlates moderately with trait social anxiety (Leary & Kowalski, 1993).

The Social Physique Anxiety Scale

Instructions: Read each item carefully and indicate how characteristic it is of you according to the following scale.

1 = Not at all characteristic of me
2 = Slightly characteristic of me
3 = Moderately characteristic of me
4 = Very characteristic of me
5 = Extremely characteristic of me

1. I am comfortable with the appearance of my physique or figure. (R)
2. I would never worry about wearing clothes that might make me look too thin or overweight. (R)
3. I wish I wasn't so uptight about my physique or figure.
4. There are times when I am bothered by thoughts that other people are evaluating my weight or muscular development negatively.
5. When I look in the mirror I feel good about my physique or figure. (R)
6. Unattractive features of my physique or figure make me nervous in certain social settings.
7. In the presence of others, I feel apprehensive about my physique or figure.
8. I am comfortable with how fit my body appears to others. (R)
9. It would make me uncomfortable to know others were evaluating my physique or figure.
10. When it comes to displaying my physique or figure to others, I am a shy person.
11. I usually feel relaxed when it's obvious that others are looking at my physique or figure. (R)
12. When in a bathing suit, I often feel nervous about how well proportioned my body is.

Note. (R) indicates that the item is reverse-scored before summing. From "The Measurement of Social Physique Anxiety" by Elizabeth A. Hart, Mark R. Leary, and W. Jack Rejeski, *Journal of Sport and Exercise Psychology*, (Vol. 1, No. 1), p. 98. Copyright 1989 by Human Kinetics Publishers. Reprinted by permission.

Interpersonal Skills

Low self-presentational efficacy may also stem from the belief that one lacks important interpersonal skills. People differ in the degree to which they behave in ways that facilitate social interactions. We all know people who seem to have a knack for responding in a poised and skillful manner. Their responses are appropriate and well timed, they communicate clearly and effectively, and their forthrightness stimulates openness and honesty in others. At the other extreme, we also know people whom others regard as socially deficient in certain respects. These individuals tend to respond inappropriately (if at all) to others, communicate ineffectively, display undesirable or annoying mannerisms, have difficulty holding up their end of conversations, and so on.

Researchers have found that observers rate socially anxious people (identified on the basis of self-report measures) as generally less socially skilled than people who are low in trait social anxiety (e.g., Arkowitz, Lichtenstein, McGovern, & Hines, 1975; Bellack & Hersen, 1979; Curran, 1977; Farrell, Mariotto, Conger, Curran, & Wallander, 1979; Monti, 1982; Twentyman & McFall, 1975). Although a few studies have not obtained differences (e.g., Clark & Arkowitz, 1975), most research concludes that observers perceive socially anxious people to be less socially skilled.

However, studies that have sought *specific* skill differences (as opposed to observers' *ratings* of general social skills) have identified few behavioral differences between high and low socially anxious subjects, and it is not clear that these constitute differences in social *skill*. For example, compared to low anxious people, socially anxious subjects speak less in conversations, look less at other interactants, nod and smile more frequently, interrupt less often, and give more indications that they are attentive to others (Arkowitz et al., 1975; Borkovec et al., 1974; Cheek & Buss, 1981; Leary, 1980; Natale, Entin, & Jaffe, 1979; Pilkonis, 1977a). Whether these findings reflect social skill differences is questionable. In fact, it could be argued that socially anxious people display *more* socially facilitative responses than socially confident people, such as greater attentiveness to other interactants. Perhaps socially anxious people are more skilled as "listeners," whereas less anxious people are more skilled as "speakers" in contingent interactions.

These behavioral data are somewhat inconsistent with the observers' ratings described earlier: Observers report that socially anxious people are low in social skill, but repeated attempts to identify skill differences have come up empty-handed. There are a number of possible reasons for this discrepancy. First, few of the behaviors examined in these studies actually indicate social skill level. For example, a low level of social participation does not, in itself, indicate poor interpersonal skills. In fact, a *high* level of participation may be socially disruptive, as in the case of the overly talkative boor who does not realize the adverse impact he or she is having on others. Similarly, neither a low nor a high amount of eye contact is necessarily inappropriate in all instances; either too much or too little eye contact may be problematic. The available behavioral data simply do not adequately address the question of social skill differences between high and low socially anxious people.

Related to this, Fischetti, Curran, and Wessberg (1977) suggested that skill deficits are not captured by the behaviors that have been studied, such as frequency of eye contact and the proportion of time people spend talking in a conversation. These kinds of measures ignore the reciprocal nature of contingent encounters. Effective social participation requires that interactants both tailor their responses to the ongoing encounter and time their contributions appropriately. Fischetti et al. (1977) found that high and low socially anxious people differ more in the timing and placement of their responses than in the frequency or duration of them.

Another explanation for the lack of congruence between observers' ratings and the objective behavioral measures of social skills is that observers may partially base their assessment of a person's social skill on overt manifestations of nervousness. That is, appearing nervous may connote low social skill. If this is the case, socially anxious people would, quite naturally, be perceived as less skilled.

A final possible explanation is that different socially anxious people have different skill deficits. The failure to detect objective behavioral skill differences between low and high socially anxious individuals shows only that the two groups do not differ systematically on a particular behavior. If each socially anxious individual has a relatively idiosyncratic pattern of behavioral difficulties, skill differences would be detected by observers but not be revealed in the analyses of specific behaviors.

According to the self-presentational approach, social skill deficits affect social anxiety indirectly by leading people to doubt that they have the interpersonal resources to convey desired impressions of themselves to others. Believing that one lacks important social skills—such as a sense of humor, the ability to carry on a conversation without faltering, or public speaking ability—may lead the individual to conclude that he or she is unlikely to make a favorable impression or to be evaluated positively in those social settings in which such skills are needed.

According to this view, the central factor is not a deficit in social skills per se, but a *self-perceived* social inadequacy. Even horribly unskilled people are unlikely to feel anxious if they fail to recognize their social limitations. On the other hand, some socially skilled and poised people may become socially anxious when they doubt that they can handle a particular encounter. People with low self-esteem, for example, may underestimate their ability to deal effectively with others and may experience social anxiety even though they are socially adept. Low and high socially anxious persons differ in their self-perceptions of social skills, with socially anxious people, particularly those high in social skill, underestimating their social skills relative to ratings provided by observers (Curran, Wallander, & Fischetti, 1980). Furthermore, socially anxious individuals are more likely than nonanxious people to assume that even successfully executed behaviors will fail to have the desired effects upon other interactants (Maddux, Norton, & Leary, 1988).

Past Experiences

Every person is his or her own personal biographer, recording—often with embellishments and distortions—his or her experiences in life. People's memories of past occurrences have a major impact on the way they deal with similar events in the future. In particular, people who have had a history of successes in interpersonal encounters can expect positive social experiences in the future, whereas those with a history of social failures (whether real or imagined) may expect negative social experiences. People who have had unsuccessful, punishing, awkward, and otherwise aversive experiences in social settings may then approach subsequent encounters with some trepidation. Such experiences lead people to doubt that they can make the kinds of impressions on others that will result in desired reactions from them, precipitating social anxiety.

Many people can point to a single, specific event that first led them to doubt their social competence. In many cases, the memory of a single traumatic experience remains powerful enough to trigger anxiety when similar situations are encountered even years later (Zimbardo, 1977). One young man reported that his problems with social anxiety and excessive embarrassability began in fifth grade when, in his words,

> "I remember becoming so embarrassingly humiliated I froze and panicked and my face grew very hot when a girl that sat across from me handed me a note and some candy. After this trauma, my peers noticed my vulnerability and teased me and made fun of me which caused me to avoid many social situations and romantic relationships in school."

In other instances, people's feelings of anxiety may derive from a series of aversive experiences over a period of time. For example, a good predictor of whether or not a person experiences audience anxiety while giving a speech is the sheer number of rewarding experiences he or she has had in such situations in the past (Paivio & Lambert, 1959). People who have had a large number of rewarding social experiences are less prone to audience anxiety than those with fewer rewarding experiences.

A mechanism by which previous experiences predispose people to social anxiety in subsequent encounters is classical conditioning. According to the classical conditioning model, fears develop when a neutral stimulus that is initially incapable of causing anxiety becomes paired or associated with stimuli that *are* capable of eliciting fear or anxiety. As a consequence of the stimuli being paired together over time, the initially neutral stimulus acquires the ability to elicit anxiety on its own.

Extending classical conditioning to the realm of social anxiety, we can see how negative experiences in social settings may condition a person to become anxious in similar situations in the future. Although a person may not have regarded certain social settings as unpleasant or anxiety arousing at some earlier time, he or she now responds to such encounters as threatening because of previous aversive experiences. Although no studies have attempted to condition social anxiety in this manner (for obvious ethical reasons), many people are able to trace their social apprehensions to a specific incident in which they had an aversive social experience (Zimbardo, 1977).

BIASES IN ASSESSMENT OF SELF-PRESENTATIONAL EFFICACY

In a perfect world, people would be relatively accurate judges of their self-presentational effectiveness. They would know precisely how others viewed them, and they would be aware of self-presentational risks and problems as they arose. As a result, they would know when all was well from a self-presentational standpoint and when to become justifiably concerned with others' impressions. However, people are not always good judges of the impressions others hold of them. Although most people are aware of the impressions they generally make on others, they are less accurate at assessing how they are perceived by particular other people (DePaulo, Kenny, Hoover, Webb, & Oliver, 1987). One reason for this is that the reactions of other individuals depend not only on the particular impressions they form of us but also on their own personality characteristics. In addition, people tend to overestimate how consistently other people perceive them. People tend to perceive their own behavior as less variable than, in fact, it really is. Thus, they think that others view them similarly across situations when others may, in reality, form different impressions of them depending on how they behave in a particular social encounter.

When people attempt to convey particular impressions, they assess their effectiveness through the feedback they receive or imagine they receive from others. People appear to compare the reactions they believe they are receiving to their internal standards. Although no research has examined such standards specifically, their presence can be inferred from the fact that people often conclude they have made "good" impressions on others, whereas at other times they believe they have made "bad" impressions. Carver and Scheier (1985, 1986) explicitly addressed the processes by which people assess the degree to which they meet their performance standards, including their self-presentational performances.

People differ greatly in the stringency of their self-presentational standards. Two individuals may both be 20 pounds overweight, but, whereas one person is mortified about being seen in swimwear at the beach (because his or her appearance does not meet his or her standards), the other is unconcerned about others' perceptions (because his or her standards regarding physical appearance are more lax). Thus, the difference in their reactions is due not to their objective appearance or even to their self-perceptions (they both recognize they are 20 pounds overweight) but rather to differences in their standards for self-evaluation. Some people hold very high standards and require very favorable impression-relevant reactions from others to be satisfied and self-approving. Others' standards are lower. They require only minimally approving feedback from others to feel satisfied with the effectiveness of their self-presentations.

The higher one's standards for assessing self-presentational efficacy, the higher the likelihood of experiencing social anxiety. A person whose standards are excessively high may often feel socially anxious, not because others' reactions are objectively unfavorable but because their reactions do not come up to his or her standards (see Bandura, 1969). In many instances, others may judge the individual quite favorably but, in the actor's eyes, not favorably enough (Nichols, 1974). Consistent with this view, people who hold unrealistically high expectations for themselves tend to score higher in trait social anxiety (Goldfried & Sobocinski, 1975).

When people evaluate themselves, they often use other people as standards for comparison. In many instances, the most useful and informative comparisons are those made in reference to others who are similar to oneself on the relevant dimensions (Festinger, 1954). Unfortunately, people sometimes evaluate themselves relative to others who are highly regarded in a particular domain, thus employing standards that are unrealistically high (Bandura, 1969). A teenage girl who compares herself to a fashion model or movie actress—even a teenage one—is likely to feel dissatisfied with her appearance, poise, and social skill. Her attempts at social interaction will always fall short of the standard she holds. As a result, she is likely to feel anxious when contemplating her self-perceived short-comings.

Although it might be expected that people who have experienced a high degree of social success in the past would be more confident and less anxious as time goes by, this is not necessarily the case. People tend to revise their standards upward as they experience success. As a result, they are no longer satisfied with the earlier level of performance and outcomes (Appley, 1971). The result of constantly revising one's standards upward with success is that many individuals who by all indications should be confident and self-assured continue to experience social anxiety because the evaluations and reactions they receive from others seldom meet their high standards (see following box).

Anxiety among the Stars

Observing from afar, people often envy the confidence and poise of professional actors and musicians who can perform in front of thousands or millions of people without apparent nervousness. On closer inspection, however, performers are often much more socially anxious than they appear.

Many professional performers, even those who have achieved superstar status, admit to experiencing stage fright before and during their performances. Stevie Nicks, formerly of Fleetwood Mac, admits that she experiences intense anxiety as a performance approaches. "My stomach gets upset. I break out in a sweat. I have asthma and it really kicks in. Everyone wonders, 'My God. Is she going to be able to pull this evening off?' " ("Drowning on Dry Land," 1994, p. 65). Carly Simon and Barbra Streisand experienced such intense anxiety on stage that they each abandoned performing live for many years. (Streisand stayed away from the stage for 27 years!) Even artists as popular as Madonna, Michael Jackson, and Luciano Pavarotti regularly experience stage fright. As Mick Jagger told the crowd at the opening concert of the Rolling Stones 1994 world tour, "You're always nervous the first night."

Some people find it difficult to understand why performers who are revered for their excellence should become so nervous.

(continued)

(continued from p. 73)

After all, these performers have demonstrated their superior ability on countless occasions for many years, have received recognition and fame far beyond what the rest of us can even imagine, and have millions of devoted fans. Yet they still become socially anxious before their performances. Why?

One reason involves the performers' perceptions of their audience's expectations. Stars at the pinnacle of their profession may believe that their fans expect every performance to be perfect. As Madonna explained after her hands trembled during her performance at the 1991 Academy Awards, "I had four minutes to be perfect, and there were three billion people watching me on TV" ("Drowning on Dry Land," 1994, p. 65). Even performers as accomplished as Pavarotti or Streisand know they cannot consistently give perfect performances. Fortunately, although people who come to see a celebrated singer, actor, or musician expect an exemplary performance, audiences are rarely astute enough to detect many of the imperfections that are obvious to the performers themselves. Furthermore, audiences are probably more forgiving of occasional flubs than the performers suspect.

Contemporary musicians and singers also worry that audiences will compare their live performances to the nearly flawless performances on their CDs, records, and tapes. (Mozart, Beethoven, Sousa, and other noted performers of earlier times did not have to face this problem.) Performers on stage rarely can achieve the perfection of their studio recordings. In the studio, performers repeat their performances until a satisfactory take is obtained, and electronic wizardry is used to correct and enhance the performance. Even though the rough edges on a live performance are compensated for by added excitement, spontaneity, and presence, the performer may worry that the audience will be disappointed in the quality of the live performance and will conclude that the performer is not really as good as he or she had appeared.

Superstars' own self-images are also at stake when they walk on stage. Should they perform poorly and convey undesired impressions, performers themselves will be forced to confront the possibility that they are not the world-class superstars they would like to believe.

People who feel nervous in front of audiences should take

(continued)

(*continued from p. 74*)

comfort from the fact that professional performers also experience stage fright. For one thing, it shows that feeling anxious does not indicate that the person is about to give a poor performance. As we've seen, people feel socially anxious when the possibility of making an undesired impression exists, but in most instances, the person's fears do not come to pass.

Second, many performers have learned to use anxiety to enhance their performances. If one views anxious arousal as energizing rather than as incapacitating, it may push the person's performance to greater heights (Alpert & Haber, 1960). In fact, some performers are concerned if they *don't* feel anxious before going on stage because a lack of anxiety often leads to a flat performance. Luciano Pavarotti, for instance, views preperformance jitters as an essential part of performing, and Stevie Nicks says that she would be worried if she didn't feel really nervous before walking out on stage.

Finally, the fact that we are often surprised to learn that our favorite actors, singers, and musicians experience stage fright shows that even intense social anxiety is not easily detected by others. This observation should make us less worried about how nervous we appear the next time we stand up in front of a group.

As we discuss in Chapter 9, counselors and clinicians often see clients whose social anxiety stems from excessively high standards for self-evaluation. Therapies based upon rational-emotive and cognitive restructuring approaches are applicable in such cases. Clients can be shown that their anxiety arises from unrealistic expectations and taught more adaptive ways to view themselves and their social worlds.

CHAPTER 5

Self-Presentational Disasters

-------◇•⊗•◇------

MOST EPISODES OF social anxiety are anticipatory in nature. Nothing in particular has happened that casts an undesired impression, but people nonetheless fear that others will not perceive them as they wish. Occasionally, however, people believe that an actual self-presentational disaster has occurred—that others have formed impressions of them that are contrary to the image they wanted to convey.

These self-presentational disasters are called predicaments: "situations in which events have undesirable implications for the identity-relevant images actors have claimed or desire to claim in front of real or imagined audiences" (Schlenker, 1980, p. 125). In everyday language, we refer to these predicaments as "humiliating" or "embarrassing." Predicaments not only cause intense anxiety (people talk of feeling embarrassed, mortified, humiliated, or downright stupid), but they seriously disrupt social encounters.

"Dear Abby" recently published a letter from a young man who, in preparation for going away for the weekend with his new girlfriend, went to a drugstore to buy condoms. Feeling decidedly uneasy as the pharmacist rang up his purchase, the fellow tried to make small talk and said something about hoping to "get lucky" that weekend. Imagine the self-presentational predicament that ensued (not to mention the acute discomfort he experienced) when, upon calling for his girlfriend at her home, he was met at the door by the pharmacist—who just happened to be the woman's father!

PREDICAMENTS

The variety of ways in which people can taint their social images seems virtually endless. Several theorists have attempted to reduce these embarrassing self-presentational predicaments to a few basic categories. Early work by E. Gross and Stone (1964), M. S. Weinberg (1968), and Sattler (1965) identified various categories of embarrassing events, but none of these frameworks provided a comprehensive catalogue of embarrassing circumstances that included the full range of situations that produce embarrassment (see also Edelmann, 1987; Sharkey & Stafford, 1990). In a recent effort to develop a taxonomy of embarrassing events, R. S. Miller (1992) asked more than 350 adolescents and young adults from various parts of the United States to describe the last time they felt embarrassed. His analyses revealed four basic categories of embarrassing situations, which are shown in Table 5.1, along with examples.

TABLE 5.1. Categories of Embarrassing Circumstances

Individual behavior
  Physical pratfalls and inept performances
    Examples: tripping; locking one's keys in the car
  Cognitive shortcomings
    Examples: forgetting an appointment; calling someone by the wrong name
  Loss of control over body or possessions
    Examples: accidentally tripping someone; spilling food on the floor
  Failures of privacy regulation
    Examples: being seen by strangers in one's underwear; walking in on someone in the bathroom
  Abashed harm-doing
    Examples: harming, inconveniencing, or disturbing others
  Conspicuousness
    Example: being the center of attention

Interactive behavior
  Awkward interaction
    Examples: lulls in the conversation; speaking to someone who doesn't speak the same language
  Team embarrassment
    Examples: one's friends become loud and unruly in a movie theatre; family member is arrested for indecent exposure

(continued on next page)

TABLE 5.1. *Continued*

Audience provocation
    Real transgression
        Examples: another person discloses a secret you told; being teased about
        one's misbehavior
    No real transgression
        Examples: others spread untrue rumors; you are made the target of a
        practical joke

Bystander behavior (empathic embarrassment)
        Examples: watching a speaker falter; seeing another student in class openly
        ridiculed by the teacher

Note. Adapted from R. S. Miller (1992, p. 193). Copyright 1992 by the Society for Personality and Social Psychology. Adapted by permission.

Individual Behavior

The first category involved embarrassing consequences of the individual's own behavior. For example, some embarrassing events involve behaviors that violate public norms (what R. S. Miller, 1992, called "normative public deficiencies"). People are likely to feel embarrassed when they are publicly inept (stalling one's car in heavy traffic), display cognitive shortcomings (misspelling the word potato), lose control over their body or possessions (being noticeably flatulent), or fail to regulate their or others' privacy (accidentally walking in on a couple engaged in amorous activities). They are also embarrassed if they accidentally hurt other people or their property ("abashed harm doing"). If you slam someone's finger in the door, spill your coffee on his pants, or step on her feet while dancing, you are likely to become embarrassed.

People also feel embarrassed when they are the center of attention or otherwise feel conspicuous. Mere conspicuousness is not in itself embarrassing, although it may make people feel self-conscious and even blush (Leary, Britt, Cutlip, & Templeton, 1992). Conspicuousness tends to lead to embarrassment primarily when the person is not sure how to act or has behaved in a way that has conveyed an undesired impression.

Interactive Behavior

A second major category of embarrassing events arises not because of the person's own behavior in isolation, but because of interactions with other people. For example, awkward interactions are often embarrassing. People sometimes feel anxious when conversations lag or become stilted, when they or others say inappropriate things, or when they have lost a coherent "script" for how to proceed in an encounter. In fact, Parrott et al. (1988) suggested that awkward interaction is the primary, if not the only, cause of embarrassment.

Another variety of interactive behavior involves "team embarrassment," in which people become embarrassed because of the behaviors of other people with whom they are associated. Parents are sometimes embarrassed by the misbehaviors of their children, children embarrassed by the behaviors of their parents, and friends embarrassed by one another's actions. Because others' perceptions of a person are affected by the people and groups with which they are affiliated, people understandably prefer to bask in reflected glory rather than to blush in reflected shame.

Audience Provocation

Embarrassing events also arise through no fault of the person whatsoever. Other people may provoke us to feel embarrassed when they tease us, reveal our personal secrets, or make us the butt of their jokes. Sometimes other people inadvertently cause us embarrassment, whereas other times people intentionally create a self-presentational predicament for us (see following box).

Why Do People Enjoy Intentionally Embarrassing Others?

Few social situations are more discomforting than being intentionally embarrassed by someone. The interesting question is why people sometimes appear to enjoy purposefully embarrassing other people.

(continued)

(*continued from p. 79*)

Ironically, one of the primary reasons people say they intentionally embarrass one another is to demonstrate or enhance the closeness of their relationship with the other person (Sharkey, 1992, 1993). Intentionally embarrassing someone can be viewed as either an extremely hostile action (intended to demean or hurt the person) or as an extremely benign one (intended to poke good-natured fun at those whom we feel comfortable enough to tease). In light of this, as long as the target of the embarrassment has no reason to think that the perpetrator acted maliciously, intentional embarrassment (within limits) can convey a sense of familiarity, liking, and closeness.

As a result, people are more likely to intentionally embarrass friends and other people they know well than they are to embarrass strangers and those they know less well. In fact, as relationships deepen, intentionally embarrassing one's friend or intimate partner may not only become accepted, but expected (Sharkey, 1991). Similarly, members of a cohesive group may freely treat one another in embarrassing ways that they would not think of treating outsiders. Even when people are not equals, as when a superior embarrasses a subordinate, the goal of good-natured embarrassment may be to show camaraderie (Sharkey & Waldron, 1990).

This use of intentional embarrassment is risky, however, because the target may interpret the perpetrator's intent as hostile rather than as friendly (Pawluk, 1989). In addition, the person who intentionally embarrasses another can reasonably expect the target of the embarrassment to reciprocate at some time in the future.

Of course, not all intentional embarrassment is benign. People also embarrass others as a sanction against inappropriate behavior or to publicly discredit a person (Sharkey, 1992). A teacher who embarrasses an unruly or inadequately prepared student in front of the class hopes to use embarrassment as a means of control. As Gibbons (1990) noted, "fear of embarrassment helps bring behavior in line with certain accepted social rules" (p. 138). Intentional embarrassment is also used to deflate the public images of those who are pretentious or self-centered. Further, people are often gratified when high achievers are cut down to size (Feather, 1989; Feather & McKee, 1993).

People also intentionally embarrass others as a means of

(*continued*)

(continued from p. 80)

establishing or maintaining their power or dominance over them (E. Gross & Stone, 1964; Sharkey, in press). Because superiors are permitted to embarrass subordinates but not vice versa, embarrassing other people is a way to demonstrate one's relative power and status both to the target of the embarrassment and to others who may be present.

Finally, some cases of intentional embarrassment seem to occur simply to satisfy the perpetrator's curiosity ("I wanted to see how she would act") or because the perpetrator thought doing so would be fun ("I enjoy embarrassing him"). In fact, some people seem to enjoy the reputation of being an "embarrassor" who can be expected to regularly poke fun at others, usually in creative ways.

Empathic Embarrassment: Bystander Behavior

The fourth and final category of embarrassing events identified by R. S. Miller (1992) involves witnessing other people's embarrassment. We've all felt empathic embarrassment (sometimes called vicarious embarrassment) when we have observed another person's self-presentational predicament (R. S. Miller, 1987). People become uncomfortable when other people convey undesired images of themselves. Many of us who have been to comedy clubs have felt the discomfort of empathic embarrassment as we have watched the painful nervousness of a comedian whose inane jokes are followed by stony silence.

Feelings of empathic embarrassment may occur for two reasons. On one hand, the feelings may be purely empathic. Just as people may feel sad simply from witnessing others' distress or happy from observing others' happiness, they sometimes experience vicarious embarrassment from seeing others who are embarrassed. On the other hand, some instances of empathic embarrassment arise because the individual feels partly responsible for creating the embarrassment. For example, the patron at a comedy club may squirm at the comedian's horrid jokes not only because of empathy for the comedian's plight but also because his or her own presence contributes to the comedian's discomfort.

It is noteworthy that we are sometimes embarrassed for other individuals who are not embarrassed themselves. Sometimes people do not even realize they are in a self-presentational predicament although, as onlookers, we realize they are making fools of themselves. In such cases, we may feel uncomfortably embarrassed even though the person in the predicament does not.

EMBARRASSMENT

The typical emotional response to a self-presentational predicament is embarrassment: an "aversive state of abashment, flusterment, and chagrin" (R. S. Miller, in press-a). For our purposes, it is useful to regard embarrassment as a special manifestation of social anxiety (see following box), specifically, social anxiety that is a reactive response to a self-presentational predicament (as opposed to an anticipatory response to a potential failure of impression management).

Researchers have been interested in the psychological features of embarrassment and in the aspects of the experience that distinguish it from other emotional reactions. Parrott and Smith (1991) examined the phenomenology of embarrassment by asking subjects to describe and rate instances of embarrassment they had experienced. In every instance, subjects reported that other people were present. Embarrassment is clearly a social emotion that is rarely experienced when people are alone.

In describing an actual embarrassing situation, most respondents reported that they had made a bad impression on other people, were unable to successfully perform their role in the interaction (or had contradicted their current role), and were unable to control or avoid the embarrassing event. Nearly half indicated that they had been subjected to ridicule, laughter, or humiliation.

Clearly, embarrassment is an aversive emotion. Parrott and Smith's (1991) respondents reported that the event made them feel foolish, inferior, or incompetent. Furthermore, they felt that they were the center of attention and wanted others to leave them alone. A high percentage of respondents also indicated that they blushed.

Theorists have debated whether embarrassment is distinguishable from shame, or whether embarrassment and shame reflect

Is Embarrassment a Form of Social Anxiety?

Most researchers have regarded embarrassment as a special type of social anxiety that occurs after a self-presentational predicament (Buss, 1980; Edelmann, 1987; Leary, 1994; R. S. Miller, 1986, in press-b; Schlenker, 1980; Schlenker & Leary, 1982). According to this view, "ordinary" social anxiety is *anticipatory* in nature, arising because of concerns that one may not make a desired impression on others. Embarrassment, in contrast, is *reactive* in that it is a response to a self-presentational failure or predicament that the person believes has already occurred.

Harris (1990) challenged the assertion that embarrassment is an anxiety state. First, he correctly noted that most analyses of anxiety view it as inherently anticipatory, a reaction to potential danger. If one accepts this conceptualization (which we do), embarrassment would seem not to qualify as an anxiety state. However, when used to describe social anxiety and embarrassment, "anticipatory" and "reactive" refer to a particular self-presentational predicament. In both cases, what people actually fear is not the predicament per se, but *the potential personal and interpersonal implications of the predicament.* Viewed in this way, both social anxiety and embarrassment are "anticipatory" in the sense that they result from the anticipation of undesired outcomes that may stem from a self-presentational failure.

Second, Harris (1990) observed, again correctly, that the physiological concomitants of anticipatory social anxiety and embarrassment differ. Social anxiety or shyness is generally associated with increased cardiovascular activity, whereas some episodes of embarrassment appear to involve decreased heart rate and blood pressure (Cutlip & Leary, 1993; Strom & Buck, 1979). Our own research showed that embarrassing events that occur suddenly, without warning, result in increased cardiovascular activity, whereas expected predicaments (that the person has had time to mentally prepare for) result in lowered activity (Leary, Rejeski, Britt, & Smith, 1994).

One possible resolution to this issue involves the distinction drawn by comparative psychologists between active and passive fear responses. Animals who are threatened may display either increased sympathetic arousal (the fight or flight reaction) or decreased arousal (the freeze and hide reaction). In both cases, the animal might be characterized as "anxious" or "afraid," but in only one is physiological arousal increased. We return to a discussion of the physiological underpinnings of social anxiety and embarrassment in Chapter 6.

different terms for the same general phenomenon. A consensus on this issue has not yet been reached, but recent research suggests that embarrassment is typically a less intense and less enduring emotion than shame. R. S. Miller and Tangney (1995) found that "whereas embarrassment resulted from surprising, relatively trivial accidents, shame occurred when foreseeable events revealed one's deep-seated flaws both to oneself and to others." Both responses involve concerns with others' evaluations, but shame results from the violation of important moral or ethical standards, whereas embarrassment reflects momentary mistakes or awkwardness.

THEORIES OF EMBARRASSMENT

Three distinct varieties of theories of embarrassment have been proposed involving (1) losses of self-esteem due to the violation of one's personal standards, (2) disrupted and awkward interactions, and (3) perceived self-presentational predicaments.

Violation of Personal Standards

One set of theories attributes embarrassment to a loss of self-esteem. Babcock (1988), for example, suggested that embarrassment results from the violation of one's personal standards:

> Embarrassment ensues when an individual finds herself acting in a way that is inconsistent with her *persona* or conception of herself. Embarrassment reflects a concern with upholding certain personal standards, not merely a concern over what others will think or what to do next. (p. 459)

In some ways, the self-esteem approach starts with the same general assumption as self-consistency theories (such as cognitive dissonance theory)—namely, that inconsistencies between one's behavior and beliefs are personally distressing. In the case of embarrassment, the inconsistency involves a discrepancy between one's standards regarding appropriate behavior and how one, in fact, has behaved.

Disrupted and Awkward Interactions

A second approach—the interactional or dramaturgical model—proposes that embarrassment occurs when interactions become awkward and disrupted (Parrott et al., 1988; Silver, Sabini, & Parrott, 1987). Smooth interaction requires that the interactants successfully maintain appropriate identities during an encounter. People are expected to cooperate in establishing a "working consensus"—an agreement about the roles that each interactant will play and the rules they will follow (Goffman, 1959). When one or more interactants are unable to continue performing their role or cannot sustain their situated identity in a particular encounter, they feel embarrassed (Parrott & Smith, 1991). Thus, according to this view, embarrassment results from a defect in the structure of the interaction more than from a revelation about any one of the interactants (see E. Gross & Stone, 1964).

Self-Presentational Predicaments

The third theory—the one we prefer—traces embarrassment to self-presentational failures. In our view, people become embarrassed when they believe they have projected undesired images of themselves to other people (R. S. Miller, 1986, in press-a, in press-b; Schlenker, 1980). Indeed, embarrassment is easily explained by the self-presentational theory of social anxiety. In terms of the two components of the theory (see Chapter 2), embarrassment occurs when an individual is motivated to make a desired impression, but believes that others have formed undesired impressions instead. Rather than reflecting anticipatory concerns about the possibility of making undesired impressions, embarrassment is *reactive* social anxiety in response to a perceived self-presentational predicament that has already occurred.

The self-presentational (or social esteem) theory easily subsumes the other two approaches. First, to the extent that the self-esteem system functions to monitor others' reactions to the individual (Leary & Baumeister, 1994; Leary & Downs, 1995), cues that connote disapproval or displeasure should not only cause embarrassment, but lower self-esteem as well. Along these lines, Modigliani (1971) proposed that embarrassment is associated with "a loss of situational self-esteem that is caused by a loss of situational-subjective-public-esteem" (p. 16). In other words, believing that one has lost esteem in others' eyes (situational-subjective-public-esteem) leads to a loss of self-esteem that results in embarrassment. Contrary to Modigliani's view, however, we view lowered self-esteem and embarrassment as coeffects of self-presentational predicaments rather than as causally related.

Furthermore, awkward, disrupted interactions often cast people in an undesirable light and create self-presentational predicaments. Not only are many instances of awkward interactions directly caused by self-presentational failures (as when one guest vomits on another), but awkwardness and a loss of poise, whatever the cause, can lead people to assume they are not making desired impressions on other interactants. Thus, in our view, awkward interactions are embarrassing because they typically involve self-presentational threats.

R. S. Miller (in press-a) directly tested two of these theories of embarrassment—the awkward interaction and self-presentational approaches—by asking college students to imagine being refused for a date for either innocuous reasons (the person had to attend class) or potentially esteem-threatening reasons (the person lied and said he or she had a class). In addition, the news of this refusal was relayed by a third party who either believed the person's reason for refusing the date or thought it was a sham. Consistent with the awkward interaction model, the awkwardness of the interaction affected students' reported embarrassment; the students indicated they would feel more embarrassed if the third party thought they were being snubbed than when the third party thought the reason for the refusal was legitimate. However, students were also embarrassed by a threatening rejection even if the third party believed the reason for the refusal (and, thus, the immediate interaction was not awkward), thus supporting a self-presentational explanation.

Although few data exist, we think that the weight of the evidence supports the self-presentational explanation of embarrassment. First, if embarrassment was caused by violations of personal standards per se, as the self-esteem theories suggest, people should regularly be embarrassed in private whenever they behave contrary to their standards. Although private violations of standards may cause people to feel guilty and to fear detection, they generally do not cause the same level of embarrassment as *public* violations. In addition, people may become embarrassed even when behaving in line with their standards if doing so portrays them in an undesired light, a fact that the self-esteem theories cannot easily explain.

Furthermore, although Miller's data appear to support both the awkward interaction and self-presentational explanations of embarrassment, we believe that his entire pattern of results can be explained by the self-presentational theory. Believing that a third party thinks one has been lied to and rejected creates a self-presentational predicament in its own right, aside from whatever awkwardness arises during the interaction itself.

Counterexamples: Conspicuousness and Overpraise

A self-presentational explanation of embarrassment may seem, on the surface, to have difficulty accounting for two common causes of embarrassment—conspicuousness and overpraise. However, we believe that the self-presentational perspective can effectively handle both of these antecedents of embarrassment.

First, many people report feeling embarrassed when they are the center of attention or otherwise feel conspicuous (Buss, 1980). As it turns out, merely being the center of attention does not seem to be the culprit, but rather being the center of attention (1) without having a cogent script regarding how to respond or (2) because one has suffered a self-presentational predicament. Merely being the focus of attention is not, in itself, embarrassing. Actors or performers on stage, lovers looking into one another's eyes, and the "life of the party" recounting a personal anecdote are each the center of others' attention, yet do not feel embarrassed.

Instances in which attention does cause embarrassment are easily handled by the self-presentational explanation. When people are the focus of others' attention but aren't sure what they should say or do, or perceive they have made an undesired impression, they are likely to suffer a self-presentational predicament and, consequently, become embarrassed. Thus, the relationship between conspicuousness and embarrassment is mediated by self-presentational concerns.

A second apparent counterexample involves overpraise. People appear embarrassed not only when they make a bad impression, but sometimes when they are complimented, honored, or otherwise recognized. Ironically, public kudos can create self-presentational difficulties. As welcome as attention and recognition may be, the person who is singled out for exemplary performance may not know how best to respond, thereby raising the spectre of conveying an undesired impression. The honoree may also worry about appearing too self-effacing on the one hand or too smug on the other. Even standing silently by as one's accomplishments are noted or as one is applauded or congratulated makes many people believe they look foolish or unpoised.

EMBARRASSABILITY

People differ in the degree to which they become embarrassed by the kinds of predicaments described above. Some people are easily and frequently embarrassed, whereas others are not affected by even major violations of social norms or shocking breaches of decorum. These traitlike differences in "a person's general susceptibility to embarrassment" are called embarrassability (Modigliani, 1968, p. 316).

Researchers have typically measured embarrassability using Modigliani's (1966) Embarrassability Scale (for reviews of psychometric data, see Edelmann, 1987; Leary, 1991). The Embarrassability Scale asks the respondent to indicate how embarrassed he or she would feel in several social situations. A few items from Edelmann's (1987, p. 121) 22-item revision of the scale include:

- You are muttering aloud to yourself in an apparently empty room when you discover someone else is there.
- You trip and fall while entering a bus full of people.
- You are talking in a small group which includes a blind person, when someone next to you unthinkingly makes a remark about everyone being "blind as a bat."

As we would expect, scores on the Embarrassability Scale correlate highly with measures of trait social anxiety, as well as with variables that predict trait social anxiety. Highly embarrassable people tend to score higher than less embarrassable people in fear of negative evaluation, public self-consciousness, and shyness (Edelmann, 1985, 1987; Leary & Meadows, 1991; R. S. Miller, in press-a; Modigliani, 1968). Embarrassability also correlates highly with skill in interpreting others' remarks and in attending to the normative appropriateness of one's behavior. Embarrassable people are also slightly more predisposed to experience negative emotions overall than less embarrassable people (R. S. Miller, in press-a). Embarrassability correlates moderately with negative affectivity—the tendency to experience unpleasant emotions (Kowalski & Cantrell, 1994).

In a study of the predictors of embarrassability, R. S. Miller (in press-a) found that, though related, embarrassability and trait social anxiety were not isomorphic. Social anxiety and embarrassability were moderately correlated, and both were related to fear of negative evaluation. However, social self-esteem and global social skill were much more strongly related to social anxiety than to embarrassability.

The possibility exists that some people are more embarrassable because they more often do embarrassing things. One study suggested this is not the case, however. Highly embarrassable people report experiencing the same sorts of self-presentational predicaments as less embarrassable people, but they are more embarrassed by them (R. S. Miller, 1992). Furthermore, people who score high in embarrassability are not only more embarrassed when they convey undesired images of themselves, but they suffer more empathic embarrassment when observing others' self-presentational predicaments (Marcus, Wilson, & R. S. Miller, 1994; Miller, 1987).

Gender Differences

Several studies show that American women are more easily embarrassed than American men. Not only do they score higher on the Embarrassability Scale, but they report feeling more embarrassed by specific embarrassing events they have experienced (R. S. Miller, 1992). The explanation of this gender difference is not clear, but at least two processes may be involved.

First, social expectations for what constitutes appropriate behavior may be more stringent for women than for men. Women may be given less latitude for performing a variety of uncouth behaviors than men, so that certain behaviors are more likely to create a self-presentational predicament for women than men. For example, it appears less appropriate for women to swear, belch, or appear obviously intoxicated than men. Extra pressures on women to attend to their physical appearance also create additional opportunities for embarrassment, as do socialized pressures to appear self-effacing. For example, the average American man is probably less embarrassed by temporary flaws in his appearance (such as tattered clothing, dishevelment, or a "bad hair day") than the average woman.

Second, during childhood and adolescence, much male humor involves teasing (if not tormenting) one's peers, and boys must develop the ability to weather direct affronts to their social images from both friends and enemies (Pearson, 1985). As a result, not only are men more accustomed to surviving events that defile their public image, but they have had more opportunities to learn ways of responding to embarrassing situations.

Cross-Cultural Differences

Edelmann and his colleagues have examined differences in the experience of embarrassment across cultures. Although embarrassment is universal, these researchers found that people from collectivist cultures are more embarrassable on average than people from individualistic cultures (Edelmann & Iwawaki, 1987; Edelmann & Neto, 1989).

Singelis and Sharkey (in press) hypothesized that cultural differences in embarrassability are due, in part, to the degree to which the self-construals of people in different cultures are independent versus interdependent. In a study of cross-cultural differences in embarrassability, Singelis and Sharkey examined predictors of embarrassability among more than 500 Euro-American and Asian American university students. They found that respondents whose self-construals were highly independent (emphasizing personal uniqueness, the pursuit of personal goals, and directness in self-expression) were less embarrassable than those whose self-construals were less individualistic. In contrast, interdependent self-construals (emphasizing fitting-in, behaving appropriately, conforming to one's status and roles, and indirect expression) were associated with greater embarrassability than less interdependent self-construals.

Presumably, these differences occur because people who see themselves as unique and independent believe that the accomplishment of their goals relies less on the good graces of others than people who see themselves as highly interdependent. In contrast, people whose self-construals are interdependent believe that their successes depend on appropriately impressing the right people. Furthermore, people with independent self-construals are simply less concerned with what other people think of them than people whose identities are tightly intermeshed with their social groups.

REMEDIAL TACTICS

People who are embarrassed by a self-presentational predicament are understandably motivated to undo whatever damage has been done to their public images. Researchers have identified three general classes of remedial behaviors: apologies, accounts, and avoidance.

Apologies

Apologies are often used as remedial tactics, particularly when one's behavior has harmed other people. Apologies can vary in complexity from a perfunctory and ritualistic "Pardon me" to full-blown apologies that express remorse or regret ("I'm sorry"), castigate oneself ("How could I be so careless?"), offer to help the injured party ("Please, let me pay for a new shirt"), and ask for forgiveness ("I hope you'll forgive me") (Schlenker & Darby, 1981). The more serious the predicament, the more extensive the apology (Schlenker, 1980).

People's apologies often appear overblown to observers. People often apologize again and again for what seem to be relatively trivial transgressions even after others have repeatedly assured them that "it's okay." Goffman (1955) suggested that people give a "worst case reading" to their self-presentational predicaments, imagining the worst possible outcomes that might result from their behavior. Apologies and other remedial strategies are based on this worst case reading. Such a tactic is not unreasonable, given that it is better to overapologize than to not apologize enough (Darby & Schlenker, 1989).

Accounts

People also attempt to undo embarrassing events through accounts, which are verbal explanations for unexpected, unacceptable, or unsatisfactory behavior that are designed to rectify a self-presentational predicament (Gonzales, Pederson, Manning, & Wetter, 1990; Schlenker, 1980; Scott & Lyman, 1968). Excuses are accounts used to minimize the person's perceived responsibility for the behavior that led to the predicament. Sometimes a person disavows *all* responsibility for the action (a defense of innocence), but more commonly the individual accepts only partial responsibility. For example, people may try to excuse their behavior by pointing out that they didn't foresee the negative consequences of their actions ("I didn't stop to think of how you'd feel"), were operating under mistaken assumptions ("Sorry, I thought you were single"), were not in full control of themselves ("I've been under a great deal of stress lately"), or were only one of several parties implicated in the image-threatening event ("I wasn't the only one involved").

In contrast, when justifications are used as accounts, the person accepts responsibility for the behavior, but denies its negative ramifications. People may justify their behavior by minimizing the importance or severity of its negative consequences ("It was only a small dent"), noting the benefits of their behavior ("At least we've learned a lesson from this"), or comparing their behavior with other, worse actions ("Thank goodness I only injured him; he could have been killed").

Avoidance

A third class of remedial tactics involves attempts to avoid providing an account at all (Scott & Lyman, 1968; Tedeschi & Riess, 1981). For example, people can use mystification by claiming there was a good reason for their behavior, but they can't tell others what it was ("If I could tell you the whole story, you would understand why I did it, but the details are confidential"). Or they can offer an empty explanation that explains virtually nothing ("I did it because I wanted to"). Laughing at one's predicament without explanation could also be viewed as an avoidance tactic. In some cases, people simply refuse to account for their behavior ("I don't have to explain my actions to you"), or physically retreat from the encounter without any response whatsoever.

Interestingly, American men and women differ in how they prefer to deal with embarrassing events. Women tend to view apologies and excuses as more appropriate tactics, whereas men seem to prefer avoidance (Cupach, Metts, & Hazelton, 1986; Petronio, 1984).

THE MALADAPTIVE SIDE OF EMBARRASSMENT

Because predicaments and the embarrassment they cause are so aversive, people generally try to avoid doing things that will prove embarrassing. In many cases, this is a good thing because it keeps our behavior within socially acceptable limits. However, in some instances, efforts to avoid embarrassment can have deleterious consequences. For example, fear of embarrassment may deter people from providing help to accident victims (Latané & Darley, 1970), introducing condoms into a sexual encounter (Leary, Tchvidjian, & Kraxberger, 1994), or offering their criticisms of obviously ill-conceived ideas in group meetings (Janis, 1982).

Although efforts to avoid embarrassment can lead to a variety of negative consequences, to demonstrate the potency and importance of embarrassment we focus here on how embarrassment may affect the quality of medical care people receive. Specifically, we discuss the influence of embarrassment on (1) reluctance to seek medical care, (2) failure to disclose medically relevant information, and (3) noncompliance with medical regimens.

Reluctance to Seek Medical Attention

Embarrassment can deter people from seeking medical attention. In some cases people find certain medical exams embarrassing, whereas in other cases they are worried that disclosure of their health problems will create a self-presentational predicament.

Embarrassment in Medical Exams

Some medical examinations and procedures cause embarrassment because they involve parts of the body that people consider private, such as the sex organs and rectal area. Many people are embarrassed by examinations of these parts of their bodies, and some postpone seeking medical attention because of their social discomfort. For example, studies of pelvic exams (Sansom, MacInerey, Oliver, & Wakefield, 1975) and mammography (Lerman, Rimer, Trock, Balshem, & Engstrom, 1990) showed that embarrassment regarding these procedures deterred women from scheduling examinations (see also Debrovner & Shubin-Stein, 1975; Domar, 1985/1986).

Most research attention along these lines involves gynecological exams. In one study, 85% of the female respondents indicated that they experienced negative emotions such as anxiety and humiliation during pelvic exams (Debrovner & Shubin-Stein, 1975). Women's discomfort in such settings is not entirely self-presentational, of course. Some fear that the exam will reveal previously undetected pathology (Hamilton & Dodge, 1981; G. Miller, 1974), and others worry that the exam itself will be painful.

Nonetheless, many girls and women find pelvic exams to be embarrassing and interpersonally awkward (Domar, 1985/1986; Millstein, Adler, & Irwin, 1984; Wheeless, 1984). One study found that 57% of the adolescent girls surveyed reported being embarrassed about undressing for pelvic exams, and 46% reported being embarrassed over the possibility that they were not sufficiently clean (Millstein et al., 1984). Not surprisingly, then, socially anxious women are less inclined to get gynecological exams than women who are less socially anxious (Kowalski & Brown, 1994). Feelings of embarrassment decline slightly with the number of pelvic exams women experience, although few women fully overcome such feelings entirely, no matter how many such exams they may have (Debrovner & Shubin-Stein, 1975).

Unfortunately, women who experience negative emotions during pelvic exams are more likely to report that the examination was painful (Millstein et al., 1984). It is not clear whether this is because anxiety increases bodily tension (thereby making the exam more difficult), anxiety increases the perception of pain, or women who normally find events more painful are understandably more anxious. Whichever the case, such data suggest that self-presentational concerns can actually increase the physical discomfort associated with gynecological examinations.

Both men and women report similar reactions to rectal examinations, such as those conducted to test for colon cancer and hemorrhoids (and, for men, prostate enlargement). In addition, some women, albeit a lower percentage, report being embarrassed by breast exams. Lerman et al. (1990) found that approximately one-third of the women in their sample reported some degree of embarrassment over having a mammogram.

From a conceptual standpoint, an interesting question is *why* patients find such exams embarrassing. The answer to this question may seem absurdly obvious, but it is not. The embarrassment that results from pelvic and rectal examinations does not fit easily into any of the three models of embarrassment described earlier. The self-presentational (or social esteem) explanation states that people become embarrassed when events have undesirable implications for the impressions they desire to claim (Edelmann, 1987; R. S. Miller, 1986, 1992; Schlenker, 1980). But why should routine medical exams, even of one's genitals, present a threat to one's social identity? Unless the patient is explicitly embarrassed by his or her physical appearance or by lack of cleanliness, it's not clear that a simple examination of one's genitals by a physician should create a self-presentational predicament. If anything, seeing a physician regularly for a Pap test or rectal exam is a socially desirable action in the eyes of medical personnel. Furthermore, patients know that their physician has performed hundreds, if not thousands, of such examinations, has seen thousands of genitals, and, presumably, is not making evaluative judgments of this particular patient's anatomy. So, why are they embarrassed?

The dramaturgical (awkward interaction) and self-esteem models fare no better as explanations of embarrassment in medical examinations. As noted earlier, the awkward interaction model (Silver et al., 1987) posits that embarrassment results from the uncertainty that follows the loss of a coherent "script" during an interaction. When people's expectancies are discomfirmed in a particular situation, they fall "out of role," become indecisive about how to proceed, and feel embarrassed. However, most patients know precisely what to expect, both their own and the physician's behaviors are strongly governed by well-learned roles, and their expectations regarding the course of the encounter are unlikely to be disconfirmed. As Emerson (1970) quipped, there "is little margin for ad-libbing during a gynecological examination" (p. 83). True, interactions during pelvic exams may be awkward, but this awkwardness seems to be the result of embarrassment and self-presentational concerns, not the cause of them.

Nor does it seem that medical embarrassment results from a loss of self-esteem (Babcock, 1988). If anything, people feel *good* about themselves for getting regular checkups. Thus, we find it difficult to imagine that people are embarrassed by medical exams because their self-esteem is threatened.

Attempts to reduce women's anxiety by having physicians explain the procedures as they occur do not generally reduce anxiety or discomfort (Domar, 1985/1986). From the self-presentational perspective, this should not be surprising. Although not understanding aspects of a pelvic exam may indeed be anxiety producing, educational interventions do little to reduce women's embarrassment during the exam. However, changes in examination procedures that decrease women's interpersonal concerns should reduce one source of the aversiveness of the procedure. In support of this, Williams and her colleagues showed that simply using a gown that more adequately covered the patient's body than the standard drape increased patient comfort (Williams, Park, & Cline, 1992).

Patients are not the only ones who are uncomfortable during pelvic and other personal exams. Many physicians express uneasiness with gynecological exams, discomfort that may further increase the patient's distress (Domar, 1985/1986). The impersonality of many physicians when performing pelvic exams may reflect a mode of coping with their own embarrassment. By maintaining an aloof, objective demeanor and avoiding explicit acknowledgment of the sexual and emotional aspects of the exam, examiners can depersonalize the encounter and reduce their own social anxiety (Tunnadine, 1980). Emerson (1970) provided a highly interesting description of the conventions by which physicians maintain the appropriate demeanor during gynecological exams.

Embarrassing Medical Conditions

People's willingness to seek medical care is affected not only by their concerns about certain medical exams, but also by their concerns with the impressions that other people will form of them if they seek medical care for particular problems. Sometimes patients are concerned about what the medical staff will think of them, whereas in other instances they are worried about how others outside the medical setting (e.g., family, friends, employers) will perceive them if they learn about their health problem.

Certain medical conditions are viewed as inherently embarrassing. Consequently, people sometimes hesitate to seek medical attention for sexually transmitted diseases, alcohol and drug abuse, sexual problems, injuries caused by embarrassing behaviors, and other difficulties that they think may create a self-presentational predicament for them. If the disorder and its symptoms are serious enough, people will eventually make their way to a physician, but any delay that results from embarrassment may affect the course of the illness as well as its prognosis.

Much has been written about the stigma of seeing a psychiatrist, psychologist, or other mental health professional. In the eyes of many, merely consulting with a psychiatrist or psychologist casts doubts on the individual's stability or sanity (Bar-Levav, 1976). Given current attitudes, this fear is not misplaced among individuals for whom seeking psychiatric care, if known by others, would jeopardize their professional or social standing. For example, business executives and politicians are often considered unfit for their positions if they have even consulted a psychotherapist. Perhaps the best known case is that of Thomas Eagleton, the Democratic vice presidential candidate in 1972, who was forced to withdraw from the race when it was learned he had seen a psychiatrist. These self-presentational concerns can lead people to avoid seeking professional help even when they know they need it.

Medical Self-Disclosure

Patients who seek medical attention may not receive adequate care if potential embarrassment makes them unwilling to discuss aspects of their lifestyle and health with the medical staff. Medical personnel often need information regarding the patient's health that, if openly disclosed, may cause the patient to feel embarrassed. As a result, patients may respond untruthfully to certain kinds of questions. For example, many patients may be reluctant to disclose information regarding their sexual practices and partners, patterns of bowel movements, alcohol and drug use, emotional problems, and other highly personal topics that might create a self-presentational predicament (e.g., Davies & Baker, 1987). Obviously, reluctance to discuss medically relevant information because of self-presentational concerns could have serious consequences for the patient's health.

In some cases, people may even fabricate responses to questions by the medical staff, underreporting unhealthy behaviors (e.g., smoking, alcohol consumption, cholesterol intake) and exaggerating healthy behaviors (e.g., exercise, nutritious eating). They may also deny symptoms that they think may cast them in a negative light (e.g., depression, anxiety, sleeplessness, relationship problems). People may also deny experiencing pain, discomfort, or other indices of weakness, underreporting the severity of their symptoms to appear strong or stoic. They may also minimize their feelings of fatigue or exertion during effortful cardiovascular tests (such as while running on a treadmill) so as not to be embarrassed (see Carver, Coleman, & Glass, 1976; Hardy, Hall, & Prestholdt, 1986).

Adherence to Medical Regimens

Fear of embarrassment can also interfere with adherence to medical regimens. When people believe that following the physician's orders may create undesired impressions in others' eyes, they may not adequately do so. People whose afflictions are otherwise invisible to others may be hesitant to do things that will bring attention to their problem.

For example, patients with insulin-dependent diabetes mellitus (IDDM) must often follow a complex regimen that involves daily insulin injections, multiple urine or blood glucose tests, and a consistent eating schedule. Some people with IDDM are reluctant to comply with such a regimen because doing so would bring unwanted attention, lead to awkward questions, or prove embarrassing (Glasgow, McCaul, & Schafer, 1986). Similarly, for the visually impaired, carrying a white cane may be viewed as a "stigma symbol" that connotes infirmity and incapacity. As a result, most visually impaired people initially resist using a cane (Wainapel, 1989). Likewise, many people who are hard of hearing refuse to wear a hearing aid because it advertises their deafness and causes others to behave differently toward them.

THE IMPORTANCE OF EMBARRASSMENT

As we discussed in Chapter 2, emotions evolved because they provided organisms with a survival and reproductive advantage. Like social anxiety more generally, embarrassment may have evolved as part of a affective–motivational system that regulates interpersonal behavior to maintain the integrity of the individual's relationships with other people (R. S. Miller & Leary, 1992). Although we may wish we never became embarrassed, our capacity for embarrassment is essential for orderly social interaction, as well as for our social well-being. As Goffman (1967) observed, "embarrassment is not an irrational impulse breaking through socially prescribed behavior but part of orderly behavior itself" (p. 111). Embarrassment (and the fear of embarrassment) keeps our behavior within the limits of propriety and prevents us from damaging our public images in ways that jeopardize our relationships with other people.

As we have seen, however, the yoke of embarrassment is so strong that people sometimes do things contrary to their own or others' best interests to avoid being embarrassed. People's concerns with others' impressions of them can be so compelling that their motivation to avoid self-presentational predicaments can overwhelm even concerns for their own safety, as when a diner in a restaurant quietly chokes to death on a piece of steak rather than create an embarrassing spectacle.

CHAPTER 6

Trait Social Anxiety and Social Phobia

———◇·❀·◇———

WATCH NEARLY ANY large group of people interacting, and you will detect wide variations in social anxiety. Some individuals seem confident and outgoing, showing few doubts about their social abilities and no signs of nervousness whatsoever. Other people appear generally poised, yet from time to time display a momentary sense of uncertainty or awkwardness. At the extreme, a few highly socially anxious individuals will seem to be constantly and painfully uncomfortable.

Furthermore, if we watch people across various social settings, we observe a degree of consistency in how a particular individual deals with different social encounters. Some people appear confident and outgoing most of the time, whereas others are characteristically anxious and shy regardless of the social context.

These emotional and behavioral tendencies can be observed across time as well. Children who are extremely fearful and inhibited in unfamiliar situations at age 2 tend to be quiet and socially avoidant at age 7 (Kagan, Reznick, & Snidman, 1988). People who were anxious and shy as children are more likely than children who were not shy to be socially anxious even 30 years later. For example, boys who were shy or socially anxious in childhood tend to marry and become fathers three years later on the average than those who were not shy. Girls who were shy were less likely to work outside the home as adults than girls who were not shy (Caspi, Elder, & Bem, 1988).

In brief, people differ in the frequency and intensity with which they experience social anxiety, and they demonstrate a certain degree of consistency in how anxious they are across social situations and over time (see following box for a description of measures of trait social anxiety). In this chapter, we examine these individual differences in social anxiety, focusing on the question of why some people are characteristically more socially anxious than others. In earlier chapters, we mentioned several personality factors that are related to the tendency to experience social anxiety; in this chapter, we focus on the source of these predisposing characteristics.

Self-Report Measures of Trait Social Anxiety

Researchers have developed several self-report measures to assess individual differences in trait social anxiety and related constructs, such as shyness. The list below provides brief descriptions of six scales that have been used most commonly in research. (The scales are listed in order of year of publication.) Leary (1991) provides a more complete description and critique of these and other measures of social anxiety and related constructs.

Social Avoidance and Distress Scale
    Location: Watson and Friend (1969)
    Item format: 28 statements answered on a true–false format
    Item content: Items assess both subjective social anxiety and the tendency to avoid social interaction.
    Reliability: KR-20 = .94

Social Anxiety Subscale of the Self-Consciousness Scale
    Location: Fenigstein, Scheier, and Buss (1975)
    Item format: Six items answered on a 5-point scale
    Item content: Items assess anxiety and inhibited behavior in several social contexts.
    Reliability: Cronbach's alpha = .70; 2-week test–retest = .73

Shyness Scale
    Location: Cheek and Buss (1981)

(continued)

(*continued from p. 102*)

Item format: Original scale contained nine items answered on 5-point scales; Cheek (1983) presented an improved 13-item version.

Item content: Items assess both subjective social anxiety and behavioral inhibition.

Reliability: 45-day test–retest = .88

Personal Report of Communication Apprehension–24
Location: McCroskey (1982)
Item format: 24 items answered on 5-point scales
Item content: Items assess social anxiety involving communication in four distinct contexts: public speaking, meetings, groups, and conversations.
Reliability: Cronbach's alpha > .75 for each subscale and > .90 for the total score

Interaction Anxiousness Scale
Location: Leary (1983c)
Item format: 15 statements answered on a 5-point scale
Item content: Unlike most other measures, the items assess subjective social anxiety independent of inhibited and avoidant behavior.
Reliability: Cronbach's alpha > .85

Social Phobia and Anxiety Inventory
Location: S. M. Turner, Beidel, Dancu, and Stanley (1989)
Item format: 32 items answered on a 7-point scale
Item content: Feelings of anxiety in specific social situations, as well as thoughts and somatic/physiological symptoms
Reliability: Cronbach's alpha > .90; test-retest > .80

IS SOCIAL PHOBIA EXTREME SOCIAL ANXIETY?

At least 1 out of 50 Americans experiences a degree of trait social anxiety sufficient to qualify for a diagnosis of social phobia (Pollard & Henderson, 1988; L. N. Robins et al., 1984). Of those clients who seek professional help for excessive anxiety, approximately 10% are diagnosed as social phobic (Marks, 1970; Sanderson, Rapee, & Barlow, 1987).

Despite the obvious similarity between trait social anxiety and social phobia, the question exists of whether social phobia is *nothing but* excessive social anxiousness. On one hand, most evidence suggests that social phobia is an extreme manifestation of "normal" social anxiety, and that the differences between trait social anxiety and social phobia are primarily a matter of degree. On the other hand, some have argued that social phobia is qualitatively distinct from social anxiousness, just as clinical depression is something other than extreme sadness.

Although the evidence is mixed (Cheek & Melchoir, 1990; S. M. Turner, Beidel, & Townsley, 1990), we see little reason to assume that social phobia is qualitatively different from trait social anxiety (Heimberg et al., 1987; Scholing & Emmelkamp, 1990). Social phobics have more intense feelings of anxiety in social situations, their attempts to avoid difficult social encounters are more desperate, and their anxiety has a more deleterious impact on their daily lives, but, as we will see, the precipitating factors and behavioral consequences of social phobia are similar to those of trait social anxiety.

Furthermore, although researchers of social phobia have rarely utilized a self-presentational approach to the problem, the description of social phobia in the DSM-IV clearly acknowledges the role of self-presentational factors, highlighting the role of social scrutiny, as well as concerns that one will behave in ways that result in humiliation or embarrassment. Thus, the self-presentational approach should help us understand social phobia (Heimberg et al., 1987; Leary & Kowalski, 1995). But, first, we begin by examining the possibility that individual differences in social anxiety (and social phobia) are due, in part, to genetic factors.

TEMPERAMENTAL UNDERPINNINGS

A temperament is a personality disposition that involves styles of behavior or emotion that are unlearned and for which evidence of a genetic component exists (Allport, 1961; Buss & Plomin, 1975).

The existence of a temperament does not imply that the person's responses may not be modified by environmental factors or affected by learning, only that he or she has inherited a physical constitution that affects behavior in specific, consistent ways. Of course, strictly speaking, behaviors, thoughts, and feelings are not inherited from one's parents. Rather, one inherits a nervous system that is structured in such a way that certain kinds of responses occur more easily or frequently than others. Thus, people do not inherit social anxiety, but rather a constitutional vulnerability to be socially anxious.

Evidence relevant to whether or not a trait has a temperamental basis is obtained primarily from studies of monozygotic (identical) and dizygotic (fraternal) twins. By examining the degree to which monozygotic versus dizygotic twins resemble one another, researchers can estimate the extent to which a certain characteristic is heritable. If a characteristic has a genetic basis, monozygotic twins (who share exactly the same genetic material) should be more similar than dizygotic twins and ordinary siblings (who share 50% of their genes).

Of course, characteristics differ in the degree to which they are affected by genetic factors. Some attributes (such as eye color) are strongly determined by genetic influences, whereas other characteristics are only weakly related to genetic factors or not inherited at all. Researchers express the degree to which a characteristic is genetically based by the heritability coefficient (h^2), which expresses the "proportion of phenotypic variance accounted for by genetic factors in a population" (Willerman, 1979, p. 106). That is, h^2 indicates the proportion of variability in a particular characteristic that is genetic. For example, if h^2 for a particular characteristic is .23, 23% of the variation we see among individuals in the characteristic is accounted for by genetic factors.

Few studies have directly examined the heritability of social anxiety or social phobia per se. Rather, researchers have focused primarily on the genetic basis of shyness and other constructs that involve both anxiety *and* behavioral inhibition or avoidance. In his research on basic personality factors, Cattell (1973) identified a personality dimension that he called the H-negative or threctic personality. Threctic people tend to be shy, timid, restrained, and sensitive to physical and social threats. They are contrasted to what Cattell referred to as paramic individuals who are adventurous, confident in interpersonal encounters, and thick-skinned. Cattell's data revealed that threctia has a heritability coefficient of .40, indicating that 40% of the variability we observe on this dimension has a genetic basis.

Other evidence of a familial basis of social anxiety comes from research showing that the first- and second-degree adult relatives of shy, fearful, inhibited infants report higher levels of social anxiety than the relatives of uninhibited children (Kagan, Snidman, Julia-Sellers, & Johnson, 1991). By itself, such findings provide little support for a genetic mechanism; after all, children may resemble their relatives not only because they share genetic material, but because they share experiences. However, Cheek and Zonderman (cited in Cheek, 1982) found that the correlation between the shyness scores for monozygotic twins was significantly greater than the correlation for dizygotic twins. Heritability estimates for shyness in excess of .50 were obtained.

Research on the twins of clients diagnosed with anxiety disorders also provides evidence for a heritable basis of trait social anxiety. The probability of one twin having an anxiety disorder if the other did was twice as high for monozygotic twins (34%) as for dizygotic twins (17%) (Torgerson, 1983).

Based on their review of several studies of shyness, Plomin and Daniels (1986) concluded that "heredity influences individual differences in shyness more than in any other personality trait" (p. 78). Although evidence of a biological basis for individual differences in social anxiety is strong, we know little about the underlying physiological mechanisms involved. One likely candidate is the degree to which people's sympathetic nervous systems respond to real or imagined threats to their well-being (Buss & Plomin, 1975).

As we discuss in Chapter 7, anxiety involves activation of the sympathetic nervous system. Apparently, some people's nervous systems activate more easily than others, and such people are more likely to experience anxiety than those whose nervous systems are slower to respond. Along these lines, Cattell (1973) suggested that the people he identified as threctic are highly sensitive to threatening situations because their sympathetic nervous systems have a lower threshold of activation.

Evidence in support of the heritability of sympathetic arousal shows that children who are inhibited or generally fearful tend to have higher heart rates than noninhibited children (Kagan et al., 1988). Inhibited children are also more likely than uninhibited children to show an increase in heart rate and muscular tension when they confront threatening situations. They also have higher levels of urinary epinephrine and salivary cortisol—hormones released in response to stress—than noninhibited children. Among adults, socially anxious clients had more spontaneous fluctuations in their resting galvanic skin response (GSR), an index of sympathetic nervous system activity, than nonanxious clients (Lader, 1967). Findings such as these led Kagan et al. (1988) to conclude that "most of the children we call inhibited belong to a qualitatively distinct category of infants who were born with a lower threshold for limbic–hypothalamic arousal to unexpected changes in the environment or novel events that cannot be assimilated easily" (p. 171).

Despite strong evidence of temperamental underpinnings for social anxiety, little evidence exists to suggest that these temperamental factors are specific to *social* anxiety. Rather, the genetic predisposition for sympathetic arousal seems to affect the tendency to experience anxiety more generally. For example, Berberian and Snyder (1982) found that infants who were temperamentally fussy and difficult tended to be more fearful and less friendly when approached by a stranger than did easygoing infants. Similarly, Scarr and Salapatek (1970) found that infants' fearfulness of a stranger was associated with general negativity, nonadaptivity, avoidance of new situations, and a low sensory threshold. Apparently, inherited predispositions toward arousability and emotionality account for some individual differences in anxiety and inhibition in social settings.

That people may inherit a low threshold for sympathetic arousal may also explain why categories of anxiety overlap so greatly. For example, although social phobics report greater fears in social situations than other types of anxious clients, a high percentage of people who have been diagnosed with nonsocial fears (such as generalized anxiety disorder, panic disorder, or agoraphobia) also experience a high level of social anxiety (Barlow, 1985; Barlow, DiNardo, Vermilyea, Vermilyea, & Blanchard, 1986; Rapee, Sanderson, & Barlow, 1988). Furthermore, although Torgerson (1983) demonstrated a familial basis of anxiety disorders, he found little evidence that particular *types* of anxiety disorders ran in families. Temperamental factors appear to contribute to the development of not only social anxiety and avoidance, but also panic reactions, agoraphobia, and other anxiety states (Kagan et al., 1988).

One of the more intriguing findings to come from studies of the heritability of social anxiety and shyness is that socially anxious people and their close relatives tend to experience certain health problems more frequently than less socially anxious people and their relatives. Specifically, the close relatives of shy, anxious children report a higher incidence of hay fever, eczema, stomach cramps, and menstrual problems than the close relatives of nonshy children! Furthermore, socially anxious adults report more problems with skin and respiratory allergies, and introversion is associated with increased susceptibility to hay fever (Bell, Jasnoski, Kagan, & King, 1990). These relationships between social anxiety (and accompanying behavioral inhibition) and physical symptoms may be due to the neurotransmitters involved in emotion. These neurotransmitters not only mediate sympathetic nervous system arousal, but they affect allergic reactions, such as those involved in hay fever. As Kagan et al. (1991) observed, "many neurochemical mediators whose levels rise both in the nasal allergic secretions and the plasma of allergic rhinitis patients during allergic reactions are also active in the limbic system as neurotransmitters or neuromodulators that affect emotional mood" (p. 338). Thus, the genetic mechanisms involved in the development of extreme shyness or social anxiety involve factors that incidentally influence vulnerability to certain allergies.

Another intriguing connection between shyness and genetic influences involves the fact that, among Caucasian children, behaviorial inhibition is disproportionately common in children with blue eyes (Rosenberg & Kagan, 1987; Rubin & Both, 1989; see following box). The basis of the link between eye color and inhibition has not been identified, but it may involve the fact that iris pigmentation is associated with the concentration of certain neurotransmitters (Rosenberg & Kagan, 1987).

Snow White, Pinocchio, and Cinderella: Are Blue-Eyed Cartoon Characters Socially Vulnerable?

Arcus (1989) raised the provocative question of whether cartoon characters also demonstrate the relationship between inhibition and eye color documented in human children (Rosenberg & Kagan, 1987; Rubin & Both, 1989). She inspected the eye color of 33 Caucasian characters in Disney animated films. Consistent with the research on children, Arcus found that characters who had blue eyes—such as Snow White, Pinocchio, Geppetto, Dopey, Cinderella, and Alice in Wonderland—were significantly more "vulnerable" than characters who were not blue-eyed—such as the evil queen in Snow White, Peter Pan, Captain Hook, and Merlin the Magician. Some exceptions existed—for example, Bashful (one of the seven dwarfs) has brown eyes—but the association was strong and significant. Arcus speculated that cartoon animators illustrate their characters based on popular stereotypes, which occasionally have some degree of validity.

Although the genetic basis of the link between eye color and inhibition is not understood at this time, if the Disney movies are to be believed, the mechanism must be strange indeed. After all, Pinocchio had blue eyes just like his "father," Geppetto, even though Pinocchio was made out of wood.

THE DEVELOPMENT OF PERSONALITY PREDISPOSITIONS

Although temperamental factors predispose some people to be more socially anxious than others, trait social anxiety is also related to personality predispositions that result from experience rather than genetics. In this section, we examine personality factors that predispose some people to be high in social anxiety. Specifically, we discuss the roots of five personal characteristics that predispose some people to be more socially anxious than others: general trait anxiety, self-consciousness, approval motivation, self-esteem, and interpersonal competence.

General Trait Anxiety

As we have seen, various types of anxiety are correlated. People who are generally anxious about one anxiety-producing stimulus tend to be more anxious than average about other things as well. In light of this, the tendency to be generally anxious may underlie some individual differences in social anxiety. For example, scores on the Interaction Anxiousness Scale correlate moderately with scores on the neuroticism scales of both the Eysenck Personality Inventory and the NEO Personality Inventory. Interaction anxiousness also correlates strongly with trait anxiety and moderately with scores on the Manifest Anxiety Scale (Leary & Kowalski, 1993).

The relationship between general trait anxiety and trait social anxiety may be due to a number of factors. First, as discussed earlier, some people's nervous systems are inherently more responsive to threat than others'. People with a reactive sympathetic nervous system will be likely to respond more quickly to all kinds of potentially threatening stimuli than people with less responsive systems.

Second, because anxiety depends on the individual's appraisal of the potential threat in a situation (Lazarus & Folkman, 1984), people who, for whatever reason, have learned to look for the worst in situations are more likely to be anxious. Thus, people who are sensitizers or pessimists are more likely to be upset about nearly everything, including how they are being regarded by other people.

Third, once people confront a threat to their physical or psychological well-being, their reaction depends in part on how they cope with the situation (C. A. Smith, 1991). Some people cope better with difficult situations of all types than other people. Individuals with poor coping skills are likely to experience greater anxiety across a broad array of situations, including social encounters. Whatever the source of the connection, people who are high in general trait anxiety tend also to be socially anxious.

Self-Consciousness

As we saw in Chapter 3, people who are high in public self-consciousness think a great deal about how they are coming across to others and, as a result, are sensitive to others' evaluations of them (Buss, 1980; Fenigstein, 1979). People who are low in public self-consciousness are less aware of and, apparently, less interested in how they are perceived and regarded by others. Given these differences in awareness of others' impressions, public self-consciousness correlates positively with social anxiety among both unselected college students and social phobics (Buss, 1980; Edelmann, 1990; Hope & Heimberg, 1988; Leary & Kowalski, 1993).

But where does public self-consciousness come from? Research on this question is limited, but evidence suggests that parental behaviors play some role. Parents who are authoritarian, strict, and demanding are more likely to have children who are high in public self-consciousness. When parents are demanding and critical, children learn to monitor their public behaviors carefully and perceive that public shortcomings often lead to punishment. Parental emphasis on achievement may also relate to public self-consciousness because it stresses that one should be concerned with others' impressions and expectations (Klonsky, Dutton, & Liebel, 1990).

Children of publicly self-conscious parents may also learn to be publicly self-conscious through modeling. Children who observe that their parents are preoccupied with others' evaluations are likely to exercise greater self-scrutiny than children whose parents are not obviously concerned with others' evaluations. When parents often express concerns with what neighbors, friends, family, and coworkers think about their income, house, car, clothing, children's behavior, or occupational prestige, children may conclude that it is important to consider others' perceptions and evaluations of oneself.

At the same time, highly self-conscious parents may instruct their children to behave in ways that will make the "right" impressions. Parents who regularly admonish their children to consider what others will think of their behavior may convey to their children that the standards for judging the appropriateness of behavior are others' reactions to it. An emphasis on the child's appearance and clothing should also help foster public self-consciousness.

Approval Motivation

As we've seen, people who are highly motivated to obtain social approval and avoid disapproval are predisposed to experience social anxiety, presumably because they are motivated to control how they are regarded by others (see Chapter 3). Trait social anxiety correlates moderately with measures of approval motivation and fear of negative evaluation (W. H. Jones et al., 1986; Leary & Kowalski, 1993).

An extensive series of longitudinal studies investigated developmental anteccdents of approval motivation (Allaman, Joyce, & Crandall, 1972). These researchers identified a set of predictors of need for approval that centered around the practices that parents use in raising their children. In general, children who scored high on a measure of approval motivation tended to have parents who used relatively harsh modes of child rearing. Compared to mothers of children who were low in need for approval, mothers of children high in need for approval tended to be less warm and affectionate, praised their children less, and punished them more. The relationship between these parental behaviors and children's need for approval was quite strong; maternal behavior predicted over 60% of the variance in need for approval scores. In addition, perceived rejection by the father was correlated with high need for approval among young men.

Allaman and colleagues (1972) concluded that parenting practices that communicate disinterest, disapproval, or rejection to the child create a generalized concern with others' evaluations and a strong desire for approval and acceptance from the parents and others. Much of the behavior of high need for approval individuals can be interpreted as attempts to obtain approval and avoid disapproval (see Strickland, 1977, for a review). Unfortunately, children of disapproving, rejecting parents not only are highly motivated to gain approval, but they are also likely to doubt that they can actually obtain it. Allaman and colleagues foreshadowed the self-presentational approach to social anxiety by noting that "a combination of high value for approval (or avoidance of disapproval), but a low expectancy of obtaining it results in apprehension in evaluative situations" (p. 1156).

Self-Esteem

Self-esteem correlates negatively with trait social anxiety of all types (Cheek & Buss, 1981; Clark & Arkowitz, 1975; Geist & Borecki,

1982; W. H. Jones, Briggs, & Smith, 1986; Leary & Kowalski, 1993; McCroskey, 1977). Not surprisingly, many of the developmental antecedents of social anxiety are similar to the antecedents of self-esteem (Klonsky et al., 1990).

The primary cause of low self-esteem appears to be a history of disapproval or rejection by family or peers. As early symbolic interactionists, such as Cooley (1902/1922), first observed, people's views of themselves depend on how they think they are regarded by other people. Thus, parents who are rejecting or indifferent toward their children tend to foster low self-esteem. Parents who are excessively authoritarian or harsh on one hand, or excessively permissive on the other, tend to have children with lower self-esteem than parents who are accepting, affectionate, firm, and involved (Baumrind, 1989; Coopersmith, 1967).

The sociometer theory of self-esteem (Leary & Downs, 1995) suggests a novel perspective on the link between rejection, self-esteem, and social anxiety. According to this theory, the self-esteem system functions as a "sociometer" that monitors the individual's behavior and the social environment (particularly others' reactions) for indications that the person may experience social disapproval or rejection. When cues connoting rejection are detected, the system alerts the individual via negative affect and motivates behavior to restore one's standing with other people. The self-esteem system may have evolved as a mechanism for minimizing the likelihood of social exclusion (Leary, 1990b; Leary & Downs, 1995; Leary, Tambor, Terdal, & Downs, 1995).

Anxiety may play a role in this process by alerting the individual when his or her social relationships are in jeopardy and providing an impetus for taking remedial action; anxiety is a common response when one's sense of inclusion and belongingness is threatened (Baumeister & Tice, 1990). Viewed in this way, social anxiety may be the affective warning system of the sociometer.

This theory readily explains why a history of rejection leads to low trait self-esteem, as well as to a propensity to experience social anxiety (Harter, 1983; Spivey, 1990). Frequent rejection results in a chronically low sense of self-regard that essentially calibrates the sociometer to be highly sensitive to interpersonal threats. Thus, a person with low self-esteem is likely to perceive the possibility of rejection where a high self-esteem person would not (Leary & Downs, 1995).

Interpersonal Competence

In Chapter 4, we explained how the tendency to experience social anxiety is inversely related to social competence. Thus, individual differences in trait social anxiety are related, in part, to individual differences in social skill.

As with most complex actions, social responses are acquired primarily through observation and modeling (Bandura, 1973). For children, the most potent models for many behaviors are parents. Parents who are not socially adroit will not provide appropriate models for their children to emulate. Not only will children of socially unskilled parents fail to observe frequent instances of skilled behaviors, but they may actually imitate examples of inappropriate, maladaptive social responses. When a child sees a parent falter nervously in social situations, use annoying or ambiguous nonverbal gestures, speak too fast or too slowly for maximal communication, or fail to provide the social cues that facilitate contingent interactions, the child will not learn skillful ways of responding and may even imitate the parent's unskilled behavior. Children of socially competent, confident, and poised parents, on the other hand, have accessible models from which to learn adaptive social responses.

In one study of the link between social difficulties in parents and their children, college students and their parents completed the Social Avoidance and Distress Scale (a measure of trait social anxiety) and the Dyadic Adjustment Scale (a measure of interpersonal competence in close relationships). Mothers' social anxiety scores correlated positively with their children's social anxiety scores and negatively with their children's interpersonal competence, suggesting that socially anxious and avoidant mothers tend to raise children who also have social difficulties. No correlations were found between fathers' and children's scores on the two measures (Filsinger & Lamke, 1983).

In addition to modeling social behavior, some parents instruct their children directly regarding important interpersonal skills. Children may be taught to converse effectively, to use appropriate nonverbal gestures, to be a good listener, to be polite, and so on.

Social behaviors require practice to make perfect. Parents who frequently talk with their children and who encourage their children to express themselves provide them with needed practice. Similarly, some parents provide opportunities for children to practice public speaking and performing at home in front of the family. Children who learn to express themselves effectively at home will carry their social skills and confidence into the outside world. Similarly, children who are exposed from an early age to a wide variety of people, places, and types of social events should develop greater confidence in their ability to handle themselves in social encounters.

SUSCEPTIBILITY TO SOCIAL ANXIETY IN SPECIFIC CONTEXTS

Some people show a tendency to become socially anxious in particular kinds of social encounters. For instance, some people are terrified by the prospect of giving a speech, but are at ease in face-to-face conversations. Other individuals become nervous and inhibited in dyadic conversations but are confident orators or performers. This fact has led some researchers to focus their attention on specific subtypes of trait social anxiety or social phobia.

As noted in Chapter 1, we regard it as misleading to view these as different "types" of social anxiety. In each case, the subjective experience of anxiety is the same, and it emerges from the same self-presentational concerns that we have discussed throughout this book. What differs is not the anxiety, but the structure of the interpersonal context that triggers the anxiety. Even so, people who are particularly prone to experience anxiety in different kinds of social situations do differ in certain ways (see Heimberg, Holt, Schneier, Spitzer, & Liebowitz, 1993). For reasons we will discuss, some people are predisposed to feel particularly anxious *in specific kinds of encounters*. In this section, we focus on five social contexts in which social anxiety is commonly experienced: interpersonal communication, interactions with the other sex, encounters in which physical appearance is salient, tests, and sport performance.

Communication Apprehension

Much of the earliest research on socially based anxieties focused on people who become highly anxious when they speak or perform in front of groups (Clevinger, 1959; Gilkinson, 1942, 1943; Paul, 1966), possibly because anxiety when speaking or performing is so common. Not only do a high percentage of otherwise normal people face the prospect of speaking in public with trepidation, but people who are diagnosed as social phobic nearly always fear, among other things, speaking in public (Pollard & Henderson, 1988). Researchers and therapists have referred to such anxieties by a number of terms, including stage fright, speech anxiety, audience anxiety, and communication apprehension. Not surprisingly, most research on this form of social anxiety has been conducted by communication researchers, as well as by psychologists and psychiatrists interested in social phobics who fear speaking in public.

James McCroskey has been a leader in the study of communication apprehension—anxiety that is associated with real or anticipated communication with other people (McCroskey, 1977). McCroskey has not only contributed a great deal to our understanding of people's communication fears (e.g., McCroskey, 1977, 1982, 1984), but has developed several widely used measures to assess communication apprehension and related constructs. Early in his research program, McCroskey (1970, 1978) constructed the Personal Report of Communication Apprehension (PRCA) to measure individual differences in communication apprehension. Although early versions of the PRCA contained items assessing anxiety experienced in interpersonal communications, small group discussions, and public speaking situations, items assessing public speaking were overrepresented on the original measure (D. T. Porter, 1979). Therefore, McCroskey (1982) constructed a new version of the scale, the Personal Report of Communication Apprehension–24 (PRCA-24) to tap anxiety in four specific types of communication contexts.

The PRCA-24 contains four subscales that measure communication apprehension in group discussions, conversations, meetings, and public speaking situations. As one would expect, people who score high on these subscales feel more anxious when they actually find themselves in these sorts of situations (Allen, Richmond, & McCroskey, 1984; McCroskey & Beatty, 1984). Furthermore, communication apprehension experienced in one context is moderately to strongly related to apprehension in other contexts. The high correlations among the four subscales suggest that communication apprehension is a general, traitlike response to communication that is largely irrespective of social context (McCroskey, Beatty, Kearney, & Plax, 1985). People who are characteristically nervous about communicating in one type of situation are also likely to be nervous about communicating in others.

Little research has been devoted specifically to the development of individual differences in communication apprehension (Comadena & Prusank, 1989), but the personological underpinnings appear to be the same as those for trait social anxiety more generally. In addition, McCroskey and Beatty (1984) hypothesized that patterns of reinforcement during childhood may be the most important contributor to communication apprehension. Children who are punished for communicating will likely develop negative reactions to communicating, whereas those who are rewarded will approach communication, if not with confidence, at least with a lack of anxiety (see Daly & Friedrich, 1981). Unfortunately, parents and teachers often regard "well-behaved" children as those who are typically quiet, thereby inadvertently reinforcing social reticence while perhaps punishing communication (Hurt, Scott, & McCroskey, 1978).

Heterosocial Anxiety

Among heterosexuals, members of the other sex appear to be particularly potent causes of social anxiety. (Presumably, homosexuals experience a similar sort of anxiety around members of their own sex; see box on page 118.) As we saw in Chapter 3, not only are many people highly motivated to make desired impressions on those of the other sex, but they often feel incapable of making the kinds of impressions they desire.

Although heterosocial interactions (social encounters with people of the other sex) cause social anxiety for most people at least occasionally, some people are particularly bothered by heterosocial situations, particularly interactions with potential romantic partners and dates with people they do not know well. In one study of nearly 4,000 randomly sampled undergraduates, 37% of the men and 25% of the women indicated that they were "somewhat" or "very" anxious about dating (Arkowitz et al., 1978).

Heterocentrism and Social Anxiety

Most research on heterosocial and dating anxiety has been clouded by inadvertent heterocentrism. Researchers who have studied people's feelings of anxiety in encounters with the other sex have rarely taken into account the sexual orientation of their subjects. If heterosocial anxiety involves concerns with the evaluations of one's desirability by members of the other sex, such concerns are likely to arise primarily, if not exclusively among heterosexuals. Gay men and lesbians should not be particularly prone to "heterosocial anxiety."

This observation has at least three implications. First, failing to account for subjects' sexual orientation in studies of heterosocial and dating anxiety may increase the error variance in the data, if not obscure the nature of the relationships among the variables under investigation.

Second, research is needed that explores the analogue of heterosocial/dating anxiety among homosexuals. Presumably, gay men and lesbians experience social anxiety in certain same-sex encounters that is at least as problematic as the anxiety experienced by heterosexuals in cross-sex encounters.

Finally, given that gay men and lesbians experience feelings analogous to heterosocial anxiety, the critical cause of heterosocial anxiety is not, as the label implies, members of the *other sex*. A more general term for the experience is needed (perhaps "relational anxiety"), along with efforts to identify its defining characteristics. Is this more general construct best characterized as a reaction to people (1) who are possible romantic partners, (2) who may provide direct or indirect evidence of one's sexual desirability, or (3) to whom one is potentially sexually attracted? A reconceptualization of so-called heterosocial or dating anxiety may illuminate interpersonal processes involved in relationships in which sexuality is salient.

Unfortunately, social anxiety can complicate cross-sex interactions. Kowalski (1993b) found that socially anxious men perceived women's behaviors as connoting greater sexual interest than men low in social anxiety. In contrast, socially anxious women attached less sexual meaning to behaviors than less anxious women.

When faced with ambiguous, anxiety producing situations, such as first dates, people fall back on readily accessible schemas which, for men, tend to be more sexual than for women. Obviously, such a disparity in perceptions of dating behaviors can lead to serious misunderstandings and even acquaintance rape (Abbey, 1987; Kowalski, 1993a).

It is important to recognize that people who are particularly prone to heterosocial anxiety also experience greater self-consciousness and social anxiety in same-sex interactions than people who are not heterosocially anxious (Himadi, Arkowitz, Hinton, & Perl, 1980; C. J. Robins, 1986). In light of this difference, research is needed that examines the degree to which trait heterosocial anxiety can be meaningfully distinguished from general social anxiousness. If we should find that most heterosocial anxiety can be accounted for by trait social anxiety, we would have to consider the possibility that so-called heterosocially anxious people are simply anxious in social settings of all sorts.

Appearance and Physique Anxiety

Some people are worried about how others regard their physical appearance. To the extent that appearance affects others' impressions of the individual, many people worry about how their physical bodies are perceived by others. People who rate their bodies less favorably tend to be more socially anxious (Hart et al., 1989). Furthermore, physique anxiety—the tendency to worry about others' perceptions of one's body's form and structure—correlates moderately with trait social anxiety (Leary & Kowalski, 1993).

As with all social anxiety, anxiety emerging from concerns with one's appearance increases with the motivation to make a desired impression (i.e., to be perceived as attractive) and with doubts that one will make the desired impression. For example, scores on the Body Self-Consciousness Scale—which measures a person's motivation to be physically attractive—correlate with both physique anxiety and trait social anxiety (Hart et al., 1989; Leary & Kowalski, 1993). Thus, people who, because of parental or peer pressure, learn to place a great deal of emphasis on their personal appearance are more prone to physique anxiety specifically and social anxiety more generally.

Some people's concerns with others' impressions of their bodies appear to be well placed. To the extent that others' perceptions are affected by one's appearance, it stands to reason that people who do not meet minimal cultural standards regarding attractiveness will be concerned about others' reactions to them. For example, people with a higher percentage of body fat tend to be more physique-anxious than people with lower body fat (Hart, 1987). Furthermore, physical exercise is associated with a decrease in physique anxiety (McAuley, Rudolph, & Lox, 1994). However, physique-anxious people may be reluctant to exercise when doing so requires that they reveal parts of their body to others (Crawford & Eklund, 1994).

People with a physical stigma may also be more prone to feelings of social anxiety. People with obvious deformities or unseemly skin problems (such as extreme acne or psoriasis) are likely to be socially anxious much of the time. Psoriasis patients score high on measures of trait social anxiety and fear of negative evaluation (Rapp & Leary, 1994). Even if they learn to discount others' negative reactions to their physical appearance, they may remain distressed by the interpersonal awkwardness they often encounter.

Test Anxiety

During the past 20 years, a large literature has developed around the construct of test anxiety. Realizing that students of all ages are troubled by sometimes paralyzing anxiety when they must take tests, researchers and therapists have studied the antecedents of test anxiety, the consequences of anxiety for students' academic performance and personal adjustment, and the effectiveness of various methods of reducing exceptionally high test anxiety (Sarason, 1980; Sarason & Sarason, 1990).

Somewhat surprisingly, few researchers have pursued the obvious connection between test anxiety and social anxiety (see, however, Beck & Emery, 1985; Sarason & Sarason, 1990). When people experience intense anxiety before or during tests, they are not, strictly speaking, afraid of the test or even of failing the test. Rather, they are usually worried primarily about the *interpersonal implications* of doing poorly on the test and specifically how their test performance will lead them to be perceived and evaluated by other people. For most students, three audiences are most salient: teachers, parents, and peers. Thus, test anxiety is, in most cases, social anxiety arising when the test-taker is motivated to convey a particular impression (of being intelligent, motivated, or a good student), but believes that his or her performance on the test will discredit the impression he or she desires to convey.

Test anxiety shares many of the same dispositional antecedents as social anxiety, many of them involving fear of failure and concerns with social evaluation (Sarason, 1980). Furthermore, like social anxiety, high test anxiety involves a tendency to be preoccupied by self-denigrating and catastrophic thoughts (Sarason & Sarason, 1990; Wine, 1971).

Although most test anxiety can be regarded as social anxiety, there are a few exceptions. For example, tests often have educational, occupational, and financial implications, as they determine the colleges we attend, the jobs we obtain, and how much money we make. In some cases, these implications have self-presentational ramifications, such as when a student worries about what others will think when his or her poor test scores prevent acceptance into medical school. Even so, some implications are not self-presentational. For example, failing to pass an exam during a job interview may mean not getting the job and having to sell one's house—an outcome with much more than self-presentational implications.

Sport Performance Anxiety

Sport performance anxiety (sometimes called competition anxiety) is yet another variant of social anxiety. People who compete against others, whether in a friendly set of weekend tennis or in the Super Bowl, often feel nervous while competing. (Quarterback Jim Kelly's teammates publicized his frequent bouts with vomiting before games leading up to the Buffalo Bills' appearance in the 1994 Super Bowl.) Stimulated by the work of Martens (1977), sport psychologists and others became interested in understanding the causes and consequences of sport performance anxiety: "a learned tendency to respond with cognitive and/or somatic state anxiety to competitive sport situations in which the adequacy of the athlete's performance can be evaluated" (Smith & Smoll, 1990, p. 421).

Although a great deal of research has investigated sport performance anxiety in many different kinds of athletes, little attention has been devoted to the question of what people are really worried about when they compete. In our view, competition and sport performance anxiety are best regarded as a variety of social anxiety that, like all social anxiety, is caused by people's concerns with how they are perceived and evaluated (Leary, 1992).

For many people, sport is an important arena in which one's ability, motivation, and personality are scrutinized and evaluated by other people. Whenever people play sports, they risk conveying unflattering images of themselves to others present. They may worry about fans, friends, teammates, coaches, opponents, and others seeing them as unskilled, incompetent, out of shape, unable to handle pressure, or, at worst, a chronic loser. Presumably, the more important it is for the person to be perceived in particular ways (or not to be perceived in particular ways) and the more the person doubts that he or she will convey the desired impressions, the more anxiety he or she will experience.

Individual differences in competition or sport performance anxiety are often measured with the Sport Competition Anxiety Test (Martens, 1977) or the Sport Anxiety Scale (R. E. Smith, Smoll, & Schutz, 1990). As one would expect, many of the psychological predictors of sport performance anxiety are the same as for social anxiety more generally, such as low self-esteem and a low expectancy of doing well (Scanlan & Passer, 1978, 1979).

Sport performance anxiety correlates negatively with indices of athletic performance, such as batting average, speed swimming, free throw shooting, and soccer performance (for a review, see R. E. Smith & Smoll, 1990). In addition, high sport performance anxiety deters many people from participating in sports; one study showed that 75% of a sample of 8- and 9-year-olds who did not participate in sports indicated that they did not because they were afraid of performing poorly or of not making the team (Orlick & Botterill,

1975). Not surprisingly, people who score high on measures of sport anxiety also enjoy sports less (Scanlan & Lewthwaite, 1986; R. E. Smith, Smoll, & Curtis, 1978).

GENDER DIFFERENCES

Which sex tends to be most socially anxious—men or women? The data are inconsistent and inconclusive. Studies have found that women score higher than men on measures of shyness (Morris, 1982), communication apprehension (McCroskey, 1982), dating anxiety (Arkowitz et al., 1978), embarrassability (Edelmann, 1987), and heterosocial anxiety (Leary & Dobbins, 1983). Others have found that men score higher than women on measures of social avoidance and distress (Glass et al., 1982; Watson & Friend, 1969) and shyness (Pilkonis, 1977b). Still others have failed to find sex differences at all (Hansford & Hattie, 1982), and approximately 50% of those diagnosed as social phobic are of each sex (S. M. Turner & Beidel, 1989). The lack of consistent sex differences in social anxiety is unusual, if not unique, among anxieties. Most other anxiety and phobic conditions are consistently more common among women.

If we consider sex differences in trait social anxiety from the self-presentational perspective, these contradictory findings are really not surprising. Men and women are socialized to possess somewhat different kinds of social competencies, to view themselves in different ways, and to be motivated to convey somewhat different images of themselves to other people (Deaux & Major, 1987). Thus, whether men or women experience greater social anxiety should depend upon the responses and self-presentations required in a particular social setting. For example, men are probably less anxious about initiating conversations (dates, sexual encounters, etc.) with the other sex and with being generally assertive than are women. They typically have had more cultural training and experience in this arena than women (although those differences are decreasing). Three of the four measures on which women score higher than men are heavily peppered with items dealing with initiating social encounters and with assertiveness.

AGE-RELATED CHANGES

Wariness in Infancy

Because people are not motivated to manage their impressions unless they are aware that they are being perceived and evaluated by others, children do not feel socially anxious until they have developed the capacity to be consciously aware of themselves and to be concerned with how they are viewed by other people. Some parents may object to this assertion, insisting that their children showed signs of being anxious in social settings long before the child was able to think about him- or herself as a social object. Even very young babies become distressed in the presence of strangers and in new situations. As early as the sixth month of life, babies frown or cry, show increased heart rate, and attempt to withdraw when strangers approach (Stroufe, 1977; Thompson & Limber, 1990). This response declines somewhat during the second year of life, but even among preschoolers, strangers are more likely than any other factor to induce shylike behavior (Zimbardo, 1977, 1981). Is this not evidence of social anxiety in the absence of self-awareness and self-presentational concern?

In babies and young children, these reactions, properly called stranger anxiety or wariness, are not evidence of preconscious social anxiety. Although these responses may occur in reaction to social factors, they are more closely related to fears of unknown objects than to social anxiety. Very young children are often fearful of new stimuli, such as unfamiliar animals, strange sounds, seemingly animate toys (such as puppets and masks), and unknown people. The cause of wariness in young children is the presence of unfamiliar or threatening stimuli (particularly those that approach the child), not interpersonal evaluation, as is the case in social anxiety (Buss, 1980; Greenberg & Marvin, 1982).

Furthermore, psychologists' penchant for focusing on aversive emotions has blinded them to the fact that the development of wariness is accompanied by increasing sociability vis à vis well-known people. As Thompson and Limber (1990) noted, "at the same time that babies are beginning to exhibit stranger wariness . . . , they also exhibit a broadened capacity for *positive* reactions to strangers and other social partners" (p. 86) In light of this, an emphasis on stranger *anxiety* among infants may be misleading.

Buss (1980) proposed that wariness in infancy, which he termed early-developing shyness, is distinct from the socially based, self-conscious variety (late-developing shyness) that emerges in later childhood. Early-developing shyness appears to be an innate reaction, although individual differences exist in its strength. Some infants demonstrate a long period of extreme fearfulness to strangers, whereas others are wary only rarely, if at all (Harmon, Morgran, & Klein, 1977). Presumably, such differences are determined in part by temperamental factors such as emotionality, inhibition, and sociability. Genetic factors play a role in the development of these temperaments; identical twins are more similar in wariness than fraternal twins (Plomin & Rowe, 1979).

This reaction can continue into adolescence and adulthood; children who are wary as infants are more likely to be wary as adults (Reznick, 1989). However, as the self emerges, the child develops the capacity for self-relevant thought and, thus, for what Buss called late-developing shyness or what we view as true social anxiety. Whereas wariness (early-developing, fearful shyness) is related to novel stimuli, true social anxiety (late-developing, self-conscious shyness) results from social scrutiny and evaluation.

True Social Anxiety

As Mead (1934), Cooley (1902/1922), and others have observed, the ability to take the perspectives of others vis-à-vis oneself is necessary for most adult social behavior, including the ability to experience social anxiety. The ability to take the viewpoint of others when thinking about oneself does not generally emerge until age four or five (Buss, 1980; Lewis, 1990). Thus, we would not expect to observe evidence of true social anxiety until at least that age. Even then, the complete complement of adult role-taking abilities involved in thinking and caring about others' reactions does not fully develop until years later.

Interestingly, children younger than age two sometimes show signs of being "self-conscious" when other people look at them, when in the presence of strangers, and even when they see their own reflection in a mirror (Buss, 1980; Lewis, Sullivan, Stanger, & Weiss, 1989). However, as we noted earlier, these reactions reflect a more primitive reaction to scrutiny or novelty than adult social anxiety. Apparently, infants react to observing their own reflection as if it were another person gazing at them.

Once children have developed the ability to view themselves as an object, they are able to contemplate how they are perceived and evaluated by others. After that, social anxiety increases with age through adolescence (Kashani, Orvaschel, Rosenberg, & Reid, 1989). Darby and Schlenker (1986) asked second-, fourth-, and seventh-grade students to read brief stories about children in social situations who were or were not motivated to get others to like them and who thought they either would or would not be successful at doing so. Among other things, the subjects were asked how uneasy and nervous the child in the story would be, and how the character might act. With increasing age, subjects became increasingly pessimistic about the character's chances of success. Compared to younger children, older children thought that the character would have more trouble communicating, would act more clumsily, and would fidget more. These data suggest that older children hold lower expectancies of success in social situations.

Older subjects also showed a greater understanding of the determinants of social anxiety. Seventh-graders understood that the characters in the stories were more likely to feel anxious when they were highly motivated to be liked. In contrast, the younger children associated greater motivation with less social anxiety and greater self-confidence, apparently assuming that children who want to do well are confident of doing so.

Adolescence is the most socially anxious period of life for most people. Not only are adolescents particularly prone to feelings of social anxiety, but people who come to be diagnosed as social phobics typically trace the onset of their problems to adolescence (Amies, Gelder, & Shaw, 1983; Marks, 1970; Scholing & Emmelkamp, 1990; S. M. Turner, Beidel, Dancu, & Keys, 1986). Furthermore, people report more episodes of embarrassment during adolescence than at any other time in life (Edelmann, 1987; Horowitz, 1962).

From the standpoint of the self-presentational theory, the increase of social anxiety in adolescence is readily explained. Although children must establish themselves in school and peer groups during childhood, during adolescence, the acceptance of peer groups becomes increasingly important. As Erikson (1950) and others observed, adolescence is characterized by an emphasis on establishing one's place in a social system outside of the family. To the extent that peer acceptance depends on being perceived in particular ways, adolescence is the time at which people first become acutely aware of the importance of the impressions they make on others. Self-consciousness appears to be curvilinearly related to age. Self-consciousness increases in late childhood to a peak in midadolescence, then declines gradually throughout middle and old age (Elkind & Bowen, 1979; Simmons, Rosenberg, & Rosenberg, 1973).

At the same time, adolescents find themselves in a large number of new roles and novel situations as they drop the behaviors and activities of childhood and take on those of young adults. Adolescents are understandably uncertain as they adopt these new roles, which lower their confidence of making the impressions they desire. And, for the first time, they face many of these new situations without being accompanied by parents or other supportive adults. The rapid bodily changes of adolescence further compound the adolescent's uncertainty and insecurity. Concurrent with these changes, one's parents and peers become increasingly intolerant of the adolescent's misbehavior. Whereas children are allowed occasional behavioral indiscretions, with age, adolescents are increasingly likely to be criticized or ridiculed for behaving inappropriately.

Thus, adolescents find themselves in the unenviable position of possessing new bodies, playing new roles, confronting novel situations, and being increasingly ridiculed and criticized. Is it any wonder, then, that adolescence is such an anxiety-prone period of life?

CHAPTER 7

Subjective Aspects of Social Anxiety: Physiology, Cognition, and Emotion

———◇◈◇———

ONE OBSTACLE THAT theorists and researchers have confronted in their attempts to understand the emotion we commonly call anxiety is that anxiety is a complex, multifaceted response that involves several psychological systems. Specifically, subjective anxiety involves three key characteristics: (1) physiological arousal, (2) apprehension regarding an impending, potentially negative outcome, and (3) aversive emotional experience. In addition, an anxious person experiences a heightened motivation to avoid or escape whatever is making him or her anxious, although he or she may or may not act on this urge.

The physiological, cognitive, and affective components must all be present for us to characterize a person's reaction as anxiety. Pure physiological arousal, such as that caused by caffeine or other stimulants, is not anxiety because it is not accompanied by cognitive dread or unpleasant affect. Nor does dread or apprehension regarding an upcoming aversive event always indicate that a person is anxious; we may greatly dread having to get up in the morning or having to go to a family get-together, yet not be anxious. Similarly, mere tension or dysphoria is not equivalent to anxiety; a person who has driven for 18 consecutive hours may feel tense, edgy, and exhausted, but we wouldn't characterize him or her as anxious. In brief, all episodes of anxiety involve a relatively distinct pattern of physiological activity, cognition, and affective feelings. To label someone as anxious we must find that the person is physiologically aroused, cognitively dreads a potentially negative event, and experiences tension and negative affect.

To this point, we have focused primarily on the antecedents of social anxiety—both aspects of the social context that make people feel anxious and the personal characteristics that predispose some people to be more socially anxious than others. Now that we understand why social anxiety occurs, we turn our attention to the experience of social anxiety itself. In this chapter, we discuss the physiological, cognitive, and affective aspects of social anxiety, as well as the effects of anxious arousal and thought on behavior. Chapter 8 then focuses on behavioral manifestations of the anxiety-based motive to avoid and escape.

PHYSIOLOGICAL AROUSAL

Whether caused by social or nonsocial factors, anxiety is accompanied by changes in the autonomic nervous system—those parts of the body that control involuntary responses involving the smooth muscles and glands, such as heart rate, respiration, and digestion.

The Sympathetic and Parasympathetic Systems

The autonomic nervous system is comprised of two branches, the sympathetic and the parasympathetic systems, both of which can be involved in anxiety reactions. These two components of the autonomic nervous system are often portrayed as mutually exclusive—only one may be operative at a time—but this is not an accurate characterization. Although the sympathetic and parasympathetic systems tend to have opposite effects (e.g., sympathetic activity increases heart rate, whereas parasympathetic activity decreases it), some emotional reactions may involve both sympathetic and parasympathetic activation.

The effects of arousal in the sympathetic nervous system have been widely studied. Activity in the sympathetic nervous system increases heart rate, respiration, blood pressure, and muscle tension. At the same time, sympathetic activity lowers activity in the gastrointestinal tract; gastric and intestinal contractions decrease, along with the production of gastric juices. The distribution of blood flow through the body is also affected. Blood flow to peripheral blood vessels, such as those in the face and hands, decreases, whereas that to the muscles and heart increases. These changes in circulation are responsible for the fact that anxious people often have cool hands and pale faces. The net effect of the changes resulting from sympathetic activity is to prepare the individual to deal with imminent threats to well-being by either escaping or directly confronting the threat. Hence, activation of the sympathetic nervous system is often called the "fight or flight" reaction.

People who feel socially anxious show clear evidence of sympathetic arousal. Episodes of social anxiety are associated with increased heart rate, respiration, galvanic skin response, and blood pressure, and with decreased hand temperature (Borkovec et al., 1974; Brodt & Zimbardo, 1981; Houtman & Bakker, 1991; Levin et al., 1993; Puigcerver, Martinez-Selva, Garcia-Sanchez, & Gomez-Amor, 1989; see, however, W. R. Miller & Arkowitz, 1977). In extreme cases, social phobics experience symptoms of intense sympathetic arousal such as those associated with panic attacks—trembling, sweating, heart palpitations, and the like (Amies et al., 1983).

Although the role of the sympathetic nervous system in anxiety reactions has been widely documented, the involvement of the parasympathetic system has been less thoroughly investigated. Activity in the parasympathetic nervous system results in effects that are largely opposite to those caused by sympathetic activity; for example, parasympathetic activation leads to lowered heart rate, blood pressure, and respiration, and to increased digestive activity. As would be expected, then, the parasympathetic nervous system is dominant (and sympathetic activity is low) when people are relaxed, calm, and contented.

However, parasympathetic activity may also accompany certain aversive emotions, including disgust, dejection, anger, and anxiety. Subjectively, a sharp drop in blood pressure leads the person to feel dizzy, weak, or wobbly. In extreme cases, excessively low blood pressure may cause the person to faint.

Frijda (1986) suggested that parasympathetic response patterns often accompany strong negative emotions in situations in which coping actions are not possible. As long as the person has viable ways of dealing with the threat, the sympathetic system remains dominant, keeping the person prepared for fight or flight. However, a sense of sullen or helpless resignation may set in once the person's behavioral options are effectively exhausted. Most commonly, an anxious individual first experiences a pure sympathetic response— increased heart rate, tension, vigilance, and other sympathetic re- actions. These symptoms may then be followed by parasympathet- ically mediated reactions that occur against the backdrop of sympathetic activity. Thus, heart pounding, the nervous person may suddenly feel unsteady (and collapse limply into a chair) as blood pressure decreases.

Recent research on animals lends additional support to the existence of two distinct types of fear responses. The *active fear response* is mediated primarily by the sympathetic nervous system and results in the fight or flight reaction discussed above. Alterna- tively, by decreasing general arousal and quieting most bodily sys- tems, the *passive fear response* prepares the animal to "freeze or hide" (so-called passive fear or atonic immobility) (Frijda, 1986; L. Ham- ilton, 1989). If we imagine a rabbit running from a predator, the sympathetic nervous system will be activated as the rabbit attempts to flee. However, on occasion a rabbit will elude a predator by hiding and remaining motionless. In such instances, activation in the parasympathetic nervous system leads to a reduction in phys- iological arousal, allowing the rabbit to remain stationary (E. N. Smith, Allison, & Crowder, 1974; E. N. Smith & Tobey, 1983).

The Case of Embarrassment

The dual involvement of the sympathetic and parasympathetic sys- tems in humans is perhaps seen most clearly in the case of embar- rassment. When embarrassed, people show signs of sympathetic arousal in some bodily systems, but responses in other systems that are consistent with parasympathetic activity. On one hand, when people are embarrassed, their hands become cooler, reflecting ef- fects of sympathetic activation (Leary et al., 1994). However, em- barrassed individuals also tend to blush, an effect opposite that of sympathetic activation, which reduces blood flow to the face, mak-

ing it pale. Furthermore, embarrassed people report feeling tense
(R. S. Miller, 1986), but their heart rate sometimes (but not always)
decelerates (Buck & Parke, 1972; Hart, 1987).

As we noted in Chapter 5, these seemingly inconsistent reactions, paired with other behaviors that often accompany embarrassment, have led some to question whether embarrassment should
even be considered a variety of social anxiety (Harris, 1990). As
MacCurdy (1930) observed, "the unhappy wretch who blushes,
averts his eyes, hangs his head, covers his face with his hands, and
wishes he might sink through the floor is hardly the picture of fear"
(p. 177). This is only true, however, if we think of fear as mediated
solely by the sympathetic nervous system. As we have seen, fear and
anxiety responses may involve the parasympathetic system as well
(Frijda, 1986).

Embarrassment, particularly passive embarrassment, appears
to involve parasympathetically mediated effects. When people who
are embarrassed respond passively (for example, by grinning stup-
idly but making no attempt to extricate themselves from their
predicament), the parasympathetic system appears to be involved.
Subjectively, embarrassment in such situations is sometimes accompanied by the sense that "all is lost" and that there is little one
can do but ride out the situation. The passive, embarrassed person
may experience a sense of helplessness or resignation, if not a
palpable feeling of visceral deflation (a "sinking" feeling). In such
situations, people tend to be tense, passive, and withdrawn while
remaining socially vigilant. Although we know of no research that
has examined physiological concomitants of a passive fear response
in humans analogous to that described above in other animals, we
conjecture that embarrassment sometimes involves such a response
(see following box).

The results of one study showed that, when an embarrassing
event was unexpected, subjects' physiological responses were predominantly sympathetic and closely resembled those of anticipatory
social anxiety. On the other hand, when subjects expected and had
time to prepare psychologically to be embarrassed, evidence of
parasympathetic involvement was obtained (Leary et al., 1994).
These data are consistent with Frijda's (1986) suggestion that parasympathetic activity is involved in passivity. People would be expected to react to unanticipated embarrassment with active attempts

to deal with the situation In contrast, people who have been fore-warned and who realize they cannot avoid or escape the embarrass-ing event may resign themselves to it.

How'd Those Butterflies Get in There?

People who feel socially anxious sometimes report having un-pleasant sensations in their stomachs, ranging from the familiar flutters of "butterflies" to cramps and nausea. Furthermore, high levels of trait anxiety are associated with gastrointestinal problems such as dyspepsia, inflammatory bowel disease, and irritable bow-el syndrome (Folks & Kinney, 1992; Fowlic, Eastwood, & Ford, 1992). These reactions are caused by the patterns of autonomic nervous system activity described above.

On one hand, activity in the sympathetic nervous system slows or stops digestion, and blood flow is channeled from the digestive tract to the brain, heart, lungs, and muscles. This slow-down in ongoing digestive processes can create unpleasant sensa-tions, including nausea.

On the other hand, parasympathetic nervous system activity increases stomach contractions and the release of gastric fluids. Little is known about why such effects sometimes occur when people are anxious, but gastrointestinal distress during emotional upset may arise from parasympathetic activity, resulting in reac-tions ranging from "butterflies" to vomiting (Frijda, 1986).

ANXIOUS COGNITIONS

When anxious, people think about the source of their fear, whether the source is nonsocial (such as snakes, thunderstorms, or hypo-dermic needles) or social (interacting with one's boss, taking tests, or speaking in public). A person who was aroused physiologically but who did not think worrisome thoughts would be characterized as agitated, aroused, or discombobulated, but not as anxious.

In the case of social anxiety, these apprehensive thoughts tend to center around three things: (1) the real or imagined evaluations and reactions of other people, (2) the potentially negative consequences of those reactions and, (3) the personal limitations and behaviors that the socially anxious person believes are creating his or her social difficulties. Whichever dominates a person's thoughts at a given time, these worrisome cognitions may tax the anxious individual's attentional capacity, diverting attention away from task-relevant information to a preoccupation with his or her self-presentational difficulties (V. Hamilton, 1975).

Apprehension

As noted, episodes of anxiety are characterized by cognitive apprehension and dread. In the case of social anxiety, these thoughts are specific to concerns regarding others' impressions and evaluations. Asendorpf (1987) found that dispositionally shy subjects had more thoughts involving fear of social evaluation during a conversation with a confederate than nonshy subjects, but that shy and nonshy participants did not differ in their fears about things that did not involve evaluation. Similarly, Halford and Foddy (1982) found that, compared to less anxious subjects, socially anxious subjects had more thoughts that involved others' disapproval of them (see also Davison & Zighelboim, 1987).

Apprehensive thoughts have also been studied in instances of test anxiety (Wine, 1971). People who experience test anxiety ruminate about how poorly they are performing and about the disastrous consequences that will result from failure (Sarason & Sarason, 1986). The result is that test-anxious students devote less attention to the test itself, producing decrements in their performance. Obviously, a student worrying about the implications of failure on the test and what parents, peers, and teachers will think if failure occurs is able to devote less attention to answering the test questions than a student who is less preoccupied with evaluative concerns.

Self-Preoccupation

The socially anxious individual's thoughts are dominated not only by worries about the source of his or her anxiety, but also by self-preoccupation with personal limitations and deficiencies (Sarason & Sarason, 1986). Social anxiety involves too much self-focused metacognition (Edelmann, 1990; Hartman, 1983) or meta-self-consciousness (Cheek & Melchoir, 1990), that is, devoting too much conscious thought to what one is thinking, feeling, and doing. Socially anxious public speakers ruminate not only about the negative evaluations of the audience but also about their own deficiencies as a speaker. They also monitor themselves very closely, looking for the feared evidence of incompetence. Each flub will be detected and agonized over. Similarly, a socially anxious adolescent on a date not only worries about the date's impressions of him or her but also castigates him- or herself for failures to respond optimally and agonizes about the aversive feelings.

The excessive self-preoccupation that accompanies social anxiety can affect cognitive processing in three ways. It (1) decreases the person's attention to environmental cues, (2) affects how the person encodes and interprets information, and (3) increases the probability of certain overt behaviors (Sarason, 1975).

First, people whose thoughts are centered on themselves are less attentive to the situation, making them less sensitive to nuances in others' behavior that convey acceptance or receptivity and less able to maintain full attention to complex tasks (Hartman, 1983; Hope, Gansler, & Heimberg, 1989). Evidence that anxious self-preoccupation interferes with the processing of task-relevant information was provided by Arnold and Cheek (1986). In their study, shy subjects made significantly more mistakes on the Stroop Color and Word Test than less shy subjects under conditions in which evaluation was salient. Presumably, the preoccupation of shy subjects interfered with their ability to think consciously about the colors versus words on the Stroop Test.

Being self-focused (i.e., in a state of objective self-awareness) not only decreases socially anxious individuals' attention to external stimuli but also increases the likelihood that they will focus specifically on *negative* characteristics of themselves. When objectively self-aware, people are more likely to notice limitations in their behavior that might lead others to form unfavorable impressions (Duval & Wicklund, 1972). Numerous studies have documented the tendency for socially anxious people to generate more negative and fewer positive thoughts about themselves than less anxious people (Cacioppo et al., 1979; Glass et al., 1982; Hartman, 1984; Heimberg, Acerra, & Holstein, 1985; Ickes, Robertson, Tooke, & Teng, 1986).

Second, self-preoccupation affects how people encode and interpret information. A socially anxious individual who is pre-occupied with thoughts of his or her social deficiencies will be more likely than a less anxious person to encode and interpret another's behavior as indicating rejection (Clark & Arkowitz, 1975). Socially anxious individuals who believe they are not coming across well are sensitized to signs of rejection and interpret even positive reactions from others in a more negative light than less anxious individuals (G. W. Bates, Campbell, & Burgess, 1990). Because socially anxious people become overly focused on others' reactions, they may become locked in a state of self-assessment from which they find it difficult to extricate themselves (Carver & Scheier, 1986). It is quite difficult *not* to think about oneself in situations in which one is motivated to make a desired impression but feels incapable of doing so.

Third, self-preoccupation affects how people behave. People who dwell on negative aspects of themselves—their deficiencies, worries, and aversive feelings—tend to be withdrawn and aloof, and minimally responsive to their surroundings. As we discuss later in the chapter, when people devote excessive attention to the source of their anxiety and to their own self-presentational difficulties, such thoughts can interfere with their ability to think and act in effective ways.

EMOTIONAL EXPERIENCE

The Experience of Social Anxiety

In everyday language, we distinguish among a very large number of emotional experiences. To the lay person, terms such as afraid, sad, angry, lonely, jealous, anxious, depressed, happy, and disgusted refer to distinct psychological states. However, behavioral scientists have had considerable difficulty agreeing upon whether these terms represent distinguishable emotions. Not only do many of these emotions share common features (for example, all involve autonomic arousal), but several tend to occur together. As a result, researchers have found it difficult to separate one emotional experience from another. In fact, at the extreme, some researchers suggest that the distinctions among various emotions are of minor importance and that all emotions are best characterized simply by the degree to which they are pleasant versus unpleasant (J. A. Russell, 1980; Watson & Tellegen, 1985).

In light of this, describing the subjective experience of all instances of social anxiety is problematic. At minimum, we can say that social anxiety is always aversive. Even when social anxiety occurs in the context of otherwise happy events (such as giving an acceptance speech for an honor received or getting married), the experience of anxiety itself is universally unpleasant. We can not imagine anyone *wanting* to feel socially anxious.

Subjectively, anxiety is experienced as a feeling of tension, agitation, and uneasiness. With increasing levels of anxiety, people are able to detect specific physiological signs of arousal (such as heart palpitations or bodily tension) that are often unpleasant. When anxious, people sometimes experience a sinking or nauseated feeling in their stomachs, or feelings of weakness or dizziness (Amies et al., 1983).

Interestingly, persons who are high in trait social anxiety may be more attuned to these kinds of physiological reactions than nonanxious persons (Johansson & Öst, 1982). In part, this may be because heightened physiological arousal increases self-focused attention (Hope et al., 1989; Wegner & Giuliano, 1980, 1983). As people become more anxiously aroused, they become increasingly self-aware, which, as we saw, further increases social anxiety. Thus, not only are people high in trait social anxiety more likely to become anxious to begin with, but they are also more likely to be aware of unpleasant physical sensations, which then lead to escalating self-awareness and anxiety.

Social anxiety is often accompanied by other emotional reactions. The most common emotional concomitant of social anxiety is depression. State social anxiety is often accompanied by feelings of dejection or depression, trait social anxiety correlates moderately with depression (Spivey, 1990), and approximately half of all social phobics demonstrate evidence of depression (Amies et al., 1983).

The nature of the connection between social anxiety and depression is not clear, however. One possibility is that depression is a consequence of a sense of learned helplessness that results from perceived self-presentational failures and the inability to effectively navigate the channels of social life (Abramson, Seligman, & Teasdale, 1978; Burns & Seligman, 1991; Gotlib, 1984). Alternatively, depression may predispose people to experience social anxiety by lowering their effectiveness in social encounters. Depressed people tend to interact less effectively than nondepressed ones, leading other people to react negatively to them (Coyne, Burchill, & Stiles, 1991). Furthermore, when depressed, people tend to interpret self-relevant information negatively, leading them to perceive others' reactions more negatively than if they were not depressed (Kuiper, Derry, & MacDonald, 1982). Although research suggests that depressed people may, in fact, be *more* accurate in their perceptions of themselves and their social worlds than nondepressed people (Alloy & Abramson, 1988), they nonetheless are more likely to perceive others' reactions as less positive. A third possibility is that depression and social anxiety are both co-effects of perceived social exclusion (Leary, 1990a; Spivey, 1990). Perceiving cues that connote rejection or exclusion elicits a variety of negative feelings, including anxiety and depression.

Escapes from Self-Presentational Worries

The aversiveness of subjective social anxiety, paired with the negative self-thoughts of socially anxious people, may help explain why people who are socially anxious or social phobic are prone to abuse alcohol and engage in other escapist behaviors (Amies et al., 1983; Smail, Stockwell, Canter, & Hodgson, 1984). As noted earlier, self-awareness, social anxiety, and physiological arousal can reciprocally affect one another. Because social anxiety entails heightened self-awareness, socially anxious persons become preoccupied with personal deficiencies and more sensitive to the negative reactions of others, leading to a further increase in social anxiety. Not surprisingly, socially anxious individuals are often motivated to escape this escalating spiral and its associated aversive emotions (Hope et al., 1989).

One way in which people blunt their self-awareness is

(continued)

(continued from p. 138)

through the use of alcohol. Many of us have been to parties where we knew virtually no one and initially felt awkward and inhibited. After a few drinks, however, those initial feelings of inhibition disappeared, being replaced by free and lively interaction (Baumeister, 1991). According to Baumeister, alcohol allows one to escape self-awareness by producing "mental narrowing" or "alcohol myopia" (Steele & Josephs, 1990). Socially anxious people at a party will, under the influence of alcohol, focus on others at the party rather than their own preoccupations, thereby reducing attention to personal deficiencies and, thus, social anxiety. Research also suggests that alcohol directly lowers self-awareness (Hull, 1981).

Thus, socially anxious people may drink to reduce their distress and increase their assertiveness. Shy men in one study were found to consume more alcohol than less shy men (Maroldo, 1983). Research has also demonstrated positive correlations between social anxiety and the expectancy that alcohol will increase social assertiveness (Leonard & Blane, 1988; O'Hare, 1990); socially anxious people are more apt to think that alcohol enhances their interpersonal effectiveness.

Not surprisingly, then, alcohol abuse is unusually high among social phobics. Many social phobics openly admit that they use alcohol to "self-medicate," often drinking before social engagements. Some explicitly attribute their alcoholism to efforts to reduce their discomfort in social situations. In fact, among socially phobic alcoholics, the onset of social phobia nearly always precedes the beginnings of their alcohol problems (Schneier, Martin, Liebowitz, Gorman, & Fyer, 1989; S. M. Turner et al., 1986).

However, the mental narrowing produced by alcohol can backfire. In the absence of external distractions, one's attention remains focused on personal shortcomings, thereby exacerbating the aversive state of self-awareness. This is why anxious and depressed people are likely to become even more anxious and depressed when they drink alone.

Alcohol is but one way in which socially anxious people may reduce aversive self-awareness. Evidence suggests, for example, that the maladaptive eating patterns of people with eating disorders may also reflect a way of diverting attention from interpersonal insecurities. As Baumeister (1991) noted, "binge eaters are acutely self-conscious about public self-presentation" (p.

(continued from p. 138)

166). Women with eating disorders tend to have a high need for approval, low self-esteem, and an intense fear of rejection, particularly rejection by men (Dunn & Ondercin, 1981; Katzman & Wolchik, 1984). By focusing so much attention and energy on eating (or, more correctly, not eating), socially insecure women can divert their attention from their interpersonal concerns. Not surprisingly, then, women with eating disorders tend to score higher in trait social anxiety than normal weight women (J. Gross & Rosen, 1988; H. M. Weinstein & Richman, 1984). In fact, one sample of women with anorexia and bulimia scored as high in social phobia as diagnosed social phobics (Bulik, Beidel, Duchmann, Weltzin, & Kaye, 1991; see also Rothenberg, 1988). Although we would not go so far as to claim that all eating disorders involve social anxiety, interpersonal concerns of the kind that underlie social anxiety are clearly pronounced in many eating disordered persons.

Misattribution

The two-factor theory of emotion proposes that, to experience an emotion, people must perceive themselves as physiologically aroused and cognitively label their arousal. Given that a person is aroused, his or her interpretation of the cause of the arousal determines the specific emotion experienced (Schachter & Singer, 1962). For example, given precisely the same state of autonomic arousal, a person interacting with jovial others may attribute the arousal to the gaiety of the situation and feel happy, whereas a person interacting with hostile others may interpret the arousal as a reaction to the negativity of the situation and feel angry. Although the two-factor theory can be questioned as a general theory of emotion (see Reisenzein, 1983), it does appear that the ways in which people label or explain their feelings can affect the emotions they experience.

To the extent this is so, people sometimes *misattribute* their arousal to something other than its actual source. For example, arousal resulting from a fearful stimulus can be misinterpreted as romantic attraction, and the arousal caused by physical exertion can be misattributed to sexual stimuli (Cantor, Zillman, & Bryant, 1975).

Of relevance to our discussion here, people may attribute

arousal emanating from a nonsocial source to interpersonal factors. For example, if a person drinks several cups of coffee prior to speaking before a large group, he or she may misattribute caffeine-induced arousal before and during the talk to concerns about the presentation. Such an attribution and its emotional consequences may then lead the person to worry about the audience's reactions, thereby creating social anxiety. Thus, some instances of social anxiety may result when arousal caused by nonsocial sources is misattributed to concerns with others' evaluations. Furthermore, misattributing one's arousal to social factors may lead not only to social anxiety but to shylike behavior as well.

Conversely, misattributing "real" social anxiety to nonsocial factors may also reduce social anxiety and its behavioral effects. A socially anxious person who misattributes his or her arousal to something other than concerns with interpersonal evaluation may actually feel and act less socially anxious. In a test of this notion, Brodt and Zimbardo (1981) had shy and nonshy women interact with a male confederate while the laboratory was bombarded by noise. Half of the subjects were told that the noise would have an arousing effect and result in increased heart rate, whereas no mention of arousal was made to the other subjects. In essence, the first group was provided with the opportunity to misattribute their social anxiety to the noise. Measures of heart rate showed that shy subjects were significantly less aroused when they believed that the noise caused arousal than when no information about the arousing effects of noise was provided. In addition, shy women who were led to misattribute their anxious arousal to the noise talked more and enjoyed the interaction more than shy women who were not provided with this explanation. In fact, shy women who were led to think that the noise was causing their inner arousal conversed as much as nonshy women! Clearly, people's attributions for their arousal in social encounters can affect both their feelings and their behavior (see Olson, 1988).

EFFECTS OF ANXIOUS AROUSAL AND THOUGHT

As we have seen, people who feel socially anxious display a characteristic pattern of physiological arousal, apprehensive thoughts, and emotional feelings. As if these subjective experiences were not bothersome enough, the physiological, cognitive, and affective concomitants of social anxiety can adversely affect the anxious person's behavior. Among other things, they can produce undesired overt signs of anxiety, cause speech dysfluencies, hamper the performance of skilled behaviors, create memory difficulties, and exacerbate sexual problems.

Arousal-Mediated Responses

The physiological responses that accompany anxiety often have effects on the individual's behavior that can be observed by others. When people feel socially anxious, they may fidgit, play with manipulatable objects such as their hair or clothes, lick their lips, squirm, tremble, stammer, and, in general, respond in ways that other people are likely to perceive as "nervous" (see Cheek & Buss, 1981; Murray, 1971; Pilkonis, 1977a; Zimbardo, 1977). These arousal-mediated or "nervous" responses are simply manifestations of the anxious individual's highly aroused state.

As noted earlier, sympathetic activity increases muscular tension that prepares the individual for fight or flight. In the case of physical danger, this response is highly adaptive. However, when the threat is interpersonal rather than physical, increased tension is not particularly helpful and may even result in less effective responses. Increased activation and tension beyond some optimal level do not increase a speaker's ability to communicate, lead an adolescent to behave more effectively on a date, or help to extricate an embarrassed individual from his or her predicament.

People who are socially anxious often worry about how others will perceive these arousal-mediated responses. Because appearing anxious is negatively valued in most cultures, people may become increasingly concerned about their public impressions when they think other people will perceive them as nervous. Of course, as their self-presentational concerns increase, they become more nervous, and the overt manifestations of their inner arousal even more obvious. This, of course, results in greater social anxiety, then in more obvious signs of nervousness, in yet greater anxiety, and so on.

Social phobics are particularly likely to experience this "fear-of-fear cycle" in which they worry not only about whatever caused them to experience social anxiety in the first place, but are also afraid *about becoming anxious* per se. Because of this fear, socially anxious people may closely monitor their bodily states for evidence that another "attack" is impending. Detection of cues indicating the onset of anxiety evokes concerns about attracting attention or falling apart, thereby precipitating the anxious reaction the person so much wishes to avoid (Nichols, 1974).

In extreme cases, social phobic individuals may worry not only about appearing nervous, but also about more extreme effects of anxious arousal. For example, nausea and other gastrointestinal effects that accompany high anxiety may produce worries about eating or vomiting. Extreme nervousness may lead people to worry about having to perform actions in which their shaking hands would be a problem, such as writing, holding one's notes for a speech, or drinking from a teacup (Trower et al., 1990).

Verbal Dysfluencies

People who are anxious or afraid often stutter, stammer, hesitate on words, repeat themselves, pause more frequently when speaking and, in general, communicate less effectively (Kasl & Mahl, 1965; Mahl, 1956; H. Porter, 1939; Schwartz, 1976). These kinds of speech dysfluencies are produced by both social and nonsocial threats. Speech dysfluencies are increased by social threats such as large audiences (H. Porter, 1939; Siegel & Haugen, 1964), the presence of authority figures (Sheehan, Hadley, & Gould, 1967), and unfavorable reactions from listeners (Hansen, 1955, cited in Van Riper, 1971). People who believe they are about to receive an electric shock (Murray, 1971; Van Riper, 1971)—a nonsocial threat—stutter more than they do without such a threat.

Anxiety appears to affect speech via three routes. First, to the extent that people who feel anxious are preoccupied by the threat and their reactions to it, they may not be able to devote sufficient attention to what they are saying. Fearful and self-deprecating thoughts may interfere with the person's natural ease of expression.

Second, people may speak less effectively when anxious because they are monitoring their speech too closely—that is, because they are engaging in excessive self-focused metacognition (Hartman, 1983; Kamhi & McOsker, 1982). Under normal circumstances, people pay little conscious attention to their speech as they talk. They rarely plan in advance what they are going to say or precisely how they will say it. However, when self-presentational concerns are high, people begin to plan their vocalizations carefully and consciously monitor what they are saying. Because people are not accustomed to attending to their speech, paying close attention can be disruptive.

A third explanation of the speech dysfluency that accompanies social anxiety involves the effects of anxious arousal on breathing. When people are highly aroused, their breathing becomes faster and more shallow; in extreme cases, people may feel breathless and nearly pant (Amies et al., 1983). In addition, anxious arousal produces tension in the throat that interferes with smooth exhalation and that tightens the muscles that control the vocal cords. The presence of epinephrine—a neurotransmitter that is released under stress—may also induce bodily trembling, resulting in a quivering voice. At the same time, sympathetic nervous system activity decreases saliva production and leads to a dry throat and mouth. Shallow respiration and general trembling, paired with a constricted throat and dry mouth, may lead people to speak less fluently (Schwartz, 1976). In fact, one of the most successful treatments for chronic stuttering involves teaching stutterers to regulate their breathing (Wagaman, Miltenberger, & Arndorfer, 1993).

Choking under Pressure

Anxiety can also interfere with the performance of other behaviors. Colloquially, we refer to people "choking under pressure" when they perform more poorly in stressful or anxiety-producing situations than we would otherwise expect (Baumeister, 1984). When a person's performance relies on fine motor skills (playing the piano, hitting a golf ball, or executing a double axle in skating), social anxiety can lead to decrements in performance (Frijda, 1986; Leary, 1992; Oxendine, 1970). For example, intercollegiate golfers who were moderate or high in competitive trait anxiety performed more poorly than golfers who were lower in competitive trait anxiety (Weinberg & Genuch, 1980).

Choking can occur either because the individual pays conscious attention to behaviors that are normally habitual and mindless or because bodily tension and minor trembling interfere with the smooth motion needed for many complex motor behaviors (Baumeister, 1984; Martens & Landers, 1972). Such effects are more likely the more concerned people are with others' impressions of them. As the motivation to impress others increases, people are more likely to pay conscious attention to their behavior and to experience the somatic manifestations of anxiety that interfere with bodily movement (Baumeister, 1984; Buss, 1980; Carver & Scheier, 1981; Leary & Kowalski, 1990; Schlenker, 1980).

Memory and Information Processing

When people feel socially anxious, they may have more difficulty remembering. As we have seen, worrisome thoughts may interfere with thinking. As a result, people who are thinking about their social images or about potentially negative social outcomes that may befall them are less likely to remember information than people who are not preoccupied by such thoughts.

Kimble and Zehr (1982) had subjects interact with another person who either could or could not see them. Subjects who could be seen by their interaction partner remembered less information about the encounter than those who could not be seen. Presumably, intrusive thoughts about the other person's impressions of them used cognitive resources that were then not available for remembering details of the encounter. Another study showed that subjects scoring high in trait social anxiety had difficulty remembering what happened while they were being scrutinized by other people, whereas subjects low in social anxiety were not affected by scrutiny (Lord, Saenz, & Godfrey, 1987).

These memory deficits may be selective, however. O'Banion and Arkowitz (1977) found that socially anxious women selectively recalled negative information provided by a confederate more accurately than nonsocially anxious women. However, level of social anxiety did not affect recall for positive information. The authors suggested that this selective attention to negative information may contribute to the tendency for socially anxious persons to generate more negative self-evaluations than nonsocially anxious individuals.

Memory deficits appear to be a function of the attention required by a particular task. Anxious people have greater difficulty remembering information about tasks that require a great deal of attention (i.e., a deeper level of cognitive processing) relative to those that require little cognitive effort. For example, few differences would be observed in the recall of an easy, structured task by socially anxious and nonanxious individuals. However, as the task becomes more complex or unstructured, requiring more conscious task-relevant attention, the memory performance of socially anxious persons decreases (Hatvany, Souza e Silva, & Zimbardo, 1979; C. E. Weinstein, Cubberly, & Richardson, 1982).

This variety of cognitive disruption may also play a role in the next-in-line effect. When people are waiting their turn to speak, they have difficulty remembering information that is presented as their turn approaches (Bond & Omar, 1990; Brenner, 1973). If, for example, a professor asks students to say a few things about themselves on the first day of class, each student is less likely to remember the name of the student who immediately preceded him or her than the student who followed. Thoughts about what one is going to say and worries about others' impressions divert the individual's full attention from other students' introductions.

In a study of the moderating effects of trait social anxiety on the next-in-line effect, Bond and Omar (1990) had subjects take turns reading words aloud then tested the subjects' recall for the words. Although subjects who were low in social anxiety remembered virtually the same number of words both before and after their turn to speak, socially anxious subjects remembered over twice as many of the words that followed their turn as preceded their turn. Furthermore, the more socially anxious a subject felt, the fewer words presented prior to the turn he or she recalled.

The effects of anxious preoccupation on cognitive processes is perhaps most troubling for people who experience test anxiety. When test anxious, people consistently have greater difficulty recalling information they have learned. Rather than devoting their full attention to the test itself, test anxious persons dwell on how poorly they may do on the test, the likely reactions of other people to what they view as inevitable failure, or other disastrous consequences of poor performance (Sarason, 1980; Wine, 1971).

As maladaptive and troubling as the cognitive effects of anxiety may seem, they may serve an important function. Specifically, anxiety focuses the organism's attention on the threat (Easterbrook, 1959). For example, a person who faces a physical threat to his or her well-being is often well served by a mental mechanism that narrows his or her focus of attention to the source of the danger. Hypervigilance in the face of threat involves a state of heightened alertness in which the person continually surveys the environment for information regarding the threat and finds it difficult to concentrate on other topics (Frijda, 1986). In the case of *physical threats*—a carnivorous predator, a marauding band, or an approaching storm—this narrowing of focus undoubtedly has survival value. The individual who ponders issues not related to the immediate situation ("What should I have for dinner?") is less likely to survive than one who focuses exclusively on the threat at hand.

The problem is that, although beneficial in the case of physical threats, cognitive preoccupation often interferes with one's behavior in interpersonal encounters. Easterbrook (1959) observed that "emotional arousal acts consistently to reduce the range of cues that an organism uses, and that the reduction in cue utilization influences actions in ways that are either organizing or disorganizing, depending on the behavior concerned" (p. 184). For example, a single-minded focus on the threatening features of a social setting (such as others' evaluations and the likely ramifications of making undesired impressions) does little to enhance the attorney's courtroom presentation, the salesperson's sales pitch, the student's test performance, or the party-goer's ease of conversation. Not only is a narrow focus on the threat itself less necessary for dealing with interpersonal difficulties than with physical dangers, but the most effective courses of action in social situations more likely involve complex cognitive processes that are hampered by hypervigilance and self-preoccupation. Fighting, hiding, and running away require fewer cognitive resources than giving an oral summation to a jury, selling a product, taking a test, or carrying on a conversation.

Sexual Performance

Social anxiety may also interfere with sexual performance. A high percentage of cases of erectile dysfunction and premature ejaculation in men and anorgasmia in women appear to be due to anxiety (Hyde, 1994). For many years, researchers and therapists believed that arousal of the sympathetic nervous system inherently inhibited sexual arousal. However, research has shown that, in many circumstances, sympathetic activity is *positively* correlated with sexual arousal (Beck & Barlow, 1984).

Recent research suggests that the effects of anxiety-inducing stimuli on sexual arousal depend, in part, on whether the person is normally sexually functional or sexually dysfunctional. For sexually functional individuals, the physiological concomitants of anxiety either have no effect on sexual arousal or actually facilitate it. For sexually dysfunctional individuals, anxiety inhibits sexual arousal (Bruce & Barlow, 1990).

This difference suggests that, contrary to what was previously assumed, the effects of anxiety on sexual performance may not be due solely to sympathetic nervous system activity. Barlow (1986; Bruce & Barlow, 1990) suggested that the inhibited sexual arousal of sexually dysfunctional persons is likely due to cognitive and attentional mechanisms rather than to physiological ones. Just as a sexually functional person can intentionally inhibit sexual arousal by thinking about distracting, nonsexual things, sexually dysfunctional people may find their sexual arousal impaired by involuntary, apprehensive cognitions such as those we described earlier. Negative thoughts about one's own appearance or performance, or about one's partner's impressions, interfere with the sexually relevant thoughts and images that facilitate sexual arousal and performance.

Furthermore, as arousal increases, people are more efficient at attending to whatever they are focusing on. Thus, sexually dysfunctional people—who are thinking about their performance, the partner's impressions of them, and the possibility of sexual failure—become increasingly focused on the consequences of sexual inadequacy. In contrast, as they become aroused, sexually functional people become increasingly attuned to the erotic stimuli in the situation.

In light of the effects of distraction and self-preoccupation on sexual arousal, it is not surprising that individuals who become worried about their sexual performance or about their partner's evaluation of them are likely to have sexual difficulties. A comparison of men who were low versus high in heterosocial anxiety showed that highly anxious men were somewhat more likely to have experienced temporary impotence and premature ejaculation than men lower in social anxiety. A similar comparison of women showed that a smaller proportion of high than low socially anxious women had experienced orgasm. Furthermore, among both men and women, socially anxious respondents rated their enjoyment of sexual encounters lower (Leary & Dobbins, 1983).

Reciprocal Effects of Impaired Behavior on Anxiety

Behavioral manifestations of anxious arousal and thought can create additional self-presentational difficulties for the socially anxious person. To the extent that the person's subjective arousal, thoughts, and feelings lead them to interact and perform less effectively, they will harbor even greater doubts about their ability to make desired impressions on other people. The anxious person who stammers, chokes under pressure, fails to remember another interactant's name, or has sexual difficulties will undoubtedly worry even more about how he or she is coming across and become increasingly socially anxious.

In addition, the behavioral effects of anxious arousal and thought may show others how anxious the person really is. Because anxiety and loss of poise are regarded negatively, people may become socially anxious because they *appear* socially anxious. In fact, the social anxiety resulting from concerns with appearing nervous may be as great as the anxiety stemming from one's initial concern with making undesired impressions. As a result, people commonly try to hide overt signs of their nervousness, as they steady their shaking hands, control their jiggling feet, force themselves to breathe slowly, and otherwise attempt to assume a facade of confidence and poise.

Some behavioral manifestations of social anxiety are more easily controlled than others. People may find it easy to hold their hands still by clasping them together or by grasping the podium but find it far more difficult to keep them from perspiring. In addition, people differ in the degree to which they are able to conceal their anxiety from others. Some people have acquired the knack of appearing poised even when highly anxious. Such people are seldom perceived as socially anxious or shy and may even be regarded as confident and extraverted (Leary & Schlenker, 1981; Zimbardo, 1977).

Because concerns with appearing nervous create additional difficulties for the socially anxious person, counselors and clinicians should inquire about the degree to which a socially anxious client is troubled by overt manifestations of nervousness. If these responses are a concern, the client may be taught tactics for reducing the degree to which his or her nervousness is apparent.

BLUSHING

We have saved what is perhaps the most interesting manifestation of social anxiety until last. Episodes of social anxiety are sometimes accompanied by increased blood flow to the face, a reaction that we commonly call blushing. In light-skinned persons, blushing is perceived as a reddening or darkening of the face, neck, ears, and upper chest (the "blush region"); in dark-skinned persons, the reaction may appear as a further darkening of the skin or not be perceptible at all.

Two distinguishable types of blushing have been suggested. The *classic* or *embarrassed blush* appears rapidly on the face, neck, and ears, and is rather uniform over the affected areas. In contrast, the *creeping blush* occurs more slowly, appearing first as splotches of red that look much like a rash on the person's upper chest, neck, or jaw. (In fact, some people mistakenly interpret their creeping blushes as a nervous rash or case of hives.) Unlike the classic blush, which appears quickly, the creeping blush spreads slowly upward, often not reaching its peak for several minutes. Even at its apex, the creeping blush typically appears splotchy rather than uniform.

The classic and creeping blushes tend to occur in somewhat different social contexts, but they both seem to arise when people believe they are being scrutinized or evaluated. On the surface, it may seem that blushing results when people have conveyed undesired impressions of themselves to others After all, people often blush in embarrassing self-presentational predicaments. This is particularly true of the classic blush, which often occurs in response to specific self-presentational predicaments or identity-threatening events.

However, people sometimes blush in situations in which their public image has not been damaged and, in fact, which may have positive implications for others' perceptions of them. People may blush when they are complimented or honored, and many blush when people sing "Happy Birthday" to them (Leary & Meadows, 1991). Clearly, such happy events provide little reason for self-presentational concerns. An adolescent talking to an attractive member of the other sex may blush even though nothing has eroded his or her social image, public speakers sometimes display a creeping blush during their presentations, and people blush when others simply stare at them. Thus, blushing does not appear to be specific to embarrassment or self-presentational failures. In fact, most instances of the creeping blush seem to occur in the absence of a specific self-presentational threat.

Undesired Social Attention

In a review of the literature on blushing, Leary and colleagues (1992) proposed that blushing is caused, not by self-presentational predicaments, but by *undesired social attention*. Although people often desire and enjoy attention from others, social attention is sometimes aversive and undesired. When others are attending to undesirable aspects of oneself, for example, their attention is understandably unwanted. Even attention that is directed toward neutral or positive aspects of oneself may be bothersome if it causes the person to become excessively self-preoccupied or if the person does not know how best to respond. People who find themselves the targets of undesired social attention often try to escape others' scrutiny, such as by averting their gaze or by leaving the situation altogether (Ellsworth & Carlsmith, 1968, 1973; Ellsworth, Carlsmith, & Henson, 1972). However, when people are unable to reduce or escape undesired social attention, blushing tends to occur.

This explanation accounts for several features of blushing. First, it explains why embarrassing predicaments often cause people to blush. People who have conveyed an undesired impression of themselves understandably prefer others to ignore them. Second, unlike explanations of blushing that emphasize the role of negative interpersonal evaluations (Darwin, 1872/1955; Harris, 1990), the undesired attention theory explains why positive events can evoke blushing. Even when being honored or praised, people may perceive the attention they are receiving as excessive and, thus, undesired. Third, this theory can account for why people sometimes blush when others stare at them, whereas at other times they do not. When others' attention is desired, as when lovers stare into one another's eyes or an actor is performing confidently on stage, blushing does not occur. However, when the staring is undesired, people often blush.

Individual Differences in Blushing Propensity

People differ in the frequency with which they blush. Whereas some people blush in many social situations, others blush only rarely. To the extent that blushing stems from concerns with undesired social attention and the evaluations other people are forming, blushing propensity should correlate with measures of people's interpersonal concerns.

In an examination of the predictors of blushing, Leary and Meadows (1991) administered the Blushing Propensity Scale, a measure of the degree to which people blush in everyday social settings, to 220 undergraduate students (see following box). As one would expect, blushing propensity scores correlated positively with embarrassability, trait social anxiety, fear of negative evaluation, and physique anxiety, and negatively with self-esteem. In addition, people high in public self-consciousness and those who tend to conform their behavior to the models provided by others were higher in blushing propensity. Not surprisingly, sensitivity to being offended by crass, uncouth, and vulgar behavior was also associated with blushing (see also Edelmann, 1990, 1991; Edelmann & Skov, 1993).

The Blushing Propensity Scale

The Blushing Propensity Scale (Leary & Meadows, 1991) is a self-report measure of people's tendency to blush in everyday social situations. Respondents indicate how often they blush in each of 14 situations. Ratings are made using a 5-point scale:

1 = I never feel myself blush in this situation
2 = I rarely feel myself blush in this situation
3 = I occasionally feel myself blush in this situation
4 = I often feel myself blush in this situation
5 = I always feel myself blush in this situation

1. When a teacher calls on me in class
2. When talking to someone about a personal topic
3. When I'm embarrassed
4. When I'm introduced to someone I don't know
5. When I've been caught doing something improper or shameful
6. When I'm the center of attention
7. When a group of people sings "Happy Birthday" to me
8. When I'm around someone I want to impress
9. When talking to a teacher or boss
10. When speaking in front of a group of people
11. When someone looks me right in the eye
12. When someone pays me a compliment
13. When I've looked stupid or incompetent in front of others
14. When I'm talking to a member of the other sex

Note. From M. R. Leary & S. Meadows, *Journal of Personality and Social Psychology,* Vol. 60, p. 256. Copyright 1991 by the American Psychological Association. Reprinted by permission of the publisher.

Blushing as an Appeasement Display

The most puzzling question about blushing is why undesired social attention should cause increased blood flow to the face. Although we have no definitive answer to this question, one possibility is that blushing evolved to diffuse certain kinds of interpersonal threats.

Most other primates, such as chimpanzees and baboons, engage in a stereotypic sequence of behaviors when threatened socially by another member of their species. Among other things, these behaviors include lowered gaze and a silly or nervous grin. When a lower status primate is threatened by a higher status one, the lower status individual invariably averts his or her eyes or looks at the dominant primate obliquely (Altmann, 1967; Van Hooff, 1972). In addition, the less dominant primate often bares its teeth in a vacant, mirthless, silly grin (Goodall, 1988; Van Hooff, 1972). These kinds of behaviors are often called appeasement displays because their effect is typically to mollify the threatening animal.

It is interesting that the two behaviors that occur during primate appeasement mirror those that occur when people blush. When people blush, they not only avert their gaze but typically find it difficult to maintain eye contact with other people even if they want to. As Darwin (1872/1955) observed, "an ashamed person can hardly endure to meet the gaze of those present so that he almost invariably casts his eyes downwards or looks askant" (pp. 320–321). Edelmann's (1990) cross-cultural data showed that respondents from every culture studied reported averting their gaze in a recent embarrassing incident they described.

Furthermore, blushing is often accompanied by a nervous or silly ("sheepish") grin that appears virtually identical to the appeasing grin of other primates. Cross-cultural studies show that embarrassed smiling occurs with some regularity in a wide range of cultures. When asked how they reacted in a recent embarrassing situation, approximately 30% of the respondents in Edelmann's cross-cultural studies reported smiling or laughing (Edelmann et al., 1989; Edelmann & Neto, 1989).

This variety of grin is paradoxical in the sense that the embarrassed person rarely feels happy, and it raises the question of why people who feel socially anxious smile. Edelmann (1990) suggested that people learn to smile when embarrassed to acknowledge to others that they recognize a predicament has occurred (a nonverbal "oops") or to mask how embarrassed they really feel. We concur that people who feel embarrassed may purposefully smile for these two reasons, but we believe that embarrassed smiling is often automatic and involuntary rather than tactical. The self-conscious, embarrassed smile may be analogous to the appeasing grin of other primates.

The fact that gaze aversion, nervous smiling, and blushing tend to occur together raises the possibility that, as in nonhuman primates, these behaviors evolved as appeasement displays among humans. This conjecture receives further support from the observation that, as with human blushing, the primary elicitor of appeasement displays among other primates is undesired social attention (appeasement is most often caused by staring; Leary et al., 1992). Consistent with the interpretation of blushing as a mechanism of appeasement, dominance is inversely related to the tendency to blush. Or, conversely, submissive persons are more likely to engage in this appeasement display (Halberstadt & Green, 1993).

Just as nonhuman appeasement displays typically lead the dominant animal to shift its attention from the appeasing one, nonverbal signs of social discomfort, including blushing, seem to reduce social attention. People typically do not continue to pay direct attention to those who are blushing, averting their gaze, nervously grinning, or otherwise appearing acutely self-conscious. To do so creates considerable discomfort not only in the target, but in the observers as well.

Furthermore, nonverbal signs of social discomfort tend to enhance others' evaluations of people who have performed embarrassing actions (Semin & Manstead, 1982). In this sense, downcast eyes, nervous grinning, and blushing may truly "appease" those who observe us behave in undesired ways. Taken together, these considerations suggest that blushing may have evolved as part of a more general appeasement display among humans. They also suggest that, at the core, so-called appeasement displays among other primates function to reduce or redirect the undesired attention of others of the species as much as to lower the incidence of agonistic aggression.

Like the blind men and the elephant, researchers have tended to focus on only one aspect of the experience of social anxiety. Some have focused on physiological aspects, some on the cognitions of socially anxious people, and some on the emotional experience of social anxiety. And, like the blind men who each grabbed hold of a different part of the elephant, these researchers have developed somewhat different conceptions of the nature of social anxiety. What is missing is an integrative perspective on how the physiological, cognitive, and affective facets of social anxiety are related.

CHAPTER 8

Interpersonal Behavior

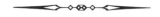

FOR MANY PEOPLE, the behaviors that accompany episodes of social anxiety are far more troubling than their subjective feelings and thoughts. They can suffer through their feelings of nervousness and trepidation, but their awkward and inhibited behaviors are more difficult to ignore. In the previous chapter, we discussed ways in which anxious arousal and thought interfere with behavior. As we will see in this chapter, not all behaviors that accompany social anxiety are direct consequences of subjective anxiety itself. Many are things that anxious people purposefully do in an attempt to make the best out of difficult interpersonal encounters. People who feel socially anxious are motivated to avoid or escape the anxiety-provoking situation and, whether they flee the situation or remain in it, try to alleviate their self-presentational difficulties. Unfortunately, these behaviors are sometimes socially maladaptive, increasing further the person's self-presentational difficulties and social anxiety.

Research on the behavioral concomitants of social anxiety is of two types. Some studies have examined the behavior of subjects exposed to experimental manipulations designed to heighten or reduce social anxiety. Other studies have examined ways in which trait social anxiety moderates behavior by investigating how people low versus high in trait social anxiety respond differently. In nearly all instances, the findings of these two research strategies converge: The behaviors observed in people exposed to situations designed to heighten anxiety are precisely those behavioral dimensions on which high and low socially anxious people differ. This is convenient, for it allows us to discuss these two bodies of research together.

In this chapter we examine the interpersonal behaviors that accompany social anxiety. We focus first on the tendency of socially anxious people to avoid and withdraw from interpersonal encounters, then turn to the tactics they use to manage the impressions that others form of them. Finally, we examine the consequences of these behaviors for the relationships of socially anxious people as well as for their personal well-being.

DISAFFILIATION

People who feel socially anxious tend to disaffiliate—behave in ways that reduce the amount of social contact they have with others. Socially anxious people tend to withdraw both physically and psychologically from social encounters. They participate less fully in ongoing interactions, speak less and for shorter periods of time, and often leave anxiety-producing situations altogether.

Social Avoidance

In the extreme case, people may disaffiliate by completely avoiding social encounters. In an investigation of the daily interactions of socially anxious and nonanxious individuals, Dodge, Heimberg, Nyman, and O'Brien (1987) asked university students to maintain a daily record of their interactions for two weeks. Compared to less anxious participants, socially anxious students reported engaging in fewer social interactions, particularly those involving unstructured casual conversations. They interacted less in classes, in their residences, and in encounters with members of the other sex. Not surprisingly, socially anxious college students date less frequently than students low in social anxiety (Arkowitz et al., 1975, 1978; Glasgow & Arkowitz, 1975; Heimberg, Harrison, Montgomery, Madsen, & Sherfey, 1980; Himadi et al., 1980; Twentyman & McFall, 1975).

College students who score high in communication apprehension tend to choose living accomodations that require them to interact less with other people (McCroskey & Leppard, 1975). For example, a student who chooses to live alone in a room at the end of a dormitory hallway could expect to engage in fewer social interactions than one who lives in a suite with several roommates. Similarly, when in a small group setting, communication apprehensives choose to sit in places that require minimal interaction with other members of the group. Socially anxious people also tend to interact with others at greater physical distances (Pilkonis, 1977a). Not surprisingly, trait social anxiety is inversely related to measures of extraversion and sociability (Cheek & Buss, 1981; Huntley, 1969; Leary, 1983a; Pilkonis, 1977b).

Social Inhibition and Withdrawal

Although socially anxious people usually prefer to avoid threatening social situations, in many instances they realize that doing so will be more damaging than helpful. When they must interact with others, individuals high in social anxiety tend to appear inhibited, reticent, and socially withdrawn. People who feel socially anxious are less likely to initiate conversations, speak less often, talk a lower percentage of the time, and take longer to respond to what others say. They also allow more silences to develop during conversations and are less likely to break conversational silences (Arkowitz et al., 1975; Borkovec et al., 1974; Borkovec, Fleischmann, & Caputo, 1973; Cheek & Buss, 1981; Daly & McCroskey, 1984; Glasgow & Arkowitz, 1975; Murray, 1971; Natale et al., 1979; Pilkonis, 1977a; Watson & Friend, 1969; Zimbardo, 1977).

The factors that make people reluctant to speak are essentially identical to those that evoke concerns with others' impressions. For example, people speak for a shorter length of time to critical, disapproving audiences than to accepting ones, and when addressing a large rather than a small group (see Murray, 1971). People are also more reluctant to perform in front of talented than less talented audiences (Brown & Garland, 1971; Knight & Borden, 1978). In addition, socially anxious individuals who hold negative expectancies regarding the outcomes of interactions have shorter conversations, speak more quietly, and engage in less eye contact with other interactants (Ammerman & Hersen, 1986; Burgio, Merluzzi, &

Pryor, 1986). DePaulo, Epstein, and LeMay (1990) found that socially anxious subjects who expected to be evaluated by an interviewer told shorter stories about themselves than anxious subjects who did not expect evaluation.

The degree to which people disaffiliate depends, in part, on whether they perceive others to be receptive to them. Not surprisingly, whether socially anxious or not, people are more withdrawn when others convey disinterest than when they appear interested (through smiling and eye contact, for example). This is a reasonable tactic; why bother interacting with people who have no interest in interacting with us? The difficulty for socially anxious people is that, relative to people low in social anxiety, they tend to perceive others to be less positive and approachable. Low and high socially anxious people are equally unlikely to initiate conversations with those who appear uninterested, but, when others signal social interest, high socially anxious people are less likely to initiate conversations (Curran, Little, & Gilbert, 1978). Socially anxious people appear reluctant to initiate interactions even when others appear receptive.

A primary way in which people withdraw from ongoing social interactions is to reduce the amount of eye contact they have with other interactants. When people feel socially anxious, they tend to look less at others and engage in less mutual eye contact with them (Cheek & Buss, 1981; Pilkonis, 1977a). Similarly, when people are embarrassed by a specific self-presentational predicament, they look at others less (Modigliani, 1971).

Three explanations can account for why people avert their gaze when anxious. First, averting one's gaze reduces the saliency of the threatening stimuli that are causing anxiety, thereby allowing a degree of psychological withdrawal while one remains physically in the encounter. Thus, averting one's gaze may reduce the individual's subjective feelings of anxiety.

Second, by giving others little eye contact, socially anxious interactants decrease the chances that others will initiate exchanges with them. People often wait until they have established eye contact before talking to someone. By refusing to establish eye contact, individuals who wish to disaffiliate discourage others from pulling them into conversations.

Third, as we discussed earlier, averted gaze may be part of an innate appeasement display. People who receive undesired social attention may avert their gaze to discourage unwanted attention and possibly to convey a sense of submission or humility (Leary et al., 1992).

Although reduced eye contact may have advantages for the socially anxious person in terms of lowering anxiety, reducing interaction, and discouraging attention, it also has drawbacks. Because people like others more who provide eye contact during conversations (Kleinke, Staneski, & Berger, 1975; LaFrance & Mayo, 1978), averting one's gaze may create a less favorable impression—the thing socially anxious people wish to avoid. Similarly, when speaking to an audience, a high level of eye contact leads to greater audience responsiveness. The speaker who does not maintain adequate eye contact will be less effective. Also, because people interpret low levels of eye contact as a cue that others are shy or nervous, failing to engage in eye contact may advertise one's discomfort to others who are present (Zimbardo, 1977).

Appropriate eye contact is also an essential aspect of conversational skill. Eye contact is involved, along with gestures and paralinguistic cues, in turn-taking during conversations. Failing to use eye contact appropriately as a turn-taking device may lead socially anxious interactants to disrupt conversations (Cappella, 1985). Such disruptions cause discomfort in other interactants, unfavorable impressions, and increased social anxiety.

Disaffiliative Firing

A writer to "Dear Abby" reported that, as she was opening the mail for her male boss, she came upon an envelope containing a book on the causes and cure of impotence. As she expected, her boss was "mortified" that she was aware of his problem. Two weeks later she was fired, being told that the boss required a secretary with greater knowledge of certain aspects of the business. However, she was convinced that she was fired because her presence in the office "was a constant reminder of his humiliation." Thus, some people reduce their social anxiety or embarrassment not by disaffiliating from a social encounter themselves but by banishing others from it.

Causes of Disaffiliation

The link between feelings of social anxiety and patterns of inhibited, withdrawn, and, occasionally, avoidant behavior is recognized by most people. In fact, it seems so natural, we rarely stop to ask why this inhibition often accompanies social anxiety. (Such inhibition should be distinguished from low sociablility; see box on page 162).

When people feel anxious for nonsocial reasons, such as when they are waiting to experience something unpleasant (such as an injection or electric shock), they prefer to be with others rather than alone (Schachter, 1959). This fact in itself indicates that anxiety per se does not lead people to disaffiliate. Why, then, do people who feel *socially* anxious avoid social encounters when possible, interact less fully when in them, and withdraw prematurely from difficult interactions? The relationship between social anxiety and disaffiliation is a complex one that may be mediated by at least five processes.

First, from a reinforcement perspective, social anxiety may punish affiliative responses, thereby reducing their frequency. When people are motivated to make a desired impression but doubt that they will do so, continued engagement in the encounter is anxiety producing; thus, continued involvement is punished. However, withdrawing from the encounter—whether partially by being reticent or fully by leaving the situation—reduces the person's anxiety. Because anxiety is inherently aversive, its removal serves as negative reinforcement for disaffiliative behaviors. (Negative reinforcement occurs when the removal of an aversive stimulus increases the frequency of the behavior that preceded its removal.) We cannot blame people for withdrawing from situations that are unpleasant.

Second, to the extent that social anxiety arises from self-presentational concerns, people who feel socially anxious may reduce their interpersonal involvement to lower their chances of making undesired impressions. For the person with self-presentational doubts, continued participation poses a notable threat, that of risking possible damage to his or her public image. By withdrawing, the person may lower the likelihood of a blatant self-presentational disaster. Thus, withdrawal and reticence may reflect

Inhibition versus Low Sociability

When discussing the withdrawal and avoidance associated with social anxiety, we must be careful to distinguish behavioral inhibition from low sociability. The difference lies in the nature of the motive that underlies a particular behavior. In the case of true avoidance or inhibition, a behavioral tendency has been impeded or checked before or during its execution. At one level the person wants to perform the behavior—to contribute to a conversation or go to a party, for example—but he or she does not do so because of competing motives (such as the motive to reduce anxiety, avoid disapproval, or protect one's social image).

Lack of interpersonal involvement also occurs, however, simply because the person is not motivated to interact. A person may not participate in a conversation or go to a party, not because he or she is inhibited, but because he or she is not motivated to perform these behaviors. Such a person may be described as unsociable, but not as avoidant or inhibited.

The disaffiliative behaviors that accompany social anxiety are primarily the result of inhibition. In most cases, socially anxious people wish they could participate more fully in social encounters, but their interpersonal concerns and accompanying anxiety deter them from doing so. In fact, some researchers suggest that, at its heart, anxiety involves a tendency toward avoidance and inhibition.

The problem for researchers is that the same behavior may result from either behavioral inhibition or from low sociability. If Woody doesn't talk much to his date, is it because he is anxious and inhibited or because he is bored and has no interest in talking to her? A full understanding of the link between social anxiety and behavior requires that we distinguish social inhibition from lack of sociability. Thus, in addition to measuring actual interpersonal behaviors, researchers should inquire regarding the degree to which participants *desire* to engage in a social encounter.

an interpersonal strategy that minimizes the person's social risk (Leary, 1990a).

A third explanation of the link between social anxiety and disaffiliation is based on the fact that, as we discussed in the previous chapter, the excessive self-preoccupation that accompanies social anxiety interferes with complex interpersonal behaviors. Socially anxious interactants may stand idly by because their attentional resources are consumed with ruminations about their social deficiencies. Unable to fully process the flow of information in the interaction, their ability to respond in a timely fashion is impeded.

A fourth process that may lead to disaffiliation involves the socially anxious person's expectancies regarding the likelihood of attaining his or her interpersonal goals. People's expectancies regarding the probability of attaining a desired goal affect the strength of their goal-directed behavior (Bandura, 1977; Carver & Scheier, 1985). People with low expectancies of successfully attaining a goal are less likely to try. As a result, people who hold low expectancies of self-presentational success are less likely to interact with others. Because socially anxious people hold lower expectancies of both their self-presentational efficacy (their ability to convey desired impressions) and their self-presentational outcome expectancy (the likelihood that particular impressions will lead to desired goals), they are less inclined to pursue social goals than less anxious people (Carver & Scheier, 1986; Leary & Atherton, 1986).

Fifth, in some cases, disaffiliation may *precede* social anxiety. People who, for whatever reason, have difficulty participating fully in an encounter may become concerned about how their lack of involvement is regarded by others present. As Goffman (1967) observed, people are obligated to convey at least an appearance of involvement in social encounters. Those who do not hold up their end of an interaction not only violate important social norms, but are unlikely to make good impressions on others. Thus, in some situations, disaffiliation leads people to feel socially anxious rather than vice versa.

An examination of the relationship between social anxiety and inhibition helps us understand why people who feel socially anxious are prone to disaffiliate. Disaffiliation is overdetermined by the factors associated with social anxiety. As "reasonable" as disaffiliation may appear from this analysis, however, being inhibited, reticent, and withdrawn can lead to further difficulties for the socially anxious person, as we discuss later in the chapter.

Individual Differences in Disaffiliation

Although withdrawal is a typical response to situations that cause social anxiety, people differ in the degree to which they disaffiliate when socially anxious. Some people are able to persist reasonably well in spite of their subjective anxiety, whereas others become quiet and withdrawn.

Along these lines, Pilkonis (1977b) distinguished between people who are "publicly shy" versus "privately shy." Publicly shy people report that they are extremely bothered by observable behaviors such as being too quiet, behaving awkwardly, and failing to respond appropriately. Privately shy people are more troubled by the subjective experience of anxiety, such as their internal arousal and apprehension about being evaluated negatively, but less so by their behavior when anxious. Not surprisingly, shyness is a greater problem for people who become very inhibited or behaviorally disrupted when anxious than for those for whom shyness is primarily an inner, personal experience. When social anxiety is accompanied by behavioral difficulties, the individual's plight is directly observable by others and creates additional difficulties.

We know little about why some people disaffiliate more than others when socially anxious. In part, the difference is due to genetic factors. As we saw in Chapter 6, behavioral inhibition in the face of novel or threatening events has an inherited basis (Reznick, 1989).

Beyond that, however, the attributions that socially anxious people make for their social difficulties may affect their willingness to participate in social encounters. People who attribute their failures to internal, stable (characterological) factors tend to abandon their pursuit of desired goals more readily than people who attribute their setbacks to unstable factors, particularly those they can control (e.g., Weiner, 1989). Because socially anxious people tend to attribute their social difficulties internally—for example, to their own lack of social ability—they may see little reason to exert much effort in their dealings with others, resulting in withdrawn and avoidant behavior (Leary, Atherton, Hill, & Hur, 1986).

SELF-PRESENTATION

Consider the plight of the person who feels nervous in an interpersonal encounter. According to the self-presentational theory, he or she is motivated to make certain impressions on other interactants but is not certain he or she will do so. If the situation is sufficiently aversive and withdrawal from the encounter is possible, the anxious individual may leave the situation entirely. If this can be accomplished easily, the person's self-presentational problems are over, at least for the moment. But what if the individual cannot leave?

We have already seen that people who feel socially anxious may partially disaffiliate by talking less, reducing eye contact, and so on. In addition, individuals in such a situation may try to protect their social images as best they can under the circumstances. Although they do not think they will make the impressions they would like to make, they still want to avoid making blatantly *undesired* impressions; they do not think they will come across as they would like, but they want to be sure they do not come across *badly*.

When socially anxious, people are likely to adopt a "protective" as opposed to an "acquisitive" self-presentational style (Arkin, 1981). Protective self-presentations involve attempts to avoid social disapproval (or losses in approval), whereas acquisitive self-presentations aim to gain approval. The socially anxious individual has been described as the prototypical type of person who is motivated to adopt a conservative, protective interpersonal style (Shepperd & Arkin, 1990). Because they are highly concerned about others' impressions, socially anxious people's self-presentational behaviors tend to be confined to relatively safe bets that carry little risk of jeopardizing their images. They are unlikely to try to portray themselves in highly attractive ways or make claims about themselves that they may have difficulty sustaining, but rely instead on conservative, low-risk self-presentations (Arkin, Lake, & Baumgardner, 1986; J. Greenberg, Pyszczynski, & Stine, 1985; Shepperd & Arkin, 1990). Much of the behavior of socially anxious people makes a great deal of sense if it is regarded as evidence of a protective self-presentational motive.

Self-Presentational Favorability

One study showed, for example, that when they expected future interaction with another person, people low in social anxiety enhanced how favorably they presented themselves to the other individual. In contrast, the self-presentations of socially anxious people were no more positive when they expected future interactions with the other individual than when they did not (J. Greenberg et al., 1985). This pattern suggests that social anxiety deters people from their normal tendency to self-enhance when they expect to interact with someone in the future. Presumably, this is because the person who harbors self-presentational doubts is unwilling to risk the consequences of making positive claims that may be contradicted in future interactions.

Similarly, the motivation to engage in protective self-presentation may partly explain why persons high in trait social anxiety typically rate themselves less positively than persons low in trait social anxiety (e.g., J. Greenberg et al., 1985; Leary, 1986b). By presenting diminished images of themselves, socially anxious people can avoid risking disapproval for being self-aggrandizing, as well as for being seen as manipulative, hypocritical, or deluded when future events contradict the image they tried to project. In addition, as long as they are not truly negative, slightly understated self-presentations may score the person points for modesty.

When they think others will have difficulty forming confident impressions of them, however, socially anxious people's self-descriptions are no less positive than people low in trait social anxiety. For example, when other events in the situation, such as distracting noise, interfere with conversation, socially anxious people take greater self-presentational risks than they otherwise would (Leary, 1986b). When they believe others may attribute their interpersonal difficulties to the situation, socially anxious individuals become less concerned with protecting their social image. Self-presentation is a less constrained and risky enterprise when the situation interferes with others' ability to form clear-cut impressions.

Another way in which people who are worried about their impressions may enhance others' perceptions of them is through monitoring and improving their physical appearance. Most people try to maintain a minimally acceptable appearance but, in extreme cases, people's efforts to look better may be maladaptive. Research shows, for example, that trait social anxiety predisposes some women to become anorexic or bulimic to achieve cultural standards of female attractiveness (Striegel-Moore, Silberstein, & Rodin, 1993).

Depth of Self-Disclosure

People who are concerned about conveying undesirable impressions of themselves can also protect their images by revealing as little of substance about themselves as possible. For example, when concerned with others' evaluations, the stories that socially anxious people recount about themselves are less revealing and focus on more commonplace events than the stories told by nonanxious individuals (DePaulo et al., 1990). Socially anxious people also express less overall information about themselves in conversations (Leary, Knight, & Johnson, 1987; Snell, 1989).

In a study that examined the relationship between social anxiety and self-disclosure, Meleshko and Alden (1993) had low and high socially anxious individuals interact with a research confederate whose own self-disclosures were either intimate or relatively superficial. People usually reciprocate the depth of others' disclosures, revealing more about themselves as others' disclosures become more intimate. However, subjects high in social anxiety communicated at moderate levels of intimacy regardless of the confederate's level of disclosure. Furthermore, whereas subjects low in social anxiety reported being motivated by acquisitive self-presentational concerns, socially anxious participants were preoccupied with self-protective behaviors.

Similarity

Overall, people like those whom they perceive to be similar to themselves more than they like those who are dissimilar. People also rate similar others as more knowledgeable, intelligent, and

adjusted than dissimilar others (Byrne, 1971). Knowing that perceived similarity increases attraction, people sometimes try to convey the impression of being similar to those they are motivated to
impress (Leary, 1995; Schlenker, 1980). In cases in which the individual is truly similar to another, he or she will simply want to
make that fact known. In other instances, people may feign similarity to increase how much others like them. The tactic of emphasizing one's similarity may be particularly useful to people who are
experiencing social anxiety because, if used discreetly, it entails little
interpersonal risk.

Related to managing the impression of similarity is conformity. Because people who conform to others' opinions and to
group norms are better liked, we might expect socially anxious
people to be more conforming. Indeed, Zimbardo (1980) presented
evidence that people who are shy are more conforming and more
easily persuaded than less shy people.

Typicality

A related protective self-presentational tactic involves conveying the
impression that one is pretty much like everybody else. Being an
average, middle-of-the-road sort of person will not usually make a
highly favorable impression, but it is not likely to make an unfavorable one either.

When discussing their attitudes publicly, socially anxious people tend to adopt neutral, defensible positions (R. G. Turner, 1977).
By doing so, people who are concerned about others' impressions
of them can reduce the possibility of arguments with others and
avoid being evaluated negatively for holding an incorrect or in-
defensible belief (see R. W. Haas & Mann, 1976). They also leave
open the option of later "changing" their attitude to conform to
others who are present, thereby scoring points for being won over
to the other person's position.

Similarly, we have unpublished data showing that socially anxious people rate themselves as more "average" on a variety of dimensions than less anxious people (that is, their ratings tend to be
closer to the mean of all subjects' ratings). Mediocrity may not be
impressive, but it is safe.

Disclaimers and Preemptive Attributions

Disclaimers are statements people make in advance of performing actions that others might interpret negatively to dispel any unfavorable impressions that might be created (Hewitt & Stokes, 1975). As such, they are used more often when people are concerned about others' impressions of them. For example, a person might hedge on his or her statements with phrases such as "I might be wrong, but it seems to me that. . ." or "I haven't really thought this through, but. . . ." Such phrases show others that the individual has no misconceptions that what he or she is saying is accurate or reasonable. If others react critically to what is said, the person can respond, "As I said, it was just a thought," allowing him or her to avoid negative reactions. Through disclaimers, people reduce some of the self-presentational risks that accompany revealing one's thoughts to others.

Closely related to disclaimers are preemptive self-serving attributions. People who are worried about the interpersonal implications of an upcoming evaluative event may offer self-serving explanations ahead of time to ward off the implications of a poor performance. For example, a person who is worried about giving a speech may comment on his or her fatigue or illness to discount the potentially negative implications of giving a poor speech. Similarly, people about to take a test may offer preemptive attributions that will help to preserve their image in case of failure, such as claiming that they are tired, ill, hung-over, inadequately prepared, or under stress (Arkin & Baumgardner, 1985). Such preemptive self-serving attributions are often called reported self-handicaps because the person who uses them is reporting, either truthfully or deceptively, that his or her behavior is impaired by the existence of a "handicap" (Baumeister & Scher, 1988; Leary & Shepperd, 1986).

INNOCUOUS SOCIABILITY

When people feel socially anxious, they often become *innocuously sociable*: While remaining engaged in the ongoing interaction, their behavior is perfectly inoffensive (Leary, 1983d). Among other things, they behave in ways that indicate their interest in and agreement with what others are saying, but offer little of themselves to the encounter. For example, shy women smile more frequently during conversations and nod their heads (as if agreeing) more often than nonshy women (Pilkonis, 1977a). People high in trait social anxiety also interrupt others less often, yet are more likely to use back-channel responses—the sounds that a listener makes to indicate that he or she is being attentive (such as "uh-huh"; Natale et al., 1979). They also ask more questions of other interactants, acknowledge others' comments more frequently, offer more confirmations (primarily agreements), and talk less about themselves than less anxious people (Leary et al., 1987).

These kinds of responses serve to convey an innocuous image of politeness, interest, and agreeableness while allowing the anxious interactant to remain only minimally involved in the encounter. Attentive listeners win friends; "He's awfully quiet, but he seems like a nice guy."

Such innocuous sociability not only projects mildly positive images of the person but also keeps the anxious individual out of the social spotlight. Smiling, nodding, and attentiveness prompt other interactants to dominate the conversation. Although having someone else monopolize the conversation is irritating to many people, it is a blessing for the person who prefers to remain silent. Asking other interactants about themselves allows the anxious person to appear interested in others, reduces the need to talk about him- or herself, prompts others to dominate the conversation, and keeps his or her own contributions safe and minimal (Efran & Korn, 1969; Leary et al., 1987).

Carried to an extreme, innocuous sociability may involve a lack of assertiveness that in fact may be quite annoying to others. Afraid of saying or doing something others might view negatively, people may refuse to express themselves openly when appropriate and may even appear to be *too* sociable and agreeable. When carried to an extreme, many of the innocuously sociable behaviors that accompany social anxiety are regarded as boring by other people. For example, people who ask excessive questions yet do not reveal an appropriate amount of information about themselves are perceived as boring (Leary, Rogers, Canfield, & Coe, 1986).

PROSOCIAL BEHAVIOR

Another way to project favorable impressions of oneself is to be seen doing helpful and thoughtful things for people. Thus, we might expect that socially anxious people go out of their way to do nice things to be evaluated positively. However, helping and favor-doing carry a certain degree of social risk. People sometimes have difficulty, for example, figuring out when helping is appropriate. It is clearly proper to help an elderly man pick up the packages he dropped in the store, but should you offer to get the attractive man or woman at the party another drink? Will he or she think you are too forward? Will he or she thank you coldly, then get the drink him- or herself? Will your friends tease you for appearing to "come on" to this person? Will you mix the drink properly? These are the kinds of questions that buzz in the heads of socially anxious people when they contemplate doing a favor for someone.

But what about when someone obviously needs help, such as in an emergency? Wouldn't the socially anxious person be first in line to help so as to make a good impression? Based upon social psychological research on prosocial behavior, the answer is probably not. A primary cause of people's failures to help in emergency situations is a concern with looking foolish or being evaluated negatively (Latané & Darley, 1970). Being helpful, even in an obvious emergency, puts the helper's behavior, characteristics, and motives under others' scrutiny. It also raises the possibility that the proffered help was inappropriate or that the individual will bungle the attempt in front of the victim and onlookers. As a result, people who are high in trait social anxiety are often *less* likely to engage in prosocial behavior than those who are low in trait social anxiety, and this is particularly true when they must break a social norm in order to help (McGovern, 1976). Even in an emergency—when extra-ordinary measures are called for and normal social conventions may not apply—socially anxious people are reluctant to behave in ways that might be construed as socially inappropriate. The potential image enhancement associated with helping is not worth the risk.

When someone *explicitly* asks for help, however, socially anx-ious people should be more likely to help because failure to do so might be regarded negatively by others. We know, for example, that people who are embarrassed are more likely to comply with others' requests for assistance than those who are not embarrassed. In some studies, subjects have been led to perform behaviors that made them look ridiculous to other subjects, such as dancing wildly to a disco record, singing "The Star-Spangled Banner" *a capella*, or pretending to throw a temper tantrum. Afterwards, subjects were asked by another student to volunteer to help on a class project by filling out a questionnaire for 30 minutes a day for a month (no small request). Compared to subjects who did not perform embarrassing behaviors, embarrassed subjects agreed to complete the questionnaire for a greater number of days (Apsler, 1975).

CONSEQUENCES OF DISAFFILIATION

In one sense, the interpersonal behaviors that accompany social anxiety can be viewed as somewhat reasonable tactics for dealing with self-presentationally difficult situations. Such behaviors help to reduce anxiety, minimize the possibility of self-presentational damage (even as they allow the person to remain physically present), and may even result in minor social rewards. Unfortunately, despite their interpersonal benefits, the inhibited and avoidant behaviors that accompany social anxiety also have negative consequences. Over time, a regular pattern of disaffiliation can lead people to suffer a number of difficulties associated with deficient interpersonal relationships. Such difficulties are, of course, more common among people high in trait social anxiety (because their withdrawal is likely to be more chronic), but even people who are otherwise low in trait social anxiety may suffer these effects when their self-presentational difficulties lead them to disaffiliate.

Impeded Relationship Development and Loneliness

People have a fundamental motive to be involved in relationships with other people (Baumeister & Leary, 1995; Baumeister & Tice, 1990; Geen, Beatty, & Arkin, 1984). Essential to the formation of interpersonal relationships is a minimal amount of social contact, accompanied by some degree of self-disclosure (Altman & Taylor, 1973). People who avoid social encounters, who have difficulty participating fully in them, or who distance themselves from others are at a disadvantage when it comes to forming friendships and romantic relationships, and in maintaining a supportive social network. As a result of their tendency to be inhibited and withdrawn, people who are prone to social anxiety often have difficulty forming and maintaining satisfying social relationships.

Three explanations can be offered for why social anxiety is associated with impeded relationship development. First, relative to nonsocially anxious persons, those high in social anxiety frequently do not avail themeselves of opportunities for social interaction (W. H. Jones & Carpenter, 1986). They date less frequently, participate less in extracurricular activities, and, in many cases, express a preference for working alone as opposed to working with others (Arkin et al., 1986; W. H. Jones & Carpenter, 1986). Dykman and Reis (1979) found that students who felt insecure selected seats on the periphery of the classroom. Thus, even when social opportunities are available, socially anxious people behave in ways unlikely to spawn friendships or even casual conversation. And, as we've seen, even in the midst of ongoing interactions, socially anxious individuals frequently distance themselves from others.

Second, because socially anxious individuals tend to interpret the reactions of others as less positive, they are more likely than nonsocially anxious persons to feel rejected even in the absence of any objective indication of exclusion (see Chapter 4). Relative to nonshy people, shy individuals report that their friends are less supportive, accepting, understanding, and attentive (W. H. Jones & Carpenter, 1986). Believing that others perceive them negatively, socially anxious individuals may behave in a less friendly manner, leading others, in turn, to respond less positively toward them. This pattern of behavioral confirmation becomes cyclical as the socially anxious person detects others' lukewarm responses and withdraws further, leading to yet less acceptance, and so on.

Third, the avoidant and inhibited behavior frequently displayed by socially anxious individuals may prompt others to exclude or avoid them. We've all had interactions in which another person fidgeted, looked around distractedly, and disclosed little about him- or herself. Although these behaviors may have simply reflected high social anxiety, we may have interpreted them as indicating disinterest, leading us to abandon interaction with this person. Consistent with this pattern, research indicates that others perceive socially anxious people to be less friendly than less anxious individuals (Cheek & Buss, 1981; W. H. Jones & Briggs, 1984; Pilkonis, 1977a).

Consistently behaving in ways that impede the formation of supportive relationships may ultimately lead socially anxious people to become chronically lonely. Several studies document a strong positive correlation between trait social anxiety and dispositional loneliness (C. A. Anderson & Harvey, 1988; Cheek & Buss, 1981; Inderbitzen-Pisaruk, Clark, & Solano, 1992; W. H. Jones, Freemon, & Goswick, 1981; Moore & Schultz, 1983).

Unfortunately, people who feel lonely engage in behaviors that further increase their likelihood of feeling socially anxious, thereby feeding yet another vicious cycle. For example, when lonely, people are highly motivated to attain others' approval and acceptance and, thus, motivated to control how they are perceived by others. Furthermore, lonely people become less trustful and more likely to perceive others as rejecting than nonlonely people (Peplau & Perlman, 1979). Thus, the stage is set for the lonely person to experience increasing social anxiety as a result of their heightened self-presentational motivation and decreased sense of self-presentational efficacy.

Lack of Experience and Skill Development

A tendency to avoid social contact may have deleterious effects on a person's social skills. "Practice makes perfect" is as true of interpersonal skills as it is of other complex behaviors. Yet people who do not fully participate in social interactions do not avail themselves of opportunities to learn and practice the skills needed for conversation, leadership, public speaking, cooperation, discussing intimate or delicate topics, and negotiation.

We discussed in Chapter 4 the fact that social anxiety is more common among people with poor interpersonal skills than those who are more socially skilled. Although most researchers have interpreted this finding in terms of the effects of poor social skills on anxiety, high anxiety may also lead to deficient skills. As social anxiety increases, people are more likely to disaffiliate, leading to social skill deficits. The effect of anxiety on the development of interpersonal skills is perhaps most evident during adolescence. Given that many skills needed for effective adult interactions and successful relationships are learned during adolescence, people whose anxiety deters them from participating in peer, social, and recreational groups miss opportunities to develop adequate skills.

Anxiety and Bashfulness in the Classroom

Surprisingly little research has examined the effects of inhibition on the educational attainment of socially anxious individuals (see, however, Gersten, 1989). In spite of the paucity of research, however, we can speculate on the negative consequences of social anxiety and inhibited behavior in educational settings.

First, as we noted, socially anxious students of all ages tend to choose seats on the periphery of the classroom. On a practical level, this seating preference would be expected to affect their participation in class discussions, their ability to attend effectively to lectures, and teachers' impressions of them as students (teachers hold different impressions of students who choose to sit in central versus peripheral positions). People who sit in the back or on the sides of a classroom are called on less frequently and participate less actively in class discussions. Furthermore, the inhibited behavior of socially anxious individuals may lead other students as well as the teacher to infer that the student is uninterested. Based on this perception alone, socially anxious students are less likely to be integrated into classroom activities.

Second, regardless of seating preference, socially anxious individuals may adopt protective self-presentational strategies that interfere with effective classroom participation. In an attempt to avoid making a negative impression by voicing an incorrect response or asking a "silly" question, socially anxious students refrain from asking or answering questions. In this way, they not only exclude themselves from class discussions but may also actively impede the learning process. If students who don't understand a particular part of the course lecture refrain from asking the instructor to elaborate, they impede their knowledge of the material and adversely affect their performance in the class.

Third, the reticence of socially anxious individuals may adversely affect class grades directly. Although the correlation between social anxiety and the overall grade-point average of college students is near zero, many classes require class participation as part of the course grade; students who fail to make an adequate contribution to the class receive lower grades. Receiving lower grades in particular classes may further impede a person's educational attainments by potentially closing off advanced educational opportunities for which high grades are required (i.e., graduate schools).

Finally, we suspect that socially anxious students are less likely than bolder students to approach the teacher on a one-on-one basis. Not only will they be less likely to seek out the teacher's help when they need it and to use resources such as academic advising, but they may be less likely to contact the teacher regarding grading errors (Friedman, 1980).

Sexual Behavior

We saw in the preceding chapter that the sympathetic arousal that accompanies social anxiety can affect sexual arousal and performance. Social anxiety is related to sexual behavior in other ways that are mediated, not by anxious arousal, but by behavioral inhibition.

People who avoid social interactions are less likely to form intimate relationships that include a sexual dimension (W. H. Jones & Carpenter, 1986; Leary & Dobbins, 1983). To the extent that satisfying sexual relationships often depend on establishing meaningful relationships with others, people who shun threatening social contacts (such as dates with potential romantic partners) are less likely to form intimate relationships that include sex. In addition, even when sexual opportunities arise, socially anxious people's concerns with others' evaluations may deter them from becoming sexually involved.

Furthermore, socially anxious people may be less likely to discuss intimate topics with their partner, including matters pertaining to sex. Compared to less anxious women, women who are socially anxious were less likely to talk about contraception with their partners (Bruch & Hynes, 1987). They were also less likely to use methods of contraception that require preplanning, such as oral contraceptives, possibly because of the social anxiety evoked by visiting a physician to obtain contraception (Leary & Dobbins, 1983).

Although mostly anecdotal, some evidence suggests that paraphilias (sexual attractions to objects and nonhuman animals) may sometimes emerge from a history of social phobia. Intense social anxiety may hinder the formation of reciprocal sexual relationships and lead to impersonal alternatives for sexual behavior (Golwyn & Sevlie, 1992).

Complaining

Complaining involves an expression of dissatisfaction, whether subjectively experienced or not, for the purpose of venting emotions or achieving interpersonal goals (Kowalski, in press). People who complain, particularly if they complain frequently, tend to be evaluated more negatively than persons who seldom express dissatisfaction (Leary, Rogers, et al., 1986). Because complaining may lead others to form negative impressions of the complainer, people who are more sensitive to the impressions that others are forming may be less likely to complain than persons less preoccupied with self-presentational concerns (Richins, 1980). If this is true, socially anxious persons would be expected to complain less frequently than individuals who are not socially anxious. Indeed, a moderate inverse correlation has been obtained between complaining and social anxiety (Kowalski & Cantrell, 1994). Part of the relationship between complaining and social anxiety may reflect the reluctance of people high in social anxiety to disclose *any* personal information about themselves. Furthermore, individuals who experience anxiety in interpersonal interactions are less likely to behave assertively in direct face-to-face confrontations (Zimbardo, 1977).

Although social anxiety appears generally associated with low complaining, socially anxious people may complain under certain circumstances. People high in social anxiety might complain if complaining allowed them to avoid the evaluative implications of a particular social encounter by withdrawing from the interaction or avoiding the situation entirely (Arkin et al., 1986). For example, a person involved in an interaction may complain about his or her social discomfort to provide an excuse for poor interaction behaviors (DeGree & Snyder, 1985; C. R. Snyder & Smith, 1986). In spite of the potentially negative ramifications of complaining in general and complaining about one's social discomfort in particular, "it may be far less pejorative to be labelled shy in comparison to such important labels as unintelligent, unattractive, etc." (C. R. Snyder & Smith, 1986, p. 166). Similarly, to avoid an encounter entirely, an individual may complain about his or her discomfort in social interactions or about other obligations he or she already has, excuses that some may view as socially acceptable (C. R. Snyder & Smith, 1986).

Taken as a whole, the interpersonal behaviors that accompany social anxiety serve three primary functions. They minimize the amount of social contact the individual has with others, they help the individual to project a minimally satisfactory public image, and they permit the individual to appear engaged in an encounter while minimizing his or her discomfort and the possibility of saying or doing something socially inept. Although these strategies are often effective in meeting these goals, they can create additional difficulties for the socially anxious individual, as we have seen. Lack of social participation may impede relationship development and result in loneliness, interfere with classroom learning, affect the quality of one's sexual relationships, and result in a lack of assertiveness (including legitimate complaining) that would promote one's well-being.

CHAPTER 9

Chasing Away the Butterflies

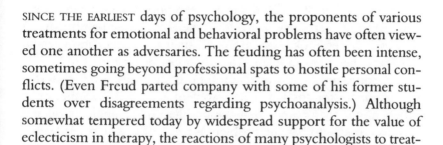

SINCE THE EARLIEST days of psychology, the proponents of various treatments for emotional and behavioral problems have often viewed one another as adversaries. The feuding has often been intense, sometimes going beyond professional spats to hostile personal conflicts. (Even Freud parted company with some of his former students over disagreements regarding psychoanalysis.) Although somewhat tempered today by widespread support for the value of eclecticism in therapy, the reactions of many psychologists to treatments that differ from their own preferred method remain adversarial.

In the research literature, we see evidence of this conflict in the implicit assumption that certain treatments are more effective than others. The research literature involving treatment effectiveness is full of studies that pit one treatment approach against another, looking for *the* best treatment for depression, alcoholism, anxiety, shame, or whatever.

Furthermore, proponents of each approach often appear determined to demonstrate the superiority of their pet therapy rather than to give all approaches a fair hearing. Failing to obtain differences among three varieties of cognitive therapy in the treatment of social anxiety led one team of researchers to quip that

> practitioners and researchers who view the cognitive-behavioral therapies as differing only in semantics will be heartened by these results. Those who harbor partisan allegiances will view these results as incomplete. (DiGiuseppe, Simon, McGowan, & Gardner, 1990, p. 143)

179

Although certain treatments may be universally effective for particular disorders, we should not expect to identify a single best treatment for trait social anxiety or phobia for two reasons. First, many theorists have suggested that the success of various psycho-therapies is partly due to "nonspecific factors" common to most, if not all, therapeutic techniques. In most types of psychotherapy and counseling, a client who is motivated to improve expends effort and time (if not money) to seek help from a trained professional who develops a supportive relationship with the client, devotes con-siderable attention to the client's well-being, and provides a credible rationale for change that creates in the client an expectation of improvement (Critelli & Neumann, 1984; Frank, 1973; Goldfried, 1980). To the extent that virtually all credible therapies possess these features, most psychological interventions will provide some benefit. Even seemingly worthless "therapies" may be effective if they include certain key components, such as a viable rationale and requiring the client to exert effort (Cooper & Axsom, 1982).

Second, and more important for our purposes, the notion that one treatment for any particular problem is universally superior to others implicitly assumes that the problem has a single cause and that everyone who has the problem is more or less alike. Although Kiesler (1966) called this "myth of uniformity" into question many years ago, many researchers continue to behave as if it were true as they continue to wage a winner-takes-all battle among psycholog-ical treatments.

Not only are there many paths to most psychological difficul-ties (and, thus, many underlying causes of a particular problem), but we might expect that different clients' personalities and back-grounds will lead them to be receptive to different treatment ap-proaches. A highly introspective client might benefit from a dif-ferent treatment than a client who was not introspective, even if they both sought treatment for the same difficulty.

TREATMENTS FOR SOCIAL ANXIETY

Despite these considerations, researchers have often pitted one treatment against another, as well as against one or more control groups, with the goal of demonstrating the superiority of one treat-

ment over another. And, like psychotherapy research more generally, research on the treatment of social anxiety and social phobia
has tended to approach treatment research as a zero-sum game in
which there can be only one winner.

The psychological treatments for social anxiety that have received the most attention from researchers fall into four general
categories: (1) *cognitive therapies* that try to change how clients think
about themselves and about social interactions, (2) *social skills training*
(including assertiveness training) that helps clients learn to interact
more adroitly, (3) *relaxation-based techniques* (including systematic
desensitization), and (4) *practice interactions* that give clients experience interacting under relatively nonthreatening conditions. In addition, research in psychiatry has examined the effectiveness of
various drug therapies for social phobia.

Rather than representing specific therapies, these categories
reflect four very broad types of treatments, and several varieties of
each of these general approaches have been developed and tested.
For example, several different cognitively based treatments for social anxiety have been examined, such as rational-emotive therapy,
systematic rational restructuring, cognitive therapy, stress inocula-
tion, and self-instructional training.

Despite scores of studies on the relative effectiveness of various treatments, no unequivocal conclusion can be drawn regarding
the overall superiority of any one treatment. Different studies have
found that different treatments are most effective, and the most
common conclusion is that two or more of the treatments under
study are more effective than no treatment but do not differ in
effectiveness from one another (e.g., DiGiuseppe et al., 1990).

Not only has the typical approach to treatment research assumed that one treatment would be superior to another, but these
studies seem to assume that the theories of social anxiety on which
the respective treatments are based are mutually exclusive, and that
demonstrating the effectiveness of a particular treatment confirms
the theoretical rationale on which the treatment is based. Although
it is seldom stated baldly, many therapists and researchers have
implicitly assumed that trait social anxiety is a product of social
skills deficits *or* of dysfunctional cognitions *or* of classical conditioning *or* whatever.

However, as we will see, the search for a single specific theory and treatment of social anxiety is based on a faulty assumption, namely, that all socially anxious people are highly anxious for the same reason. As we have seen throughout the book, individuals who regularly experience a high degree of social anxiety are not a homogeneous group. Although all cases of social anxiety are pre-cipitated by factors that motivate people to make certain impres-sions on others or lead them to doubt they will do so, the *specific* factors involved differ from case to case (and, for that matter, from situation to situation for a given person). Some people are bothered by high social anxiety because they unrealistically strive for approval and acceptance from everyone, others may have very low self-esteem, still others may perceive (quite accurately) that they are deficient in certain social skills, and so on. On the surface, each of these individuals appears to have the same problem—each is so-cially anxious—but an erroneous assumption of homogeneity hides important differences among them that have implications for treat-ment.

From the perspective of the self-presentational theory, trait social anxiety is best regarded as a second-order personality variable. In other words, individual differences in the tendency to experience social anxiety occur because of individual differences in other, more basic personality characteristics related to self-presentational con-cerns. Although all socially anxious people are concerned with how they present themselves to others, a variety of attributes may pre-dispose certain individuals to be motivated to control the impres-sions they make on others or to harbor doubts they can do so. Further, these specific differences have important implications be-cause treatments for trait social anxiety will be most effective when they are tailored to the personality dispositions associated with a particular individual's self-presentational worries.

The treatment literature involving social anxiety (including shyness, speech anxiety, dating anxiety, and so on) is quite ex-tensive, and we make no effort to provide a comprehensive review. Rather, our goal is to discuss existing treatments for social anxiety within the self-presentational framework. In our view, treatments for social anxiety are effective, for the most part, because they (1) lower self-presentational motivation, (2) increase self-presenta-tional efficacy, or (3) lower anxiety directly (through relaxation or drug therapy). Readers who are interested in more complete reviews of treatment studies, comparisons of treatment effectiveness, and critiques of treatment models are referred to Goldfried (1979), Glass and Shea (1986), and Heimberg, Liebowitz, Hope, and Schneier (1995).

SELF-PRESENTATIONAL MOTIVATION

As we have seen, some people experience social anxiety because they are highly motivated to control how they are viewed by others even in situations where others' perceptions of them make little difference. These socially anxious people should be helped by treatments that reduce the degree to which they are motivated to impression-manage.

Lowering Self-Preoccupation

As we saw in Chapter 3, social anxiety is more common among people who are high in self-consciousness. People who are publicly self-conscious spend a great deal of time thinking about others' impressions of them. As a result, they are typically more aware of their social images, more concerned with the impressions others form, and more likely to feel socially anxious (Buss, 1980; Fenigstein, 1979; Leary, 1983c). In light of this, A. T. Beck and Emery (1979) proposed that socially anxious clients be taught to "decenter"—to challenge the assumption that they are the center of attention and always being evaluated by other people. Not only do socially anxious people soon realize that others are not really scrutinizing them, but, in beginning to think consciously about other people's reactions in a social situation, their attention is shifted away from their own concerns and feelings.

Although the role of excessive self-consciousness in social anxiety has been recognized for some time, few attempts have been made to devise treatments tailored specifically for the overly self-conscious individual (see Alden & Cappe, 1986). However, such treatments have been utilized in the test-anxiety literature with marked success. Treatments that teach test-anxious students to direct their attention away from themselves and toward the task at hand not only reduce test anxiety, but improve students' test performance (see Wine, 1980, for a review).

We might expect that training socially anxious clients to be less self-focused would similarly reduce their apprehension and allow them to interact less self-consciously. Lowering a person's self-consciousness should not only reduce anxiety, but allow him or her to pay more attention to the ongoing interaction, thereby facilitating social behavior. One way of reducing self-consciousness might be to teach clients to adopt the strategy of explicitly focusing on other interactants. Instructing socially anxious people simply to "find out as much as you can" about other interactants significantly reduced anxiety in one study (Leary, Kowalski, & Bergen, 1988). Not only does focusing on others lead people to direct their attention outwardly, but they have an all-purpose agenda to guide their behavior in ambiguous and unstructured encounters (see Pilkonis, 1977a).

Alden and Cappe (1986) also tried a "decentering" treatment with shy clients, using human relations training to teach them to focus more directly on other interactants. Although the treatment was effective in reducing shyness, evidence that the effect was mediated by changes in self-consciousness was mixed. Further, because human relations training is a multifaceted program, we are unable to determine which components were responsible for reducing shyness. Nevertheless, this research highlights the importance of self-focused attention in social anxiety and calls for further work that explores ways of reducing the degree to which socially anxious people are characteristically self-focused.

Reducing Approval Motivation

A second reason that some people are exceptionally motivated to manage their impressions is that they have a very high need for social approval and/or a strong fear of disapproval. As we have seen, trait social anxiety correlates highly with the importance people place on obtaining social approval (Goldfried & Sobocinski, 1975; Watson & Friend, 1969) and with the degree to which they are concerned with being evaluated negatively (Leary, 1983c; Leary, Barnes, & Griebel, 1986). Desirous of obtaining approval or avoiding disapproval, they are constantly concerned with the appropriateness and acceptability of their self-presentations.

The individual whose concern with approval is excessively high might benefit from cognitive therapies designed to reduce the importance placed on others' evaluations (see Glass & Shea, 1986). Most treatments of this sort can be traced to rational-emotive therapy (Ellis, 1962), in which the therapist questions the client's "irrational belief" that it is imperative to be loved and accepted by everyone. More recent cognitive restructuring techniques achieve the same goal by teaching clients to identify and modify their assumptions about the importance of others' evaluations and the belief that "other people's approval of me is crucial to my sense of self-worth" (A. T. Beck, 1976; A. T. Beck & Emery, 1979, 1985; Meichenbaum, 1977). In either case, the outcome is the same: Social anxiety is reduced by decreasing the importance people place on making impressions on others (A. T. Beck & Emery, 1979; DiGiuseppe et al., 1990; Kanter & Goldfried, 1979; Meichenbaum et al., 1971).

SELF-PRESENTATIONAL EFFICACY

Some people may be socially anxious not because they are unusually motivated to manage their impressions but because they believe they seldom are able to make satisfactory impressions on others. However, this belief may arise for a number of different reasons, each requiring a somewhat different treatment approach.

Increasing Interpersonal Competence

We saw in Chapter 4 that people with poor interpersonal skills are more likely to experience social anxiety than socially skilled people. From the perspective of the self-presentational theory, the link between social skills and social anxiety exists for two related reasons. First, people who perceive they have social skill problems are likely to expect they will make unsatisfactory impressions on others. In addition, people with inadequate interpersonal skills often mismanage their interactions with others, leading to awkwardness and, occasionally, social rejection. As a result, the socially unskilled person comes to dread interpersonal encounters.

Although the connection between interpersonal skills and social anxiety is weak, social skills training is effective in enhancing social behavior and reducing social anxiety (Curran, 1977; W. H. Jones, Hobbs, & Hockenbury, 1982; Wlazlo, Schroeder-Hartwig, Hand, Kaiser, & Munchau, 1990). Social skills training involves several components, including observation and modeling of socially skilled targets, direct instruction, self-evaluation of one's own behavior on videotape, role playing, and behavior rehearsal (practice interactions with corrective feedback). Skills training seems to be particularly effective when clients have the opportunity to practice their newly-learned skills *in vivo*, that is, in real interactions (Wlazlo et al., 1990).

Proponents of skills training have assumed that skills training works because clients develop more effective ways of interacting, but no evidence supports this explanation. In our view, social skills training is effective in reducing social anxiety primarily because it increases the individual's confidence that he or she will come across more acceptably. If this is so, the skills targeted for remediation should generally be ones that the client believes will help him or her make better impressions on other people (Leary & Atherton, 1986). Clients should be consulted regarding their perceived self-presentational deficiencies and "impression management training" tailored to the client's particular difficulties.

Furthermore, for skills training to reduce social anxiousness, the client must perceive that the newly acquired skills do, in fact, enhance his or her image in others' eyes. Changes in behavior that are not accompanied by changes in how the client thinks he or she is viewed by others are not likely to lower anxiety. In addition, it is important that clients attribute the improvement in their interpersonal effectiveness to themselves (Alden, 1987).

Social skills training should be effective chiefly with socially anxious people who have skills deficits. If this sounds too commonsensical to mention, keep in mind that some researchers (and practitioners) have used skills training without regard to the actual source of the individual's anxiety. Research by Öst, Jerremalm, and Johansson (1981) and by Trower, Yardley, Bryant, and Shaw (1978) demonstrated that skills training was particularly effective in reducing anxiety for subjects who were identified beforehand as having difficulty behaving skillfully in threatening social encounters.

Providing Experience

Giving socially anxious people the opportunity to practice interacting can reduce anxiety and improve social behavior even without explicit skills training (Arkowitz et al., 1978; Martinson & Zerface, 1970). For example, in some studies researchers have arranged a series of practice dates, each with a different dating partner, for college students with intense dating anxiety (Christensen & Arkowitz, 1974; Christensen, Arkowitz, & Anderson, 1975). Such practice dates significantly reduced social anxiety and increased social activity, and such changes were still evident up to 15 months later. A similar study that provided practice interactions with people of the same sex improved same-sex friendships as well (Royce & Arkowitz, 1978).

Studies of the effectiveness of real-life practice have not identified the process by which mere practice reduces social anxiety. At least three processes may be involved. First, practice techniques may help to reduce anxious clients' conditioned anxiety by allowing them to interact under relatively nonthreatening conditions (Arkowitz, 1977; Galassi & Galassi, 1979). By associating social interaction with positive outcomes, the previously anxious individual begins to experience more pleasant affect in social encounters.

A second possibility is suggested by research showing that, over time, *in vivo* exposure to fear-provoking situations reduces anxiety. Simply inducing anxious clients to repeatedly confront anxiety-producing situations can reduce anxiety even without skills training (see Scholing & Emmelkamp, 1990).

A third explanation is that practice interactions give clients increased confidence that they can interact successfully while conveying a minimally desirable impression. Unless they are extremely dysfunctional, most socially anxious people can interact with others well enough to derive pleasure from their social encounters *if* they are not chronically preoccupied about how others are perceiving and evaluating them. Many socially anxious people have developed the habit of avoiding and fleeing social interactions at the first sign of anxiety, so that they do not learn that the dire consequences they expect usually do not materialize. Practice interactions in relatively nonthreatening encounters may provide experience combined with positive feedback that reduces their self-presentational worries.

Eliminating Uncertainty

Social anxiety is heightened in situations that are novel, unstructured, and ambiguous, in interactions with strangers, and for individuals who are less adept at monitoring and controlling their self-presentations. In each of these instances, the individual lacks a cogent plan for responding. Uncertainty about how to respond and doubt about the best self-presentations to foster in a given encounter result from not having viable social plans or scripts to guide one's behavior. When people do not have confidence in their scripts for an encounter, they are likely to doubt that they will be able to make the impressions upon others they desire.

This suggests that social anxiety caused by response uncertainty can be reduced by providing people with the information they need to formulate appropriate plans and scripts (Schlenker & Leary, 1982). In many cases, simply briefing people regarding what they can expect in novel situations should reduce uncertainty and social anxiety. Knowing what to expect on one's first date, on a job interview, at a professional convention, in an oral examination, or at a business meeting should provide rough but useful guidelines.

Similarly, teaching people how they should behave in a novel situation or role should reduce uncertainty. Much of the anguish of adolescence could be minimized if parents, teachers, and older siblings took it upon themselves to prepare children and adolescents for new roles and situations. Too often we learn our social scripts and interpersonal skills through trial and error.

Pilkonis (1977a) suggested that dispositionally shy people could be taught to set their own "interaction agenda" in ambiguous and unstructured social settings. Rather than waiting insecurely for others to make the first interpersonal move, people could develop all-purpose scripts for use in encounters in which response uncertainty would otherwise be high. By taking an active role in structuring the encounter, the individual is able to respond more confidently. Socially anxious people can be shown that individuals who seem most at ease conversing with strangers are not generally performing any great interpersonal feat. Rather, they are simply providing their own structure to the conversation by asking questions or directing the conversational topics. Their confidence and poise arise, in part, from the fact that they are in control. These same individuals often become reticent and inhibited when they are not in control of the encounter and must respond in accordance with others' behavior.

For individuals who "never know what to say," one solution would be to teach them to structure ambiguous situations in ways that best suit them—to impose their own preplanned script upon the interaction. One all-purpose option for unstructured situations, for example, might be to find out as much as possible about other interactants. Stipulating such a goal in advance provides a framework for responding in unstructured situations. Armed with a specific plan, the person will never be paralyzed by social uncertainty. In addition, as we noted earlier, finding out about other interactants keeps the focus of attention off oneself and on other interactants while allowing the anxious individual to acquire information about the other that will allow him or her to respond in the most facilitative fashion possible.

Not only may the individual who provides structure to otherwise awkward interactions be regarded favorably, but the tack of trying to learn about other interactants in particular presents one in a very favorable light. Socially anxious people should realize that, as Dale Carnegie noted (1936), the person you are talking to "is a hundred times more interested in himself and his wants and his problems than he is in you and your problems" (p. 88). Interactants who show interest in others are regarded as friendly, sociable, and likeable.

Raising Self-Esteem

Treatments focused on raising self-esteem have been used to reduce problems ranging from teenage pregnancy to test anxiety to aggression (Mecca, Smelser, & Vasconcellos, 1989). In many cases, these efforts have been misguided. Despite the fact that low self-esteem is associated with a variety of emotional and behavioral problems, high self-esteem is not a panacea for psychological problems. In fact, misplaced or undeserved self-esteem may create additional dysfunction (Baumeister, Smart, & Boden, 1994).

In the case of social anxiety, therapies that focus on self-esteem seem most appropriate for clients who do, in fact, have unrealistically negative views of themselves. Low self-esteem contributes to social anxiety because people with low self-esteem are likely to doubt that they will make the impressions they desire on other people. Furthermore, they may believe that they will be unable to cope with difficult social situations that may arise. Thus, social anxiety should decrease to the extent that perceptions of inadequacy and inefficacy are replaced with perceptions of worth and self-efficacy.

People's perceptions of themselves can be changed either directly through cognitive interventions or indirectly by providing them with successful experiences. In pure cognitively based approaches, clients are taught to recognize and challenge negative, limiting, unrealistic self-thoughts when they occur. After recognizing the self-thoughts that cause them to feel anxious in social encounters, they learn to ask themselves whether these thoughts are, in fact, supported by objective "evidence." What evidence do they have that other people think they're stupid? What evidence is there that they are less socially capable than most other people? Does the evidence actually indicate they are really a less desirable, attractive, or worthwhile person than most other people?

Often, clients are taught to use their feelings of anxiety as a cue that maladaptive thoughts are occurring. Thus, anxiety itself is transformed from something to be feared to a mere cue reflecting the occurrence of irrational or maladaptive self-thoughts.

Clients are also helped by concrete evidence that they are regarded positively by others. An interesting example of a therapeutic approach based on this effect was provided by Haemmerlie and Montgomery (1982, 1984; Haemmerlie, 1983; Montgomery & Haemmerlie, 1987). Researchers provided students who experienced a high degree of social anxiety with a series of "positively biased" social interactions. Under the guise of a study of dyadic interaction, students who had scored high on a measure of hetero-social anxiety interacted in 10- to 12-minute interactions with a research assistant of the other sex. The assistant had been instructed simply to carry on a friendly, positive, and natural conversation. Each participant interacted with 12 different assistants over a two-day period.

Compared to those in control conditions, participants who experienced a series of positively biased interactions subsequently reported greater self-confidence and lower anxiety on self-report measures. Furthermore, they were less anxious in an interaction with yet another assistant and interacted more skillfully in it. More-over, these treatment gains were maintained for at least six months, during which men in the treatment group had more dates than those in the control group! Although ethical issues arise in trying to implement this kind of treatment in clinical settings (see Mon-tgomery & Haemmerlie, 1987), these studies suggest that a few doses of positive interaction can go a long way toward raising self-esteem and lowering social anxiety.

Whether cognitive or behavioral, for esteem-based treatments to be maximally effective, they must affect clients' self-evaluations on dimensions they believe are related to their ability to make desired impressions. Simply raising global self-esteem ("I am a good and worthy person") is unlikely to have much impact. Social anxiety is usually related to concerns specifically about one's inter-personal attributes (see Efran & Korn, 1969).

One caveat regarding self-esteem is in order. In our view, treatments designed to raise self-esteem should be undertaken only to the extent that the person's unflattering self-image is inaccurate. In many cases, people with low self-esteem *see themselves accurately*. For the client who truly lacks essential conversational skills, for example, modifying the client's self-image without helping to im-prove his or her maladaptive behaviors does the client a disservice.

LOWERING ANXIETY

Some treatments are directed at lowering social anxiety directly by decreasing the client's level of anxiety or arousal.

Relaxation and Systematic Desensitization

Cue-Controlled Relaxation

The simplest variety of this form of treatment is relaxation training. People can learn strategies that allow them, with practice, to lower their anxiety on demand. For example, in cue-controlled relaxation, clients are first trained in progressive muscle relaxation: a lengthy sequence of tensing and relaxing specific muscle groups to induce a state of muscular relaxation.

After the person has learned to relax, he or she is taught to pair a specific cue word (such as "calm") with being in a relaxed state (Bernstein & Borkovec, 1973). After many pairings, the cue word itself comes to produce relaxation. Cue-controlled relaxation has been used effectively to reduce not only social anxiety (such as stage fright), but other sources of anxiety as well (Grimm, 1980; Lent, Russell, & Zamostny, 1981; Sweeney & Horan, 1982).

Systematic Desensitization

Historically, systematic desensitization has been the most commonly used behavioral treatment for anxiety of all sorts, including social anxiety (Kanter & Goldfried, 1979). Dozens of studies have shown that systematic desensitization reduces high levels of social anxiety (e.g., Bander, Steinke, Allen, & Mosher, 1975; Curran, 1975; Curran & Gilbert, 1975; Kanter & Goldfried, 1979; Kirsch & Henry, 1979; Kondas, 1967; Meichenbaum et al., 1971; Paul, 1966; Paul & Shannon, 1966).

Some evidence suggests that systematic desensitization is particularly effective when the person's anxiety involves a relatively circumscribed set of social situations. For example, systematic desensitization is quite effective in reducing public speaking anxiety (B. A. Berger, Richmond, Baldwin, & McCroskey, 1984).

Although the effectiveness of systematic desensitization was originally explained in terms of classical conditioning (Wolpe, 1958), desensitization may work via cognitive routes as well. For example, systematic desensitization may give people a sense of control over the feared object or event as well as over their reactions to it (Goldfried, 1980). Lowering clients' anxiety via systematic desensitization may also reduce or eliminate the degree to which they use their feelings of anxiety as a cue that something is amiss. People often interpret feelings of anxiety as an indication that the situation is threatening and that they are unable to deal with the threat (Bandura, 1977). Indeed, anxiety may have evolved as a subjective signal to warn people of threats to their well-being (Baumeister & Tice, 1990). Lowering anxiety essentially eliminates one cue people use to infer that stimuli are dangerous. As a result, helping clients to relax may actually reduce the degree to which they perceive interpersonal encounters as threatening.

Pharmacological Interventions

Just as proponents of various therapeutic approaches within psychology have found themselves at odds, psychologists have sometimes been at odds with psychiatrists over the the merits of the behavioral versus medical model in understanding and treating emotional and behavioral problems. Should psychological difficulties be treated psychologically through talk therapy, skills training, counseling, and the like, or should they be treated medically by administering drugs that modify the functioning of the client's nervous system? Although some hard-core advocates of each position remain, most mental health professionals seem to believe that certain problems are best handled psychologically, whereas others are best handled pharmaceutically.

Several drugs have been shown to be moderately effective in reducing symptoms of social phobia (see Schneier, 1991). For example, monoamine oxidase (MAO) inhibitors, such as phenelzine, are particularly effective in reducing generalized social phobia (Liebowitz, Fyer, Gorman, Campeas, & Levin, 1986; Liebowitz et al., 1988). However, MAO inhibitors have a number of undesirable side effects, including low blood pressure, weight gain, drowsiness, and stomach upset. The most serious side effects of MAO inhibitors are life-threatening interactions with foods that contain high concentrations of certain amines, which must be eliminated from the diet. A quick look at foods containing tyramine shows that this is no easy task: bananas, yogurt, cheese, alcoholic beverages, sausage, meat tenderizer, and all foods that have been aged, pickled, or fermented. Furthermore, MAO inhibitors interact with a number of medications, including many decongestants and bronchial inhalers.

Beta-blockers, such as propranolol, may be particularly useful for specific forms of social phobia, such as speech or performance anxiety (Liebowitz et al., 1988). Beta-blockers limit autonomic

---

Paradoxical Therapy for Blushing

Although many different treatments are effective in reducing social anxiety, therapists have been much less successful in helping chronic blushers reduce how much they blush. The particular difficulty with blushing is that it is not under volitional control. People can neither blush on demand, nor can they will themselves to stop blushing. In fact, it appears that the harder a person tries to keep from blushing, the more he or she will blush. The observation that consciously trying to inhibit a blush increases blushing had led to the suggestion that, conversely, people may be able to impede the onset of a blush by purposefully *trying* to blush.

In a case study of paradoxical treatment for blushing, Lamontagne (1978) instructed a 25-year-old chronic blusher to stop fighting his symptoms of blushing when they arose. In addition, he was told to try to blush as much as possible for three 10-minute periods each day for a month. At his weekly therapy session, he was supposed to convince the therapist that there had been absolutely no improvement in his blushing. Severe blushing episodes decreased from 28 during the month preceding treatment (i.e., approximately one per day) to no more than two occurrences per month in the six months following treatment. In fact, after three months, the client reported that "his phobia was cured and that his nightmare was over" (p. 306). Timms (1980) and Boeringa (1983) also reported successfully treating chronic blushing through paradoxical therapy.

Research has shown that certain other emotional and behavioral problems also disappear when people intentionally engage in the problematic response. For example, insomniacs fall asleep more quickly when they are told to try to remain awake. However, the reasons for the effectiveness of paradoxical treatment are not well-understood (see Leary & Miller, 1986; Tennen & Affleck, 1991, for a review of research on paradox-based treatments).

arousal and, thus, the somatic symptoms of anxiety (such as sweating, trembling, blushing, and palpitations). Several studies have shown that a single dose of a beta-blocker administered 45 to 60 minutes before a threatening public performance significantly lowered anxiety in persons with speech or musical performance anxiety (see Scholing & Emmelkamp, 1990).

Benzodiazepines, such as diazepam, are also prescribed for social phobia. Although this class of antianxiety medications (which includes Xanax) has been widely investigated as a treatment for anxiety, their effects on social phobia have not been adequately assessed in controlled studies (Scholing & Emmelkamp, 1990). Even so, many therapists believe that benzodiazepines may be taken on an "as-needed" basis when the person feels anxious or on a regular schedule. The primary side effect of these drugs appears to be drowsiness.

The issue yet to be addressed is when the use of pharmacological treatments for social phobia is warranted. In cases in which excessive anxiety has a clear physiological basis, medical intervention may be indicated. As we've seen, some people possess an inherited predisposition to be excessively anxious, and it seems reasonable to prescribe agents that lower sympathetic reactivity in such cases. However, when socially anxious clients clearly possess characteristics that predispose them to episodes of social anxiety—such as excessive need for approval, low self-esteem, or poor social skills—prescribing medications seems to us a "Band-aid approach" that fails to address the real source of the person's interpersonal difficulties.

RELATIVE EFFECTIVENESS OF VARIOUS TREATMENTS

As we noted at the outset of this chapter, most research on the effectiveness of various treatments for social anxiety has pitted one therapeutic approach against another. Yet, despite dozens of studies, few clear conclusions can be drawn about the relative effectiveness of the treatments that have been developed. Even so, two general conclusions emerge.

Multimodal Treatments

One such conclusion that emerges from the research is that, in head-to-head tests, the most effective treatments for social anxiety and phobia tend to be those that combine features of two or more treatment models. For example, Glass and Shea (1986) described a cognitive-behavioral intervention for social anxiety that used both social skills training and cognitive restructuring. Heimberg and his colleagues have developed an effective cognitive-behavioral treatment package for social phobics that includes exercises designed to help clients identify problem thoughts, practice in simulated interactions involving fear-provoking social encounters, cognitive restructuring exercises, and homework assignments involving real-life interactions (Heimberg, Becker, Goldfinger, & Verilyea, 1985; Heimberg, Dodge, Hope, Kennedy, & Zollo, 1990; Heimberg, Salzman, Holt, & Blendell, 1993). P. R. Gross (1989) described a three-pronged multimodal therapy that involved cognitive components (rational-emotive therapy and cognitive restructuring), behavioral components (assertion training, communication skills training, behavioral practice), and physiological components (relaxation training and systematic desensitization).

Multimodal treatments such as these appear to be maximally effective for at least two reasons. First, although we have identified several discrete sources of trait social anxiety and the treatment approaches that may be most effective for each, many socially anxious people have difficulties in several of these areas. This may be particularly likely for people whose anxiety is so debilitating that they meet the diagnostic criteria for social phobia. Given that many socially anxious people are troubled by more than one source of anxiety, treatments that attack social anxiety on multiple fronts are more likely to be effective than those that target a single antecedent.

Second, as we have seen, all socially anxious people are not anxious for the same reason (or set of reasons). Thus, in any sample of socially anxious or social phobic subjects, some are likely to be particularly bothered by high impression motivation, some are likely to have low self-esteem, some are likely to have social skills problems, and so on. Given this state of affairs, a multimodal treatment that targets several areas for improvement will, on the average, have a greater effect *on the group* as a whole than any particular treatment that focuses on only one area. A different "mechanism of change" is responsible for the improvement of each subgroup of socially anxious clients (Wlazlo et al., 1990, p. 191), but the overall effect is that a multimodal treatment will be superior to any particular unimodel one.

Client–Treatment Matching

The fact that not all socially anxious people are anxious for precisely the same reasons suggests yet another consideration for treatment. To be maximally effective, treatment should be matched to the specific nature of a particular client's interpersonal difficulties. For example, a person who is truly socially inept requires a different treatment program than one who is socially skilled but excessively worried about what others think. Social skills training would be expected to improve the social ability and self-confidence of the inept individual, but have minimal effect on the person who already has good social skills (Curran & Gilbert, 1975).

Two forms of client–treatment matching can be identified. The first, which is not particularly relevant here, involves matching treatment to some other aspect of a client's personality or to the client's "predisposition for various methods" (Glass & Arnkoff, 1982). For example, Malkiewich and Merluzzi (1980) tested whether socially anxious clients differing in conceptual level responded differently to treatments that provided a high or low degree of structure (systematic desensitization versus cognitive restructuring), but found no effects of client–treatment matching on this variable. However, DiLoreto (1971) found that rational-emotive therapy and client-centered therapy were differentially effective for introverts versus extraverts in reducing social anxiety.

Of more relevance and interest for our purposes is the second type of client–treatment matching. In this variety, the treatment approach is tailored to either the presumed source of a socially anxious client's difficulty or to some specific manifestation of the problem. Öst et al. (1981) used an interesting application of client–treatment matching to examine the relative effectiveness of social skills training and relaxation training on two categories of social phobic clients. They divided a sample of social phobics into "physiological reactors" and "behavioral reactors" based on physiological and behavioral measurements obtained during an interpersonal encounter. Their results showed that physiological reactors, who showed high arousal during the interaction, responded better to relaxation training than skills training. In contrast, the behavioral reactors, who displayed inadequate interpersonal behavior during the encounter, improved more with social skills training.

R. T. Gross and Fremouw (1982) classified speech-anxious subjects according to whether they were characterized by physiological or cognitive aspects of anxiety, then exposed them to treatments based on either progressive relaxation or cognitive restructuring. Although the effects were weak, evidence suggested that relaxation training was less effective for people who experienced few physiological symptoms of anxiety but a multitude of cognitive symptoms.

The idea of client–treatment matching applies not only to notably different therapeutic approaches (such as systematic desensitization vs. social skills training), but to different incarnations of the same general approach. As we noted, there are several variations of cognitive therapy—rational-emotive therapy, self-statement modification, cognitive problem-solving, and so on—each of which may be differentially effective for different clients. Furthermore, specific variations of these therapies may focus on different aspects of the client's problem.

Finally, treatment for social anxiety and phobia should take into account other client characteristics that may promote or interfere with treatment effectiveness. Heimberg et al. (1987) reported the results of a study showing that social phobics who scored high on measures of depression showed less improvement from cognitive-behavioral therapy than less depressed social phobics. The authors attributed the difference to the lower motivation, energy, and optimism of the highly depressed clients.

Although based on only a few studies, evidence supports the superiority of treatments based on client–treatment matching. Clearly, a great deal of research is needed to identify the client variables that moderate the effectiveness of various treatments for social anxiety, as well as the measures of these variables that are most useful in clinical settings.

Socially Anxious Children: A Neglected Population

Virtually all research on therapy for social anxiety and social phobia has been conducted using adult samples, particularly samples of young adults (specifically, college students). Although much attention has been devoted to nonsocial fears in childhood (such as fears of animals, the dark, and medical and dental procedures), little attention has been devoted to the treatment of childhood *social* fears (Comadena & Prusank, 1989; Francis & Ollendick, 1990).

Not only does social anxiety occur in children (J. C. Anderson, Williams, McGee, & Silva, 1987; Last, Strauss, & Francis, 1987), but evidence suggests that high social anxiety is related to many of the same kinds of interpersonal problems in childhood as experienced by socially anxious adults. Socially anxious and shy children tend to have more problems with their peers, avoid social encounters, talk to adults (including teachers) less, and experience greater loneliness (Crick & Ladd, 1993; Gersten, 1989; Zimbardo, 1981). Furthermore, a high percentage of children who regularly avoid going to school (so-called "phobic school refusers") meet the criteria for a diagnosis of social phobia (Francis, Strauss, & Last, 1987). Apparently, many children who experience a great deal of social anxiety try to avoid school because of their discomfort interacting with teachers and classmates (Pennebaker, Hendler, Durrett, & Richards, 1981).

Considering the extensive social, cognitive, and emotional differences between children and adults, we must question whether the treatments that are most effective for socially anxious adults are also effective for socially anxious children. This seems to be a ripe area for future research.

SELF-HELP APPROACHES

Books and audiotapes designed to assist the lay public in dealing with a wide assortment of personal problems have become common in recent years, and self-help products for the remediation of social anxiety and shyness are no exception (e.g., Cheek, 1989a; Girodo, 1978; Markaway, Carmen, Pollard, & Flynn, 1992; G.

Phillips, 1980; Powell, 1979; Zimbardo, 1977). Interestingly, little attention has been paid to the question of whether self-help books and tapes really help people with their problems and, if so, how the improvements compare to conventional therapies.

In the only published study to examine the effects of self-administered therapy for social anxiety, Vestre and Judge (1989) evaluated the relative effectiveness of self-administered rational-emotive therapy on social anxiety compared to therapist-assisted therapy, a minimal-contact control group, and a no-treatment control group. The findings regarding the effectiveness of the self-administered treatment were mixed. Although more effective than no treatment, the self-administered therapy was less effective than group therapy and the minimal-contact control condition.

We would not be surprised to find that self-help books and tapes are helpful for some people, and certainly more helpful on average than doing nothing. However, they are unlikely to be as generally effective as seeing a flesh-and-blood counselor or psychotherapist. Here is another area in which research is needed. We may be approaching a day in which authors of self-help books and tapes will evaluate the usefulness of their products in helping people to deal with their problems in living.

THE SOCIAL–CLINICAL INTERFACE: A CONCLUDING COMMENT

Beginning in the early 1980s, many researchers and practitioners became involved in drawing explicit connections between social and clinical psychology. Although the role of interpersonal factors in the development and treatment of emotional and behavioral problems has been recognized for many years (e.g., Adler, 1930; Carson, 1969; Frank, 1973; Sullivan, 1947), psychologists interested in interpersonal processes (primarily social psychologists) and those interested in dysfunctional behavior (primarily clinical, counseling, school, and other "practicing" psychologists) historically have paid scant attention to one another's work.

However, fueled by the publication of a new journal (*Journal of Social and Clinical Psychology*) and several books that demonstrated the relevance of social psychological perspectives to emotional and behavioral problems (Brehm, 1976; Leary & Miller, 1986; Maddux, Stoltenberg, & Rosenwein, 1987; Weary & Mirels, 1982), increasing efforts were made to draw explicit connections between these two fields (see C. R. Snyder & Forsyth, 1991, for an overview). Given that social anxiety is inherently and unambiguously interpersonal in nature, theory and research in social anxiety was particularly appropriate for cross-fertilization of this type, and we have seen many attempts to integrate social psychological and clinical perspectives in efforts to understand and treat social anxiety.

We urge future researchers, whatever their area of formal training, to cast the widest possible net when developing hypotheses, conducting research, and designing treatments vis à vis social anxiety. As we have seen, social anxiety is a multifaceted phenomenon, and a full understanding of its causes, concomitants, consequences, and treatments requires a multifaceted approach involving many subspecialties of behavioral science.

References

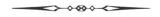

Abbey, A. (1987). Misperceptions of friendly behavior as sexual interest: A survey of naturally occurring incidents. *Psychology of Women Quarterly, 11,* 173–194.

Abramson, L. Y., Seligman, M. E. P., & Teasdale, J. D. (1978). Learned helplessness in humans: Critique and reformulation. *Journal of Abnormal Psychology, 87,* 49–74.

Adler, A. (1930). Individual psychology. In C. Murchinson (Ed.), *Psychologies of 1930* (pp. 395–405). Worcester, MA: Clark University Press.

Ainsworth, M. D. S. (1989). Attachments beyond infancy. *American Psychologist, 44,* 709–716.

Alden, L. (1987). Attributional responses of anxious individuals to different patterns of social feedback: Nothing succeeds like improvement. *Journal of Personality and Social Psychology, 52,* 100–106.

Alden, L., & Cappe, R. (1986). Interpersonal process training for shy clients. In W. H. Jones, J. M. Cheek, & S. R. Briggs (Eds.), *Shyness: Perspectives on research and treatment* (pp. 343–355). New York: Plenum Press.

Allaman, J. D., Joyce, C. S., & Crandall, V. C. (1972). The antecedents of social desirability response tendencies of children and young adults. *Child Development, 43,* 1135–1160.

Allen, J., Richmond, V. P., & McCroskey, J. C. (1984). Communication and the chiropractic profession. *Journal of Chiropractic, 21,* 25–30.

Alloy, L. B., & Abramson, L. Y. (1988). Depressive realism: Four theoretical perspectives. In L. B. Alloy (Ed.), *Cognitive processes in depression* (pp. 223–265). New York: Guilford Press.

Allport, G. W. (1961). *Pattern and growth in personality.* New York: Holt, Rinehart & Winston.

Alpert, R., & Haber, R. N. (1960). Anxiety in academic achievement situations. *Journal of Abnormal and Social Psychology, 61,* 207–215.

Altman, I., & Taylor, D. (1973). *Social penetration: The development of interpersonal relations.* New York: Holt, Rinehart & Winston.

Altmann, S. A. (1967). The structure of primate communication. In S. A. Altmann (Ed.), *Social communication among primates* (pp. 55–59). Chicago: University of Chicago Press.

American Psychiatric Association. (1994). *Diagnostic and statistical manual of mental disorders* (4th ed.). Washington, DC: Author.

Amies, P. L., Gelder, M. G., & Shaw, P. M. (1983). Social phobia: A comparative clinical study. *British Journal of Psychiatry, 142,* 174–179.

Ammerman, R. T., & Hersen, M. (1986). Effects of scene manipulation on role-play test behavior. *Journal of Psychopathology and Behavioral Assessment, 8,* 55–67.

Anderson, C. A., & Harvey, R. J. (1988). Discriminating between problems in living: An examination of measures of depression, loneliness, shyness, and social anxiety. *Journal of Social and Clinical Psychology, 6,* 482–491.

Anderson, J. C., Williams, S., McGee, R., & Silva, P. A. (1987). DSM-III disorders in preadolescent children. *Archives of General Psychology, 44,* 69–76.

Appley, M. H. (1971). *Adaptation-level theory.* New York: Academic Press.

Apsler, R. (1975). Effects of embarrassment on behavior toward others. *Journal of Personality and Social Psychology, 32,* 145–153.

Arcus, D. (1989). Vulnerability and eye color in Disney cartoon characters. In J. S. Reznick (Ed.), *Perspectives on behavioral inhibition* (pp. 291–298). Chicago: University of Chicago Press.

Arkin, R. M. (1981). Self-presentation styles. In J. T. Tedeschi (Ed.), *Impression management theory and social psychological research* (pp. 311–333). New York: Academic Press.

Arkin, R. M., & Baumgardner, A. H. (1985). Self-handicapping. In J. H. Harvey & G. Weary (Eds.), *Basic issues in attribution theory and research* (pp. 169–202). New York: Academic Press.

Arkin, R. M., Lake, E. A., & Baumgardner, A. H. (1986). Shyness and self-presentation. In W. H. Jones, J. M. Cheek, & S. R. Briggs (Eds.), *Shyness: Perspectives on research and treatment* (pp. 189–204). New York: Plenum Press.

Arkowitz, H. (1977). Measurement and modification of minimal dating behavior. In M. Hersen, R. M. Eisler, & P. M. Miller (Eds.), *Progress in behavior modification* (Vol. 5, pp. 1–62). New York: Academic Press.

Arkowitz, H., Hinton, R., Perl, J., & Himadi, W. (1978). Treatment strategies for dating anxiety in college men based on real-life practice. *Counseling Psychologist, 7,* 41–46.

Arkowitz, H., Lichtenstein, E., McGovern, K., & Hines, P. (1975). The behavioral assessment of social competence in males. *Behavior Therapy, 6,* 3–13.

Arnold, A. P., & Cheek, J. M. (1986). Shyness, self-preoccupation, and the Stroop Color and Word Test. *Personality and Individual Differences, 7,* 571–573.

Asendorpf, J. B. (1987). Videotape reconstruction of emotions and cognitions related to shyness. *Journal of Personality and Social Psychology, 53,* 542–549.

Asendorpf, J. (1994). *Two kinds of social anxiety and their relation to impression monitoring.* Unpublished manuscript, Max Planck Institute, Munich, Germany.

Babcock, M. K. (1988). Embarrassment: A window on the self. *Journal for the Theory of Social Behaviour, 18,* 459–483.

Backman, C., Secord, P., & Pierce, J. (1963). Resistance to change in self-concept as a function of consensus among significant others. *Sociometry, 26,* 102–111.

Bander, K. W., Steinke, G. V., Allen, G. J., & Mosher, D. L. (1975). Evaluation of three dating-specific treatment approaches for heterosexual dating anxiety. *Journal of Consulting and Clinical Psychology, 43,* 259–265.

Bandura, A. (1969). *Principles of behavior modification.* New York: Holt, Rinehart & Winston.

Bandura, A. (1973). *Social learning theory.* Englewood Cliffs, NJ: Prentice-Hall.

Bandura, A. (1977). Self-efficacy: Toward a unifying theory of behavioral change. *Psychological Review, 84,* 191–215.

Barash, D. P. (1977). *Sociobiology and behavior.* New York: Elsevier.

Barber, V. (1939). Studies in the psychology of stuttering: XV. Chorus reading as a distraction in stuttering. *Journal of Speech Disorders, 4,* 371–383.

Bar-Levav, R. (1976). The stigma of seeing a psychiatrist. *American Journal of Psychotherapy, 30,* 473–480.

Barlow, D. H. (1985). The dimensions of anxiety disorders. In A. H. Tuma & J. D. Maser (Eds.), *Anxiety and the anxiety disorders* (pp. 479–500). Hillsdale, NJ: Erlbaum.

Barlow, D. H. (1986). Causes of sexual dysfunction: The role of anxiety and cognitive interference. *Journal of Consulting and Clinical Psychology, 54,* 140–148.

Barnes, B. D., Mason, E., Leary, M. R., Laurent, J., Griebel, C., & Bergman, A. (1988). Reactions to social vs self-evaluation: Moderating effects of personal and social identity orientations. *Journal of Research in Personality, 22,* 513–524.

Bates, G. W., Campbell, I. M., & Burgess, P. M. (1990). Assessment of articulated thoughts in social anxiety: Modification of the ATSS procedure. *British Journal of Clinical Psychology, 29,* 91–98.

Bates, H. D. (1971). Factorial structure and MMPI correlates of a fear survey in a clinical population. *Behaviour Research and Therapy, 9,* 355–360.

Baumeister, R. F. (1982). A self-presentational view of social phenomena. *Psychological Bulletin, 91,* 3–26.

Baumeister, R. F. (1984). Choking under pressure: Self-consciousness and paradoxical effects of incentives on skillful performance. *Journal of Personality and Social Psychology, 46,* 610–620.

Baumeister, R. F. (1991). *Escaping the self: Alcoholism, spirituality, masochism, and other flights from the burden of selfhood*. New York: Basic Books.

Baumeister, R. F., & Leary, M. R. (1995). The need to belong: Desire for interpersonal attachments as a fundamental human motivation. *Psychological Bulletin, 117*, 497–529.

Baumeister, R. F., & Scher, S. J. (1988). Self-defeating behavior patterns among normal individuals: Review and analysis of common self-destructive tendencies. *Psychological Bulletin, 104*, 3–22.

Baumeister, R. F., Smart, L., & Boden, J. M. (in press). Relation of threatened egotism to violence and aggression: The dark side of high self-esteem. *Psychological Review*.

Baumeister, R. F., & Tice, D. M. (1990). Anxiety and social exclusion. *Journal of Social and Clinical Psychology, 9*, 165–195.

Baumrind, D. (1989). Rearing competent children. In W. Damon (Ed.), *Child development today and tomorrow* (pp. 349–378). San Francisco: Jossey-Bass.

Beck, A. T. (1976). *Cognitive therapy and the emotional disorders*. New York: International Universities Press.

Beck, A. T., & Emery, G. (1979). *Cognitive therapy of anxiety and phobic disorders*. Philadelphia: Center for Cognitive Therapy.

Beck, A. T., & Emery, G. (1985). *Anxiety disorders and phobias: A cognitive perspective*. New York: Basic Books.

Beck, J. G., & Barlow, D. H. (1984). Current conceptualizations of sexual dysfunction: A review and an alternative perspective. *Clinical Psychology Review, 4*, 363–378.

Bell, I. R., Jasnoski, M. L., Kagan, J., & King, D. S. (1990). Is allergic rhinitis more frequent in young adults with extreme shyness? *Psychosomatic Medicine, 52*, 517–525.

Bellack, A. S., & Hersen, M. (Eds.). (1979). *Research and practice in social skills training*. New York: Plenum Press.

Berberian, K. E., & Snyder, S. S. (1982). The relationship of temperament and stranger reaction for younger and older infants. *Merrill-Palmer Quarterly, 28*, 79–94.

Berger, B. A., Richmond, V. P., Baldwin, H. J., & McCroskey, J. C. (1984). *Reducing communication apprehension: Is there a best way?* Paper presented at the annual meeting of the Eastern Communication Association, Philadelphia.

Berger, S. E., Levin, P., Jacobsen, L. I., & Milham, J. (1977). Gain approval or avoid disapproval: Comparison of motive strengths in high need for approval scorers. *Journal of Personality, 45*, 458–468.

Bernstein, D. A., & Allen, G. J. (1969). Fear survey schedule (II): Normative data and factor analyses based upon a large college sample. *Behaviour Research and Therapy, 7*, 403–407.

Bernstein, D. A., & Borkovec, T. D. (1973). *Progressive relaxation training*. Champaign, IL: Research Press.

Berscheid, E., & Walster, E. (1974). Physical attractiveness. In L. Berkowitz

(Ed.), *Advances in experimental social psychology* (Vol. 7, pp. 158–215), New York: Academic Press.

Boeringa, J. A. (1983). Blushing: A modified behavioral intervention using paradoxical intention. *Psychotherapy: Theory, Research, and Practice, 20,* 441–444.

Bond, C. F., Jr., & Omar, A. S. (1990). Social anxiety, state dependence, and the next-in-line effect. *Journal of Experimental Social Psychology, 26,* 185–198.

Borkovec, T. D., Fleischmann, D. J., & Caputo, J. A. (1973). The measurement of anxiety in an analogue social situation. *Journal of Consulting and Clinical Psychology, 44,* 157–161.

Borkovec, T. D., Stone, N., O'Brien, G., & Kaloupek, D. (1974). Identification and measurement of a clinically relevant target behavior for analogue outcome research. *Behavior Therapy, 5,* 503–513.

Braun, P. R., & Reynolds, D. J. (1969). A factor analysis of a 100–item fear survey inventory. *Behaviour Research and Therapy, 7,* 399–402.

Breck, B. E., & Smith, S. H. (1983). Selective recall of self-disclosure traits by socially anxious and nonanxious females. *Social Behavior and Personality, 11,* 71–76.

Brehm, S. S. (1976). *The application of social psychology to clinical practice.* Washington, DC: Hemisphere.

Brenner, M. (1973). The next-in-line effect. *Journal of Verbal Learning and Verbal Behavior, 12,* 320–323.

Brewer, M. B. (1991). The social self: On being the same and different at the same time. *Personality and Social Psychology Bulletin, 17,* 475–482.

Brodt, S. E., & Zimbardo, P. G. (1981). Modifying shyness-related social behavior through symptom misattribution. *Journal of Personality and Social Psychology, 41,* 437–449.

Brown, B. R., & Garland, H. (1971). The effects of incompetency, audience acquaintanceship, and anticipated evaluative feedback on face-saving behavior. *Journal of Experimental Social Psychology, 7,* 490–502.

Brownell, K. D. (1991). Personal responsibility and control over our bodies: When expectation exceeds reality. *Health Psychology, 10,* 303–310.

Bruce, T. J., & Barlow, D. H. (1990). The nature and role of performance anxiety in sexual dysfunction. In H. Leitenberg (Ed.), *Handbook of social and evaluation anxiety* (pp. 357–384). New York: Plenum Press.

Bruch, M. A., & Hynes, M. J. (1987). Heterosocial anxiety and contraceptive behavior. *Journal of Research in Personality, 21,* 343–360.

Buck, R. W., & Parke, R. D. (1972). Behavioural and physiological response to the presence of a friendly or neutral person in two types of stressful situations. *Journal of Personality and Social Psychology, 24,* 143–153.

Bulik, C. M., Beidel, D. C., Duchmann, E., Weltzin, T. E., & Kaye, W. H. (1991). An analysis of social anxiety in anorexic, bulimic, social phobic, and control women. *Journal of Psychopathology and Behavioral Assessment, 13,* 199–211.

Burgio, K. L., Glass, C. R., & Merluzzi, T. V. (1981). The effects of social anxiety and videotape performance feedback on cognitions and self-evaluations. *Behavioral Counseling Quarterly, 1*, 288–301.

Burgio, K. L., Merluzzi, T. V., & Pryor, J. B. (1986). Effects of performance expectancy and self-focused attention on social interaction. *Journal of Personality and Social Psychology, 50*, 1216–1221.

Burns, M. O., & Seligman, M. E. P. (1991). Explanatory style, helplessness, and depression. In C. R. Snyder & D. R. Forsyth (Eds.), *Handbook of social and clinical psychology* (pp. 267–284). New York: Pergamon Press.

Buss, A. H. (1980). *Self-consciousness and social anxiety*. San Francisco: Freeman.

Buss, A. H., & Plomin, R. (1975). *A temperament theory of personality development*. New York: Wiley.

Bylina, J. M. (1991). *The relationship between self-consciousness, social anxiety, and sociability*. Paper presented at the annual meeting of the American Psychological Association, San Francisco.

Byrne, D. (1971). *The attraction paradigm*. New York: Academic Press.

Cacioppo, J. T., Glass, C. R., & Merluzzi, T. V. (1979). Self-statements and self-evaluations: A cognitive response analysis of heterosocial anxiety. *Cognitive Therapy and Research, 3*, 249–262.

Cantor, J., Zillman, D., & Bryant, J. (1975). Enhancement of experienced sexual arousal in response to erotic stimuli through misattribution of unrelated residual excitation. *Journal of Personality and Social Psychology, 32*, 69–75.

Cappella, J. N. (1985). Production principles for turn-taking rules in social interaction: Socially anxious vs. socially secure persons. *Journal of Language and Social Psychology, 4*, 193–212.

Carnegie, D. (1936). *How to win friends and influence people*. New York: Simon & Schuster.

Carson, R. C. (1969). *Interaction concepts of personality*. Chicago: Aldine.

Carver, C. S., Coleman, A. E., & Glass, D. G. (1976). The coronary-prone behavior pattern and the suppression of fatigue on a treadmill test. *Journal of Personality and Social Psychology, 33*, 460–466.

Carver, C. S., & Scheier, M. F. (1981). *Attention and self-regulation: A control-theory approach to human behavior*. New York: Springer-Verlag.

Carver, C. S., & Scheier, M. F. (1985). Aspects of self and the control of behavior. In B. R. Schlenker (Ed.), *The self and social life* (pp. 146–174). New York: McGraw-Hill.

Carver, C. S., & Scheier, M. F. (1986). Analyzing shyness: A specific application of broader self-regulatory principles. In W. H. Jones, J. M. Cheek, & S. R. Briggs (Eds.), *Shyness: Perspectives on research and treatment* (pp. 173–185). New York: Plenum Press.

Caspi, A., Elder, G. H., Jr., & Bem, D. J. (1988). Moving away from the world: Life-course patterns of shy children. *Developmental Psychology, 24*, 824–831.

Cattell, R. B. (1946). *Description and measurement of personality.* New York: World Book.

Cattell, R. B. (1973). *Personality and mood by questioning.* San Francisco: Jossey-Bass.

Chaleby, K. (1987). Social phobia in Saudis. *Social Psychiatry, 22,* 167–170.

Cheek, J. M. (August, 1982). Shyness and self-esteem: A personological perspective. In M. R. Leary (Chair), *Recent research in social anxiety.* Symposium presented at the annual meeting of the American Psychological Association, Washington, DC.

Cheek, J. M. (1989a). *Conquering shyness.* New York: Dell.

Cheek, J. M. (1989b). Identity orientations and self-interpretation. In D. M. Buss & N. Cantor (Eds.), *Personality psychology* (pp. 275–285). New York: Springer-Verlag.

Cheek, J. M., & Briggs, S. R. (1982). Self-consciousness and aspects of identity. *Journal of Research in Personality, 16,* 401–408.

Cheek, J. M., & Buss, A. H. (1981). Shyness and sociability. *Journal of Personality and Social Psychology, 41,* 330–339.

Cheek, J. M., & Melchoir, L. A. (1990). Shyness, self-esteem, and self-consciousness. In H. Leitenberg (Ed.), *Handbook of social and evaluation anxiety* (pp. 47–82). New York: Plenum Press.

Cherry, E. C. (1953). Some experiments on the recognition of speech with one and two ears. *Journal of the Acoustical Society of America, 25,* 975–979.

Christensen, A., & Arkowitz, H. (1974). Preliminary report on practice dating and feedback as a treatment for college dating problems. *Journal of Counseling Psychology, 21,* 92–95.

Christensen, A., Arkowitz, H., & Anderson, J. (1975). Practice dating as a treatment for college dating inhibitions. *Behaviour Research and Therapy, 13,* 321–331.

Clark, J. V., & Arkowitz, H. (1975). Social anxiety and self-evaluation of interpersonal performance. *Psychological Reports, 36,* 211–221.

Clevinger, T. A. (1959). A synthesis of experimental research in stage fright. *Quarterly Journal of Speech, 45,* 134–145.

Comadena, M. E., & Prusank, D. T. (1989). Communication apprehension in children. In J. F. Nussbaum (Ed.), *Life-span communication: Normative processes* (pp. 79–91). Hillsdale, NJ: Erlbaum.

Comer, R. J., & Piliavin, J. A. (1972). The effects of physical deviance upon face-to-face interaction: The other side. *Journal of Personality and Social Psychology, 23,* 33–39.

Comrey, A. L. (1965). Scales for measuring compulsion, hostility, neuroticism, and shyness. *Psychological Reports, 16,* 697–700.

Cooley, C. H. (1922). *Human nature and the social order* (rev. ed.). New York: Scribner. (Original work published 1902)

Cooper, J., & Axsom, D. (1982). Effort justification in psychotherapy. In G. Weary & H. L. Mirels (Eds.), *Integrations of clinical and social psychology* (pp. 214–230). New York: Oxford University Press.

Coopersmith, S. (1967). *The antecedents of self-esteem*. San Francisco: W. H. Freeman.

Cosmides, L., Tooby, J., & Barkow, J. H. (1992). Introduction: Evolutionary psychology and conceptual integration. In J. H. Barlow, L. Cosmides, & J. Tooby (Eds.), *The adapted mind: Evolutionary psychology and the generation of culture* (pp. 3–15). New York: Oxford University Press.

Cox, W. J., & Kenardy, J. (1993). Performance anxiety, social phobia, and setting effects in instrumental music students. *Journal of Anxiety Disorders, 7*, 49–60.

Coyne, J. C., Burchill, S. A. L., & Stiles, W. B. (1991). An interactional perspective on depression. In C. R. Snyder & D. R. Forsyth (Eds.), *Handbook of social and clinical psychology* (pp. 327–349). New York: Pergamon Press.

Crawford, S., & Eklund, R. C. (1994). Social physique anxiety, reasons for exercise, and attitudes toward exercise settings. *Journal of Sport and Exercise Psychology, 16*, 70–82.

Crick, N. R., & Ladd, G. W. (1993). Children's perceptions of their peer experiences: Attributions, loneliness, social anxiety, and social avoidance. *Developmental Psychology, 29*, 244–254.

Critelli, J. W., & Neumann, K. F. (1984). The placebo: Conceptual analysis of a construct in transition. *American Psychologist, 39*, 32–39.

Crowne, D. P., & Marlowe, D. (1964). *The approval motive: Studies in evaluative dependence*. New York: Wiley.

Crozier, W. R. (1979). Shyness as a dimension of personality. *British Journal of Social and Clinical Psychology, 18*, 121–128.

Cupach, W. R., Metts, S., & Hazelton, V., Jr. (1986). Coping with embarrassing predicaments: Remedial strategies and their perceived utility. *Journal of Language and Social Psychology, 5*, 181–200.

Curran, J. P. (1975). An evaluation of a skills training program and a systematic desensitization program in reducing dating anxiety. *Behaviour Research and Therapy, 13*, 65–68.

Curran, J. P. (1977). Skills training as an approach to the treatment of heterosexual-social anxiety: A review. *Psychological Bulletin, 84*, 140–157.

Curran, J. P., & Gilbert, F. S. (1975). A test of the relative effectiveness of a systematic desensitization program and an interpersonal skills training program with date anxious subjects. *Behavior Therapy, 6*, 510–521.

Curran, J. P., Little, L. M., & Gilbert, F. S. (1978). Reactivity of males of differing heterosexual social anxiety to female approach and nonapproach cue conditions. *Behavior Therapy, 9*, 961.

Curran, J. P., Wallander, J. L., & Fischetti, M. (1980). The importance of behavioral and cognitive factors in heterosexual-social anxiety. *Journal of Personality, 48*, 285–292.

Cutlip, W. D., & Leary, M. R. (1993). Anatomic and physiological bases of social blushing: Speculations from neurology and psychology. *Behavioral Neurology*, *6*, 181–185

Daly, J. A., & Friedrich, G. (1981). The development of communication apprehension: A retrospective analysis and contributing correlates. *Communication Quarterly*, *29*, 243–255.

Daly, J. A., & McCroskey, J. C. (1984). *Avoiding communication: Shyness, reticence, and communication apprehension*. Beverly Hills, CA: Sage.

Darby, B. W., & Schlenker, B. R. (1986). Children's understanding of social anxiety. *Developmental Psychology*, *22*, 633–639.

Darby, B. W., & Schlenker, B. R. (1989). Children's reactions to transgressions: Effects of the actor's apology, reputation, and remorse. *British Journal of Social Psychology*, *28*, 353–364.

Darwin, C. (1955). *The expression of the emotions in man and animals*. New York: Philosophical Library. (Original work published 1872)

Davies, J. B., & Baker, R. (1987). The impact of self-presentation and interviewer bias effects on self-reported heroin use. *British Journal of Addiction*, *82*, 907–912.

Davison, G. C., & Zighelboim, V. (1987). Irrational beliefs in the articulated thoughts of college students with social anxiety. *Journal of Rational-Emotive Therapy*, *5*, 238–254.

Deaux, K. (1992). Personalizing identity and socializing self. In G. M. Breakwell (Ed.), *Social psychology of identity and the self-concept* (pp. 9–33). London: Surrey University Press.

Deaux, K., & Major, B. (1987). Putting gender into context: An interactive model of gender-related behavior. *Psychological Review*, *94*, 369–389.

Debrovner, C., & Shubin-Stein, R. (1975). Psychological aspects of vaginal examinations. *Medical Aspects of Human Sexuality*, *9*, 163–164.

DeGree, C. E., & Snyder, C. R. (1985). Adler's psychology (of use) today: Personal history of traumatic life events as a self-handicapping strategy. *Journal of Personality and Social Psychology*, *48*, 1512–1519.

DePaulo, B. M., Epstein, J. A., & LeMay, C. S. (1990). Responses of the socially anxious to the prospect of interpersonal evaluation. *Journal of Personality*, *58*, 623–640.

DePaulo, B. M., Kenny, D. A., Hoover, C., Webb, W., & Oliver, P. (1987). Accuracy of person perception: Do people know what kinds of impressions they convey? *Journal of Personality and Social Psychology*, *52*, 303–313.

DiGiuseppe, R., McGowan, L., Simon, K., & Gardner, F. (1990). A comparative outcome study of four cognitive therapies in the treatment of social anxiety. *Journal of Rational-Emotive and Cognitive-Behavior Therapy*, *8*, 129–146.

DiLoreto, A. O. (1971). *Comparative psychotherapy*. Chicago: Aldine.

Dixon, J. J., de Monchaux, C., & Sandler, J. (1957). Patterns of anxiety: An analysis of social anxieties. *British Journal of Medical Psychology*, *30*, 102–112.

Dodge, C. S., Heimberg, R. G., Nyman, D., & O'Brien, G. T. (1987).

Daily heterosocial interactions of high and low socially anxious college students: A diary study. *Behavior Therapy, 18*, 90–96.

Domar, A. D. (1985/1986). Psychological aspects of the pelvic exam: Individual needs and physician involvement. *Women and Health, 10*, 75–89.

Drowning on dry land. (1994, May 23). *Newsweek*, pp. 64–66.

Dunn, P. K., & Ondercin, P. (1981). Personality variables related to compulsive eating in college women. *Journal of Clinical Psychology, 37*, 43–49.

Duval, S., & Wicklund, R. A. (1972). *A theory of objective self-awareness*. New York: Academic Press.

Dykman, B., & Reis, H. T. (1979). Personality correlates of classroom seating position. *Journal of Educational Psychology, 71*, 346–354.

Easterbrook, J. A. (1959). The effect of emotion on cue utilization and the organization of behavior. *Psychological Review, 66*, 183–201.

Edelmann, R. J. (1985). Individual differences in embarrassment: Self-consciousness, self-monitoring, and embarrassability. *Personality and Individual Differences, 6*, 223–230.

Edelmann, R. J. (1987). *The psychology of embarrassment*. New York: Wiley.

Edelmann, R. J. (1990). Chronic blushing, self-consciousness, and social anxiety. *Journal of Psychopathology and Behavioral Assessment, 12*, 119–127.

Edelmann, R. J. (1991). Correlates of chronic blushing. *British Journal of Clinical Psychology, 20*, 177–178.

Edelmann, R. J., Asendorpf, J., Contarello, A., Zammuner, V., Georgas, J., & Villanueva, C. (1989). Self-reported expression of embarrassment in five European countries. *Journal of Cross-Cultural Psychology, 20*, 357–371.

Edelmann, R. J., & Iwawaki, S. (1987). Self-reported expression and consequences of embarrassment in the United States and Japan. *Psychologica: An International Journal of Psychology in the Orient, 30*, 205–211.

Edelmann, R. J., & Neto, F. (1989). Self-reported expression and consequences of embarrassment in Portugal and U.K. *International Journal of Psychology, 24*, 351–366.

Edelmann, R. J., & Skov, V. (1993). Blushing propensity, social anxiety, anxiety sensitivity, and awareness of bodily sensations. *Personality and Individual Differences, 14*, 495–498.

Efran, J. S., & Korn, P. R. (1969). Measurement of social caution: Self-appraisal, role playing, and discussion behavior. *Journal of Consulting and Clinical Psychology, 33*, 78–83.

Elkind, D., & Bowen, R. (1979). Imaginary audience behavior in children and adolescents. *Developmental Psychology, 15*, 38–44.

Elliott, G. C. (1984). Dimensions of the self-concept: A source of further distinctions in the nature of self-consciousness. *Journal of Youth and Adolescence, 13*, 285–306.

Ellis, A. (1962). *Reason and emotion in psychotherapy*. New York: Lyle Stuart.

Ellsworth, P. C., & Carlsmith, J. M. (1968). Effects of eye contact and verbal content on affective response to a dyadic interaction. *Journal of Personality and Social Psychology, 10,* 15–20.

Ellsworth, P. C., & Carlsmith, J. M. (1973). Eye contact and gaze aversion in an aggressive encounter. *Journal of Personality and Social Psychology, 28,* 280–292.

Ellsworth, P. C., Carlsmith, J. M., & Henson, A. (1972). The stare as a stimulus to flight in human subjects: A series of field experiments. *Journal of Personality and Social Psychology, 21,* 302–311.

Emerson, J. P. (1970). Behavior in private places: Sustaining definitions of reality in gynecological examinations. In H. P. Dreitzel (Ed.), *Recent sociology* (Vol. 2, pp. 74–97). New York: Macmillan.

Endler, N. S., Hunt, J., & Rosenstein, A. J. (1962). An S-R inventory of anxiousness. *Psychological Monographs, 79* (Whole No. 17), 1–33.

Feather, N. T. (1989). Attitudes toward the high achiever: The fall of the tall poppy. *Australian Journal of Psychology, 41,* 239–267.

Feather, N. T., & McKee, I. R. (1993). Global self-esteem and attitudes toward the high achiever for Australian and Japanese students. *Social Psychology Quarterly, 56,* 65–76.

Feingold, A. (1992). Good-looking people are not what we think. *Psychological Bulletin, 111,* 304–341.

Fenigstein, A. (1979). Self-consciousness, self-attention, and social interaction. *Journal of Personality and Social Psychology, 37,* 75–86.

Fenigstein, A., Scheier, M. F., & Buss, A. H. (1975). Public and private self-consciousness: Assessment and theory. *Journal of Consulting and Clinical Psychology, 43,* 522–527.

Festinger, L. (1954). A theory of social comparison processes. *Human Relations, 7,* 117–140.

Filsinger, E. F., & Lamke, L. K. (1983). The lineage transmission of interpersonal competence. *Journal of Marriage and the Family, 45,* 75–80.

Fischetti, M., Curran, J. P., & Wessberg, H. W. (1977). A sense of timing: A skill deficit in heterosexual-socially anxious males. *Behavior Modification, 45,* 75–80.

Fishbein, M., Middlestadt, S. E., Ottati, V., Strauss, S., & Ellis, A. (1988). Medical problems among ICSOM musicians: Overview of a national survey. *Medical Problems of Performing Artists, 3,* 1–8.

Folks, D. G., & Kinney, F. C. (1992). The role of psychological factors in gastrointestinal conditions: A review pertinent to DSM-IV. *Psychosomatics, 33,* 257–270.

Fowlie, S., Eastwood, M. A., & Ford, M. J. (1992). Irritable bowel syndrome: The influence of psychological factors on the symptom complex. *Journal of Psychosomatic Research, 36,* 169–173.

Francis, G., & Ollendick, T. H. (1990). Behavioral treatment of social anxiety. In E. L. Feindler & G. R. Kalfus (Eds.), *Adolescent behavior therapy handbook* (pp. 127–145). New York: Springer.

Francis, G., Strauss, C. C., & Last, C. G. (1987, November). *Social anxiety in school phobic adolescents*. Paper presented at the meeting of the Association for Advancement of Behavior Therapy, Boston.

Frank, J. D. (1973). *Persuasion and healing: A comparative study of psychotherapy* (rev. ed.). Baltimore: Johns Hopkins University Press.

Fremouw, W. J., Gross, R., Monroe, J., & Rapp, S. (1982). Empirical subtypes of performance anxiety. *Behavioral Assessment, 4*, 179–193.

Frey, D., Stahlberg, D., & Fries, A. (1986). Information seeking of high- and low-anxiety subjects after receiving positive and negative self-relevant feedback. *Journal of Personality, 54*, 694–703.

Friedman, P. G. (1980). *Shyness and reticence in students*. Washington, DC: National Education Association.

Friend, R. M., & Gilbert, J. (1973). Threat and fear of negative evaluation as determinants of locus of social comparison. *Journal of Personality, 41*, 328–340.

Frijda, N. H. (1986). *The emotions*. New York: Cambridge University Press.

Funder, D. C., & Colvin, C. R. (1988). Friends and strangers: Acquaintanceship, agreement, and the accuracy of personality judgment. *Journal of Personality and Social Psychology, 55*, 149–158.

Galassi, J. P., & Galassi, M. D. (1979). Modification of heterosocial skills deficits. In A. S. Bellack & M. Hersen (Eds.), *Research and practice in social skills training* (pp. 131–138). New York: Plenum Press.

Garcia, S., Stinson, L., Ickes, W., Bissonnette, V., & Briggs, S. R. (1991). Shyness and physical attractiveness in mixed-sex dyads. *Journal of Personality and Social Psychology, 61*, 35–49.

Geen, R. G., Beatty, W. W., & Arkin, R. M. (1984). *Human motivation: Physiological, behavioral, and social approaches*. Boston: Allyn & Bacon.

Geist, C. R., & Borecki, S. (1982). Social avoidance and distress as a predictor of perceived locus of control and level of self-esteem. *Journal of Clinical Psychology, 38*, 611–613.

Gersten, M. (1989). Behavioral inhibition in the classroom. In J. S. Reznick (Ed.), *Perspectives on behavioral inhibition* (pp. 71–91). Chicago: University of Chicago Press.

Gibbons, F. X. (1990). The impact of focus of attention and affect on social behavior. In W. R. Crozier (Ed.), *Shyness and embarrassment* (pp. 119–143). New York: Cambridge University Press.

Gilbert, P., & Trower, P. (1990). The evolution and manifestation of social anxiety. In W. R. Crozier (Ed.), *Shyness and embarrassment* (pp. 144–177). New York: Cambridge University Press.

Gilkinson, H. (1942). Social fears as reported by students in college speech classes. *Speech Monographs, 9*, 141–160.

Gilkinson, H. (1943). A questionnaire study of the causes of social fears among college speech students. *Speech Monographs, 10*, 74–83.

Girodo, M. (1978). *Shy? (You don't have to be!)*. New York: Pocket Books.

Glasgow, R., & Arkowitz, H. (1975). The behavioral assessment of male and female social competence in dyadic heterosexual interactions. *Behavior Therapy, 6*, 488–498.

Glasgow, R. E., McCaul, K. D., & Schafer, L. C. (1986). Barriers to regimen adherence among persons with insulin-dependent diabetes. *Journal of Behavioral Medicine*, *9*, 65–77.

Glass, C. R., & Arnkoff, D. B. (1982). Think cognitively: Selected issues in cognitive assessment and therapy. In P. C. Kendall (Ed.), *Advances in cognitive-behavioral research and therapy* (Vol. 1, pp. 35–71). New York: Academic Press.

Glass, C. R., Gottman, J. M., & Shmurak, S. (1976). Response acquisition and cognitive self-statement modification approaches to dating-skills training. *Journal of Counseling Psychology*, *23*, 520–526.

Glass, C. R., Merluzzi, T. V., Biever, J. L., & Larsen, K. H. (1982). Cognitive assessment of social anxiety: Development and validation of a self-assessment questionnaire. *Cognitive Therapy and Research*, *6*, 37–56.

Glass, C. R., & Shea, C. A. (1986). Cognitive therapy for shyness and social anxiety. In W. H. Jones, J. M. Cheek, & S. R. Briggs (Eds.), *Shyness: Perspectives on research and treatment* (pp. 315–327). New York: Plenum Press.

Goffman, E. (1955). On facework. *Psychiatry*, *18*, 213–231.

Goffman, E. (1959). *The presentation of self in everyday life*. New York: Doubleday.

Goffman, E. (1967). *Interaction ritual*. New York: Doubleday.

Goldfried, M. R. (1979). Anxiety reduction through cognitive-behavioral intervention. In P. C. Kendall & S. D. Hollon (Eds.), *Behavioral intervention: Theory, research, and procedures* (pp. 117–151). New York: Academic Press.

Goldfried, M. R. (1980). Toward the delineation of therapeutic change principles. *American Psychologist*, *35*, 991–999.

Goldfried, M. R., & Sobocinski, D. (1975). Effect of irrational beliefs on emotional arousal. *Journal of Consulting and Clinical Psychology*, *43*, 504–510.

Golwyn, D. H., & Sevlie, C. P. (1992). Paraphilias, nonparaphilic sexual addictions, and social phobia. *Journal of Clinical Psychiatry*, *53*, 9.

Gonzales, M. H., Pederson, J. H., Manning, D. J., & Wetter, D. W. (1990). Pardon my gaffe: Effects of sex, status, and consequence severity on accounts. *Journal of Personality and Social Psychology*, *58*, 610–621.

Goodall, J. (1988). *In the shadow of man* (rev. ed.). Boston: Houghton Mifflin.

Gotlib, I. H. (1984). Depresssion and general psychopathology in university students. *Journal of Abnormal Psychology*, *93*, 19–30.

Gough, H. G., & Thorne, A. (1986). Positive, negative, and balanced shyness: Self-definitions and reactions of others. In W. H. Jones, J. M. Cheek, & S. R. Briggs (Eds.), *Shyness: Perspectives on research and treatment* (pp. 205–225). New York: Plenum Press.

Greenberg, J., Pyszczynski, T., & Stine, P. (1985). Social anxiety and anticipation of future interaction as determinants of the favorability of self-presentation. *Journal of Research in Personality*, *19*, 1–11.

216 References

Greenberg, M. T., & Marvin, R. S. (1982). Reactions of preschool children to an adult stranger: A behavioral systems approach. *Child Development*, *53*, 481–490.
Gregorich, S. E., Kemple, K., & Leary, M. R. (1986). Fear of negative evaluation and reactions to information regarding others' performances. *Representative Research in Social Psychology*, *16*, 15–27.
Grimm, L. G. (1980). The evidence of cue-controlled relaxation. *Behavior Therapy*, *11*, 283–293.
Gross, E., & Stone, G. P. (1964). Embarrassment and the analysis of role requirements. *American Journal of Sociology*, *70*, 1–15.
Gross, J., & Rosen, J. C. (1988). Bulimia in adolescents: Prevalence and psychological correlates. *International Journal of Eating Disorders*, *7*, 51–61.
Gross, P. R. (1989). Multimodal therapy for generalized and social anxieties: A pilot study. *Behavioral Psychotherapy*, *17*, 316–322.
Gross, R. T., & Fremouw, W. J. (1982). Cognitive restructuring and progressive relaxation for treatment of empirical subtypes of speech-anxious subjects. *Cognitive Therapy and Research*, *6*, 429–436.
Guilford, J. P., & Guilford, R. B. (1936). Personality factors S, E, and M, and their measurement. *Journal of Psychology*, *2* 109–127.
Haas, H. T., & Maehr, M. L. (1965). Two experiments in the concept of self and the reaction of others. *Journal of Personality and Social Psychology*, *1*, 100–105.
Haas, R. G., & Mann, R. W. (1976). Anticipatory belief change: Persuasion or impression management? *Journal of Personality and Social Psychology*, *34*, 105–111.
Haemmerlie, F. M. (1983). Heterosocial anxiety in college females: A biased interactions treatment. *Behavior Modification*, *7*, 611–623.
Haemmerlie, F. M., & Montgomery, R. L. (1982). Self-perception theory and unobtrusively biased interactions: A treatment for heterosocial anxiety. *Journal of Counseling Psychology*, *29*, 362–370.
Haemmerlie, F. M., & Montgomery, R. L. (1984). Purposefully biased interactions: Reducing heterosocial anxiety through self-perception theory. *Journal of Personality and Social Psychology*, *47*, 900–908.
Halberstadt, A. G., & Green, L. R. (1993). Social attention and placation theories of blushing. *Motivation and Emotion*, *17*, 53–64.
Halford, K., & Foddy, M. (1982). Cognitive and social skills correlates of social anxiety. *British Journal of Clinical Psychology*, *23*, 17–28.
Hamilton, L. (1989). Fight, flight, or freeze: Implications of the passive fear response for anxiety and depression. *Phobia Practice and Research Journal*, *2*, 17–27.
Hamilton, M., & Dodge, E. (1981). Pelvic examination: Patient safety and comfort. *JOGN-Nursing*, *10*, 334–345.
Hamilton, V. (1975). Socialization anxiety and information processing: A capacity model of anxiety-induced performance deficits. In I. G.

Sarason & C. Spielberger (Eds.), *Stress and anxiety* (pp. 45–68). New York. Wiley.

Hansford, B. C., & Hattie, J. A. (1982). Communication apprehension: An assessment of Australian and United States data. *Applied Psychological Measurements, 6,* 225–233.

Hardy, C. J., Hall, E. G., & Prestholdt, P. H. (1986). The mediational role of social influence in the perception of exertion. *Journal of Sport Psychology, 8,* 88–104.

Harmon, R. J., Morgran, G. A., & Klein, R. P. (1977). Determinants of normal variation in infants' negative reactions to unfamiliar adults. *Journal of the American Academy of Child Psychiatry, 16,* 670–683.

Harris, P. R. (1990). Shyness and embarrassment in psychological theory and ordinary language. In W. R. Crozier (Ed.), *Shyness and embarrassment* (pp. 59–86). New York: Cambridge University Press.

Hart, E. A. (1987). *Social physique anxiety in college females.* Unpublished master's thesis, Wake Forest University.

Hart, E. A., Leary, M. R., & Rejeski, W. J. (1989). The measurement of social physique anxiety. *Journal of Sport and Exercise Psychology, 11,* 94–104.

Harter, S. (1983). Developmental perspectives on the self-system. In E. M. Hetherington (Ed.), *Handbook of child psychology: Vol. 4. Socialization, personality, and social development* (pp. 275–386). New York: Wiley.

Hartman, L. M. (1983). A metacognitive model of social anxiety: Implications for treatment. *Clinical Psychology Review, 3,* 435–456.

Hartman, L. M. (1984). Cognitive components of social anxiety. *Journal of Clinical Psychology, 40,* 137–139.

Hatfield, E., & Rapson, R. L. (1990). Passionate love in intimate relationships. In B. Moore & A. Isen (Eds.), *Affect and social behavior* (pp. 126–151). Cambridge: Cambridge University Press.

Hatvany, N., Souza e Silva, M. C., & Zimbardo, P. (1979). *Shyness and recall deficits: The relationship between attention and arousal.* Unpublished manuscript, Stanford University.

Hayes, D., & Ross, C. E. (1987). Concern with appearance, health beliefs, and eating habits. *Journal of Health and Social Behavior, 28,* 120–130.

Heimberg, R. G., Acerra, M. C., & Holstein, A. (1985). Partner similarity mediates interpersonal anxiety. *Cognitive Therapy and Research, 9,* 443–453.

Heimberg, R. G., Becker, R. E., Goldfinger, K., & Verilyea, J. A. (1985). Treatment of social phobia by exposure, cognitive restructuring and homework assignments. *Journal of Nervous and Mental Disease, 173,* 236–245.

Heimberg, R. G., Dodge, C. S., & Becker, R. E. (1987). Social phobia. In L. Michelson & L. M. Ascher (Eds.), *Anxiety and stress disorders: Cognitive-behavioral assessment and treatment* (pp. 280–309). New York: Guilford Press.

Heimberg, R. G., Dodge, C. S., Hope, D. A., Kennedy, C. R., & Zollo, L. J. (1990). Cognitive behavioral group treatment for social phobia: Comparison to a credible placebo control. *Cognitive Therapy and Research, 14,* 1–23.

Heimberg, R. G., Harrison, D. F., Montgomery, D., Madsen, C. H., & Sherfey, J. A. (1980). Psychometric and behavioral analysis of a social anxiety inventory: The Situation Questionnaire. *Behavioral Assessment, 2,* 403–415.

Heimberg, R. G., Liebowitz, M., Hope, D., & Schneier, F. (Eds.). (1995). *Social phobia: Diagnosis, assessment, and treatment.* New York: Guilford Press.

Heimberg, R. G., Salzman, D. G., Holt, C. S., & Blendell, K. A. (1993). Cognitive-behavioral group treatment for social phobia: Effectiveness at five-year followup. *Cognitive Therapy and Research, 17,* 325–339.

Hewitt, J. P., & Stokes, R. (1975). Disclaimers. *American Sociological Review, 40,* 1–11.

Himadi, W., Arkowitz, H., Hinton, R., & Perl, J. (1980). Minimal dating and its relationship to other social problems and general adjustment. *Behavior Therapy, 11,* 345–352.

Holt, C. S., Heimberg, R. G., Hope, D. A., & Liebowitz, M. R. (1992). Situational domains of social phobia. *Journal of Anxiety Disorders, 6,* 63–77.

Hope, D. A., Gansler, D. A., & Heimberg, R. G. (1989). Attentional focus and causal attributions in social phobia: Implications from social psychology. *Clinical Psychology Review, 9,* 49–60.

Hope, D. A., & Heimberg, R. G. (1988). Public and private self-consciousness and social phobia. *Journal of Personality Assessment, 52,* 626–639.

Horowitz, E. (1962). Reported embarrassment memories of elementary school, high school, and college students. *Journal of Social Psychology, 56,* 317–325.

Houtman, I. L. D., & Bakker, F. C. (1991). Individual differences in reactivity to and coping with the stress of lecturing. *Journal of Psychosomatic Research, 35,* 11–24.

Hull, J. G. (1981). A self-awareness model of the causes and effects of alcohol consumption. *Journal of Abnormal Psychology, 90,* 586–600.

Huntley, J. R. (1969). *An investigation of the relationships between personality and types of instructor criticism in the beginning speech-communication course.* Unpublished doctoral dissertation, Michigan State University.

Hurt, H. T., Scott, M. D., & McCroskey, J. C. (1978). *Communication in the classroom.* Reading, MA: Addison-Wesley.

Hyde, J. S. (1994). *Understanding human sexuality* (5th ed.). New York: McGraw-Hill.

Ickes, W., Robertson, E., Tooke, W., & Teng, G. (1986). Naturalistic social cognition: Methodology, assessment, and validation. *Journal of Personality and Social Psychology, 51,* 66–82.

Inderbitzen-Pisaruk, H., Clark, M. L., & Solano, C. H. (1992). Correlates of loneliness in midadolescence. *Journal of Youth and Adolescence, 21,* 151–167.

Ishiyama, F. I. (1984). Shyness: Anxious social sensitivity and self-isolating tendency. *Adolescence, 19,* 903–911.

Izard, C. E. (1977). *Human emotions.* New York: Plenum Press.

Jackson, J. M., & Latané, B. (1981). All alone in front of those people: Stage fright as a function of number and type of co-performers and audience. *Journal of Personality and Social Psychology, 40,* 73–85.

Janis, I. L. (1982). *Victims of groupthink* (2nd. ed.). Boston: Houghton-Mifflin.

Johansson, J., & Öst, L. G. (1982). Perception of autonomic reactions and actual heart rate in phobic patients. *Journal of Behavioral Assessment, 4,* 133–143.

Jones, E. E., & Gerard, H. B. (1967). *Foundations of social psychology.* New York: Wiley.

Jones, E. E., & Goethals, G. R. (1972). Order effects in impression formation: Attribution context and the nature of the entity. In E. E. Jones, Kanouse, D. E., Kelley, H. H., Nisbett, R. E., Valins, J., & Weiner, B. (Eds.), *Attribution: Perceiving the causes of behavior* (pp. 27–46). Morristown, NJ: General Learning Press.

Jones, E. E., & Pittman, T. S. (1982). Toward a general theory of strategic self-presentation. In J. Suls (Ed.), *Psychological perspectives on the self* (Vol. 1, pp. 231–262). Hillsdale, NJ: Erlbaum.

Jones, W. H., & Briggs, S. R. (1984). The self-other discrepancy in social shyness. In R. Schwarzer (Ed.), *The self in anxiety, stress, and depression* (pp. 93–107). Amsterdam: North Holland.

Jones, W. H., Briggs, S. R., & Smith, T. G. (1986). Shyness: Conceptualization and measurement. *Journal of Personality and Social Psychology, 51,* 629–639.

Jones, W. H., & Carpenter, B. N. (1986). Shyness, social behavior, and relationships. In W. H. Jones, J. M. Cheek, & S. R. Briggs (Eds.), *Shyness: Perspectives on research and treatment* (pp. 227–238). New York: Plenum Press.

Jones, W. H., Cheek, J. M., & Briggs, S. R. (1986). *Shyness: Perspectives on research and treatment.* New York: Plenum Press.

Jones, W. H., Freemon, J. E., & Goswick, R. A. (1981). The persistence of loneliness: Self and other determinants. *Journal of Personality, 49,* 27–48.

Jones, W. H., Hobbs, S. A., & Hockenbury, D. (1982). Loneliness and social skill deficits. *Journal of Personality and Social Psychology, 42,* 682–689.

Jones, W. H., & Russell, D. (1982). The Social Reticence Scale: An objective instrument to measure shyness. *Journal of Personality Assessment, 46,* 629–631.

Kagan, J., Reznick, J. S., & Snidman, N. (1988). Biological bases of childhood shyness. *Science, 240,* 167–171.

Kagan, J., Snidman, N., Julia-Sellers, M., & Johnson, M. O. (1991). Temperament and allergic symptoms. *Psychosomatic Medicine, 53*, 332–340.

Kamhi, A. G., & McOsker, T. G. (1982). Attention and stuttering: Do stutters think too much about speech? *Journal of Fluency Disorders, 7*, 309–321.

Kanter, N. J., & Goldfried, M. R. (1979). Relative effectiveness of rational restructuring and self-control desensitization in the reduction of interpersonal anxiety. *Behavior Therapy, 10*, 472–490.

Karno, M., Golding, J. M., Bunam, A., Hough, R. L., Escober, J. I., Wells, K. M., & Bouer, R. (1989). Anxiety disorders among Mexican Americans and non-Hispanic whites in Los Angeles. *Journal of Nervous and Mental Disease, 177*, 202–209.

Kashani, J. H., Orvaschel, H., Rosenberg, R. K., & Reid, J. C. (1989). Psychopathology in a community sample of children and adolescents: A developmental perspective. *Journal of the American Academy of Child and Adolescent Psychiatry, 28*, 701–706.

Kasl, S. V., & Mahl, G. F. (1965). The relationship of disturbances and hesitations in spontaneous speech to anxiety. *Journal of Personality and Social Psychology, 1*, 425–433.

Katzman, M. A., & Wolchik, S. A. (1984). Bulimia and binge eating in college women: A comparison of personality and behavioral characteristics. *Journal of Consulting and Clinical Psychology, 52*, 423–428.

Kiesler, D. J. (1966). Some myths of psychotherapy research and the search for a paradigm. *Psychological Bulletin, 65*, 110–136.

Kimble, C. E., & Zehr, H. D. (1982). Self-consciousness, information load, self-presentation, and memory in a social situation. *Journal of Social Psychology, 118*, 39–46.

Kirsch, I., & Henry, D. (1979). Self-desensitization and meditation in the remediation of public speaking anxiety. *Journal of Consulting and Clinical Psychology, 47*, 536–541.

Kleck, R. E., Ono, H., & Hastorf, A. H. (1966). The effects of physical deviance on face-to-face interaction. *Human Relations, 19*, 425–436.

Kleinke, C. L., Staneski, R. A., & Berger, D. E. (1975). Evaluation of an interviewer as a function of interviewer gaze, reinforcement of subject gaze, and interviewer attractiveness. *Journal of Personality and Social Psychology, 31*, 115–122.

Klonsky, B. G., Dutton, D. L., & Liebel, C. N. (1990). Developmental antecedents of private self-consciousness, public self-consciousness, and social anxiety. *Genetic, Social, and General Psychology Monographs, 116*, 273–297.

Knight, M. L., & Borden, R. J. (1978, August). *Performer's affect and behavior: Relationships with audience size and expertise.* Paper presented at the annual meeting of the American Psychological Association, Toronto.

Kondas, O. (1967). Reduction of examination anxiety and "stage-fright" by group desensitization and relaxation. *Behaviour Research and Therapy, 5,* 275 281.

Kowalski, R. M. (1993a). Inferring sexual interest from behavioral cues: Effects of gender and sexually-relevant attitudes. *Sex Roles, 29,* 13–31.

Kowalski, R. M. (1993b). Interpreting behaviors in mixed-gender encounters: Effects of social anxiety and gender. *Journal of Social and Clinical Psychology, 12,* 239–247.

Kowalski, R. M. (in press). Complaints and complaining: Antecedents, functions, and consequences. *Psychological Bulletin.*

Kowalski, R. M., & Brown, K. J. (1994). *Psychosocial barriers to cervical cancer screening: Concerns with self-presentation and social evaluation. Journal of Applied Social Psychology, 24,* 941–958.

Kowalski, R. M., & Cantrell, C. C. (1994). *Individual differences in the propensity to complain.* Unpublished manuscript, Western Carolina University.

Kowalski, R. M., & Chapple, T. (1994). *Effects of the social stigma of menstruation on impression motivation: Facilitator or inhibitor?* Unpublished manuscript, Western Carolina University.

Kowalski, R. M., & Leary, M. R. (1990). Strategic self-presentation and the avoidance of aversive events: Antecedents and consequences of self-enhancement and self-depreciation. *Journal of Experimental Social Psychology, 26,* 322–336.

Kowalski, R. M., & Wolfe, R. (1994). Collective identity orientation, patriotism, and reactions to national outcomes. *Personality and Social Psychology Bulletin, 20,* 533–540.

Kuiper, N. A., Derry, P. A., & MacDonald, M. R. (1982). Self-reference and person perception in depression: A social cognition perspective. In G. Weary & S. L. Mirels (Eds.), *Integrations of clinical and social psychology* (pp. 79–103). New York: Oxford University Press.

Lader, M. H. (1967). Palmar skin conductance measures in anxiety and phobic states. *Journal of Psychosomatic Research, 11,* 271–281.

LaFrance, M., & Mayo, C. (1978). *Moving bodies.* Monterey, CA: Brooks/Cole.

Lamontagne, Y. (1978). Treatment of erythrophobia by paradoxical intention. *The Journal of Nervous and Mental Disease, 166,* 304–306.

Landy, F. J., & Gaupp, L. A. (1971). A factor analysis of the Fear Survey Schedule—III. *Behaviour Research and Therapy, 9,* 89–93.

Last, C. G., Strauss, C. C., & Francis, G. (1987). Comorbidity among childhood anxiety disorders. *Journal of Nervous and Mental Disease, 175,* 726–730.

Latané, B. (1981). The psychology of social impact. *American Psychologist, 36,* 343–356.

Latané, B., & Darley, J. (1970). *The unresponsive bystander: Why doesn't he help?* New York: Appleton-Century-Crofts.

Latané, B., & Harkins, S. (1976). Cross-modality matches suggest anticipated stage fright a multiplicative function of audience size and status.

Perception and Psychophysics, 20, 482–488.

Lazarus, R. S., & Folkman, S. (1984). *Stress, appraisal, and coping.* New York: Springer.

Leary, M. R. (1980). *The social psychology of shyness: Testing a self-presentational model.* Unpublished doctoral dissertation, University of Florida.

Leary, M. R. (1983a). A brief version of the Fear of Negative Evaluation Scale. *Personality and Social Psychology Bulletin, 9,* 371–376.

Leary, M. R. (1983b). The conceptual distinctions are important: Another look at communication apprehension and related constructs. *Human Communication Research, 10,* 305–312.

Leary, M. R. (1983c). Social anxiousness: The construct and its measurement. *Journal of Personality Assessment, 47,* 66–75.

Leary, M. R. (1983d). *Understanding social anxiety: Social, personality, and clinical perspectives.* Beverly Hills, CA: Sage.

Leary, M. R. (1986a). Affective and behavioral components of shyness: Implications for theory, measurement, and research. In W. H. Jones, J. M. Cheek, & S. R. Briggs (Eds.), *Shyness: Perspectives on research and treatment* (pp. 27–38). New York: Plenum Press.

Leary, M. R. (1986b). The impact of interactional impediments on social anxiety and self-presentation. *Journal of Experimental Social Psychology, 22,* 122–135.

Leary, M. R. (1990a). Anxiety, cognition, and behavior: In search of a broader perspective. In M. Booth-Butterfield (Ed.), *Communication, cognition, and anxiety* (pp. 39–44). Newbury Park, CA: Sage.

Leary, M. R. (1990b). Responses to social exclusion: Social anxiety, jealousy, loneliness, depression, and low self-esteem. *Journal of Social and Clinical Psychology, 9,* 221–229.

Leary, M. R. (1991). Social anxiety, shyness, and related constructs. In J. Robinson, P. Shaver, & L. Wrightsman (Eds.), *Measures of personality and social psychological attitudes* (pp. 161–194). New York: Academic Press.

Leary, M. R. (1992). Self-presentational processes in exercise and sport. *Journal of Sport and Exercise Psychology, 14,* 339–351.

Leary, M. R. (1993). The interplay of private self-processes and interpersonal factors in self-presentation. In J. Suls (Ed.), *Psychological perspectives on the self* (Vol. 4, pp. 127–155). Hillsdale, NJ: Erlbaum.

Leary, M. R. (1995). *Self-presentation: Impression management and interpersonal behavior.* Madison, WI: Brown & Benchmark.

Leary, M. R., & Atherton, S. (1986). Self-efficacy, anxiety, and inhibition in interpersonal encounters. *Journal of Social and Clinical Psychology, 4,* 256–267.

Leary, M. R., Atherton, S. C., Hill, S., & Hur, C. (1986). Attributional mediators of social inhibition and avoidance. *Journal of Personality, 54,* 188–200.

Leary, M. R. Barnes, B. D., & Griebel, C. (1986). Cognitive, affective, and attributional effects of potential threats to self-esteem. *Journal of Social and Clinical Psychology, 4,* 461–474.

Leary, M. R., & Baumeister, R. F. (1994). *The nature and function of the self-esteem motive.* Unpublished manuscript, Wake Forest University.

Leary, M. R., Britt, T. W., Cutlip, W. D., & Templeton, J. L. (1992). Social blushing. *Psychological Bulletin, 112,* 446–460.

Leary, M. R., & Dobbins, S. E. (1983). Social anxiety, sexual behavior, and contraceptive use. *Journal of Personality and Social Psychology, 45,* 1347–1354.

Leary, M. R., & Downs, D. L. (1995). Intepersonal functions of the self-esteem motive: The self-esteem system as a sociometer. In M. Kernis (Ed.), *Efficacy, agency, and self-esteem.* New York: Plenum Press.

Leary, M. R., Knight, P. D., & Johnson, K. A. (1987). Social anxiety and dyadic conversation: A verbal response analysis. *Journal of Social and Clinical Psychology, 5,* 34–50.

Leary, M. R., & Kowalski, R. M. (1990). Impression management: A literature review and two-component model. *Psychological Bulletin, 107,* 34–47.

Leary, M. R., & Kowalski, R. M. (1993). The Interaction Anxiousness Scale: Construct and criterion-related validity. *Journal of Personality Assessment, 61,* 136–146.

Leary, M. R., & Kowalski, R. M. (1995). The self-presentation model of social phobia. In R. Heimberg, M. Liebowitz, D. Hope, & F. Schneier (Eds.), *Social phobia: Diagnosis, assessment, and treatment.* New York: Guilford Press.

Leary, M. R., Kowalski, R. M., & Bergen, D. J. (1988). Interpersonal information acquisition and confidence in first encounters. *Personality and Social Psychology Bulletin, 14,* 68–77.

Leary, M. R., Kowalski, R. M., & Campbell, C. (1988). Self-presentational concerns and social anxiety: The role of generalized impression expectancies. *Journal of Research in Personality, 22,* 308–321.

Leary, M. R., & Meadows, S. (1991). Predictors, elicitors, and concomitants of social blushing. *Journal of Personality and Social Psychology, 60,* 254–262.

Leary, M. R., & Miller, R. S. (1986). *Social psychology and dysfunctional behavior.* New York: Springer-Verlag.

Leary, M. R., Rejeski, W. J., Britt, T. W., & Smith, G. E. (1994). *Physiological differences between embarrassment and social anxiety.* Manuscript under editorial review, Wake Forest University.

Leary, M. R., Rogers, P. A., Canfield, R. W., & Coe, C. (1986). Boredom in interpersonal encounters: Antecedents and social implications. *Journal of Personality and Social Psychology, 51,* 968–975.

Leary, M. R., & Schlenker, B. R. (1981). The social psychology of shyness: A self-presentation model. In J. T. Tedeschi (Ed.), *Impression management theory and social psychological research* (pp. 335–358). New York: Academic Press.

Leary, M. R., & Shepperd, J. A. (1986). Behavioral self-handicaps versus self-reported handicaps: A conceptual note. *Journal of Personality and Social Psychology, 51,* 1265–1268.

Leary, M. R., Tambor, E. S., Terdal, S. K., & Downs, D. L. (1995). Self-esteem as an interpersonal monitor: The sociometer hypothesis. *Journal of Personality and Social Psychology, 68,* 518–530.

Leary, M. R., Tchvidjian, L. R., & Kraxberger, B. E. (1994). Self-presentation can be hazardous to your health: Impression management and health risk. *Health Psychology, 13,* 1–10.

Leary, M. R., Wheeler, D. S., & Jenkins, T. D. (1986). Aspects of identity and behavioral preference: Studies of occupational and recreational choice. *Social Psychology Quarterly, 49,* 11–18.

Lehrer, P. M., & Woolfolk, R. L. (1982). Self-report assessment of anxiety: Somatic, cognitive, and behavioral modalities. *Behavioral Assessment, 4,* 167–177.

Lent, R. W., Russell, R. K., & Zamostny, K. P. (1981). Comparison of cue-controlled desensitization, rational restructuring, and a credible placebo in the treatment of speech anxiety. *Journal of Consulting and Clinical Psychology, 49,* 235–243.

Leonard, K. E., & Blane, H. T. (1988). Alcohol expectancies and personality characteristics in young men. *Addictive Behaviors, 13,* 353–357.

Lerman, C., Rimer, B., Trock, B., Balshem, A., & Engstrom, P. F. (1990). Factors associated with repeat adherence to breast cancer screening. *Preventive Medicine, 19,* 279–290.

Levin, A. P., Saoud, J. B., Strauman, T., Gorman, J. M., Fyer, A. J., Crawford, R., & Liebowitz, M. R. (1993). Responses of "generalized" and "discrete" social phobics during public speaking. *Journal of Anxiety Disorders, 7,* 207–221.

Lewis, M. (1990). Social knowledge and social development. *Merrill-Palmer Quarterly, 36,* 93–116.

Lewis, M., Sullivan, M. W., Stanger, C., & Weiss, M. (1989). Self development and self-conscious emotions. *Child Development, 60,* 146–156.

Liebowitz, M. R., Fyer, A. J., Gorman, J. M., Campeas, R., & Levin, A. P. (1986). Phenelzine in social phobia. *Journal of Clinical Psychopharmacology, 6,* 93–98.

Liebowitz, M. R., Gorman, J. M., Fyer, A. J., Campeas, R., Levin, A. P., Sandberg, D., Hollander, E., Papp, L., & Goetz, D. (1988). Pharmacotherapy of social phobia: An interim report of a placebo-controlled comparison of phenelzine and atenolol. *Journal of Clinical Psychiatry, 49,* 252–257.

Lindskold, S., & Propst, L. R. (1981). Deindividuation, self-awareness, and impression management. In J. T. Tedeschi (Ed.), *Impression management theory and social psychological research* (pp. 201–222). New York: Academic Press.

Lord, C. G., Saenz, D. D., & Godfrey, D. K. (1987). Effects of perceived scrutiny on participant memory for social interaction. *Journal of Ex-*

perimental Social Psychology, 23, 498–517.

Lucock, M. P., & Salkovskis, P. M. (1988). Cognitive factors in social anxiety and its treatment. *Behaviour Research and Therapy, 26,* 297–302.

MacCurdy, J. T. (1930). The biological significance of blushing and shame. *British Journal of Psychology, 21,* 174–182.

Maddux, J. E., Norton, L. W., & Leary, M. R. (1988). Cognitive components of social anxiety: An investigation of the integration of self-presentation theory and self-efficacy theory. *Journal of Social and Clinical Psychology, 6,* 180–190.

Maddux, J. E., Stoltenberg, C. D., & Rosenwein, R. (1987). *Social processes in clinical and counseling psychology.* New York: Springer-Verlag.

Mahl, G. F. (1956). Disturbances and silences in the patient's speech in psychotherapy. *Journal of Abnormal and Social Psychology, 53,* 1–15.

Mahone, E. M., Bruch, M. A., & Heimberg, R. G. (1993). Focus of attention and social anxiety: The role of negative self-thoughts and perceived positive attributes of the other. *Cognitive Therapy and Research, 17,* 209–224.

Malkiewich, L. E., & Merluzzi, T. V. (1980). Rational restructuring versus desensitization with clients of diverse conceptual level: A test of client-treatment matching model. *Journal of Counseling Psychology, 27,* 453–461.

Marcus, D. K., Wilson, J. R., & Miller, R. S. (1994). *Is embarrassment in the eye of the beholder or the face of the beheld?* Unpublished manuscript, Sam Houston State University.

Markaway, B. G., Carmen, C. N., Pollard, C. A., & Flynn, T. (1992). *Dying of embarrassment.* Oakland, CA: New Harbinger.

Marks, I. M. (1969). *Fears and phobias.* London: Heinemann.

Marks, I. M. (1970). The classification of phobic disorders. *British Journal of Psychiatry, 116,* 377–386.

Markus, H. (1980). The self in thought and memory. In D. M. Wegner & R. R. Vallacher (Eds.), *The self in social psychology* (pp. 102–130). New York: Oxford University Press.

Maroldo, G. K. (1983). *The effects of shyness interventions on college drinking.* Unpublished manuscript, Texas Lutheran College.

Martens, R. (1977). *Sport competition anxiety test.* Champaign, IL: Human Kinetics.

Martens, R., & Landers, D. M. (1972). Evaluation potential as a determinant of coaction effects. *Journal of Experimental Social Psychology, 8,* 347–359.

Martinson, W. D., & Zerface, J. P. (1970). Comparison of individual counseling and a social program with nondaters. *Journal of Counseling Psychology, 17,* 36–40.

McAuley, E., Rudolph, D. L., & Lox, C. L. (1994). *Relationship among body image, exercise, sex, and aging: An impression management perspective.* Unpublished manuscript, University of Illinois.

McCroskey, J. C. (1970). Measures of communication-bound anxiety. *Speech Monographs, 37*, 269–277.

McCroskey, J. C. (1975). *Validity of the PRCA as an index of oral communication apprehension*. Paper presented at the meeting of the Speech Communication Association, Houston.

McCroskey, J. C. (1977). Oral communication apprehension: A summary of recent history and research. *Human Communication Research, 4*, 78–96.

McCroskey, J. C. (1978). Validity of the PRCA as an index of oral communication apprenhension. *Communication Monographs, 45*, 192–203.

McCroskey, J. C. (1982). Oral communication apprehension: Reconceptualization and a new look at measurement. In M. Burgoon (Ed.), *Communication yearbook 6*. Beverly Hills, CA: Sage.

McCroskey, J. C. (1984). The communication apprehension perspective. In J. A. Daly & J. C. McCroskey (Eds.), *Avoiding communication: Shyness, reticence, and communication apprehension* (pp. 13–38). Beverly Hills, CA: Sage.

McCroskey, J. C., & Beatty, M. J. (1984). Communication apprehension and accumulated communication state anxiety experiences: A research note. *Communication Monographs, 51*, 79–84.

McCroskey, J. C., Beatty, M. J., Kearney, P., & Plax, T. G. (1985). The content validity of the PRCA-24 as a measure of communication apprehension across communication contexts. *Communication Quarterly, 33*, 165–173.

McCroskey, J. C., & Leppard, T. (1975). *The effects of communication apprehension on nonverbal behavior*. Paper presented at the annual convention of the Eastern Communication Association, New York.

McGovern, L. P. (1976). Dispositional social anxiety and helping behavior under three conditions of threat. *Journal of Personality, 44*, 84–97.

Mead, G. H. (1934). *Mind, self, and society*. Chicago: University of Chicago Press.

Mecca, A. M., Smelser, N. J., & Vasconcellos, J. (Eds.) (1989). *The social importance of self-esteem*. Berkeley, CA: University of California Press.

Meichenbaum, D. H. (1977). *Cognitive behavior modification*. New York: Plenum Press.

Meichenbaum, D. H., Gilmore, J. B., & Fedoravicius, A. (1971). Group insight versus group desensitization in treating speech anxiety. *Journal of Consulting and Clinical Psychology, 36*, 410–421.

Meleshko, K. G. A., & Alden, L. E. (1993). Anxiety and self-disclosure: Toward a motivational model. *Journal of Personality and Social Psychology, 64*, 1000–1009.

Miller, G., (1974). The gynecological exam as a learning experience. *Journal of the American College Health Association, 23*, 163–164.

Miller, L. C., Barrett, C. L., & Hampe, E. (1974). Phobias in children in a prescientific era. In A. Davids (Ed.), *Child personality and psychotherapy: Current topics* (Vol. 1). New York: Wiley.

Miller, L. C., Barrett, C. L., Hampe, E., & Noble, H. (1972). Factor structure of childhood fears. *Journal of Consulting and Clinical Psychology*, *39*, 264–268.

Miller, R. S. (1986). Embarrassment: Causes and consequences. In W. H. Jones, J. M. Cheek, & S. R. Briggs (Eds.), *Shyness: Perspectives on research and treatment* (pp. 295–311). New York: Plenum Press.

Miller, R. S. (1987). Empathic embarrassment: Situational and personal determinants of reactions to the embarrassment of another. *Journal of Personality and Social Psychology*, *53*, 1061–1069.

Miller, R. S. (1992). The nature and severity of self-reported embarrassing circumstances. *Personality and Social Psychology Bulletin*, *18*, 190–198.

Miller, R. S. (in press-a). On the nature of embarrassability: Shyness, social skill, and social-evaluation. *Journal of Personality*.

Miller, R. S. (in press-b). *Understanding embarrassment: Poise and peril in social interaction*. New York: Guilford Press.

Miller, R. S., & Leary, M. R. (1992). Social sources and interactive functions of emotion: The case of embarrassment. In M. Clark (Ed.), *Emotion and social behavior* (pp. 202–221). Beverly Hills, CA: Sage.

Miller, R. S., & Tangney, J. P. (1995). Differentiating embarrassment and shame. *Journal of Social and Clinical Psychology*, *13*, 273–287.

Miller, W. R., & Arkowitz, H. (1977). Anxiety and perceived causation in social success and failure experiences: Disconfirmation of an attribution hypothesis in two experiments. *Journal of Abnormal Psychology*, *36*, 665–668.

Millstein, S. G., Adler, N. E., & Irwin, C. E. Jr. (1984). Sources of anxiety about pelvic examinations among adolescent females. *Journal of Adolescent Health Care*, *5*, 105–111.

Modigliani, A. (1966). *Embarrassment and social influence*. Unpublished doctoral dissertation, University of Michigan, Ann Arbor.

Modigliani, A. (1968). Embarrassment and embarrassability. *Sociometry*, *31*, 313–326.

Modigliani, A. (1971). Embarrassment, facework, and eye-contact: Testing a theory of embarrassment. *Journal of Personality and Social Psychology*, *17*, 15–24.

Montgomery, R. L., & Haemmerlie, F. M. (1982). Self-report and behavioral measures with heterosocially anxious subjects. *Psychological Reports*, *50*, 1219–1222.

Montgomery, R. L., & Haemmerlie, F. M. (1987). Self-perception theory and heterosocial anxiety. In J. E. Maddux, C. D. Stoltenberg, & R. Rosenwein (Eds.), *Social processes in clinical and counseling psychology* (pp. 139–153). New York: Springer-Verlag.

Monti, P. M. (1982, August). Multi-modal measurement of anxiety and social skills in a behavioral role-play test. In M. R. Leary (Chair), *Recent research in social anxiety*. Symposium presented at the annual meeting of the American Psychological Association, Washington, DC.

Moore, D., & Schultz, N. R. (1983). Loneliness at adolescence: Correlates, attributions, and coping. *Journal of Youth and Adolescence, 12,* 95–100.

Morris, C. G. (1982). *Assessment of shyness.* Unpublished manuscript, University of Michigan, Ann Arbor.

Murray, D. C. (1971). Talk, silence, and anxiety. *Psychological Bulletin, 75,* 244–260.

Natale, M., Entin, E., & Jaffe, J. (1979). Vocal interruptions in dyadic communication as a function of speech and social anxiety. *Journal of Personality and Social Psychology, 37,* 865–878.

Neiger, S., Atkinson, L., & Quarrington, B. (1981). A factor analysis of personality and fear variables in phobic disorders. *Canadian Journal of Behavioral Science, 13,* 336–348.

Nichols, K. A. (1974). Severe social anxiety. *British Journal of Medical Psychology, 74,* 301–306.

O'Banion, K., & Arkowitz, H. (1977). Social anxiety and selective memory for affective information about the self. *Social Behavior and Personality, 5,* 321–328.

O'Hare, T. M. (1990). Alcohol expectancies and social anxiety in male and female undergraduates. *Addictive Behaviors, 15,* 561–566.

Olson, J. M. (1988). Misattribution, preparatory information, and speech anxiety. *Journal of Personality and Social Psychology, 54,* 758–767.

Orlick, T. D., & Botterill, C. (1975). *Every kid can win.* Chicago: Nelson-Hall.

Öst, L. G., Jerremalm, A., & Johansson, J. (1981). Individual response patterns and the effects of different behavioral methods in the treatment of social phobia. *Behaviour Research and Therapy, 19,* 1–16.

Oxendine, J. B. (1970). Emotional arousal and motor performance. *Quest, 13,* 23–32.

Paivio, A., & Lambert, W. E. (1959). Measures and correlates of audience anxiety ("stagefright"). *Journal of Personality, 27,* 1–17.

Parrott, W. G., Sabini, J., & Silver, M. (1988). The roles of self-esteem and social interaction in embarrassment. *Personality and Social Psychology Bulletin, 14,* 191–202.

Parrott, W. G., & Smith, S. F. (1991). Embarrassment: Actual vs. typical cases, classical versus prototypical representations. *Cognition and Emotion, 5,* 467–488.

Paul, G. L. (1966). *Insight versus desensitization in psychotherapy.* Stanford: Stanford University Press.

Paul, G. L., & Shannon, D. T. (1966). Treatment of anxiety through systematic desensitization in therapy groups. *Journal of Abnormal Psychology, 71,* 124–135.

Pawluk, C. J. (1989). Social construction of teasing. *Journal for the Theory of Social Behaviour, 19,* 145–167.

Pearson, J. C. (1985). *Gender and communication.* Dubuque, IA: William C. Brown.

Pennebaker, J. W., Hendler, C. S., Durrett, M. E., & Richards, P. (1981).

Social factors influencing absenteeism due to illness in nursery school children. *Child Development, 52*, 692–700.

Peplau, L. A., & Perlman, D. (1979). Toward a social psychological theory of loneliness. In M. Cook & G. Wilson (Eds.), *Love and attraction*. New York: Pergamon Press.

Petronio, S. (1984). Communication strategies to reduce embarrassment: Differences between men and women. *Western Journal of Speech Communication, 48*, 28–38.

Phillips, G. M. (1968). Reticence: Pathology of the normal speaker. *Speech Monographs, 35*, 39–49.

Phillips, G. (1980). *Help for shy people*. Englewood Cliffs, NJ: Spectrum.

Phillips, K. A. (1991). Body dysmorphic disorder: The distress of imagined ugliness. *American Journal of Psychiatry, 148*, 1138–1149.

Pilkonis, P. A. (1977a). The behavioral consequences of shyness. *Journal of Personality, 45*, 596–611.

Pilkonis, P. A. (1977b). Shyness, public and private, and its relationship to other measures of social behavior. *Journal of Personality, 45*, 585–595.

Plomin, R., & Daniels, D. (1986). Genetics and shyness. In W. H. Jones, J. M. Cheek, & S. R. Briggs (Eds.), *Shyness: Perspectives on research and treatment* (pp. 63–80). New York: Plenum Press.

Plomin, R., & Rowe, D. C. (1979). Genetic and environmental etiology of social behavior in infancy. *Developmental Psychology, 15*, 62–72.

Plutchik, R. (1980). *Emotion: A psychoevolutionary synthesis*. New York: Harper & Row.

Pollard, C. A., & Henderson, J. G. (1988). Four types of social phobia in a community sample. *Journal of Nervous and Mental Disease, 176*, 440–445.

Porter, D. T. (1979). Communication apprehension: Communication's last artifact? In D. Nimmo (Ed.), *Communication yearbook 3* (pp. 241–259). New Brunswick, NJ: Transaction Books.

Porter, H. (1939). Studies in the psychology of stuttering: XIV. Stuttering phenomena in relation to size and personnel of audience. *Journal of Speech Disorders, 4*, 323–333.

Powell, B. (1979). *Overcoming shyness: Practical scripts for everyday encounters*. New York: McGraw-Hill.

Pozo, C., Carver, C. S., Wellens, A. R., & Scheier, M. F. (1991). Social anxiety and social perception: Construing others' reactions to the self. *Personality and Social Psychology Bulletin, 17*, 355–362.

Puigcerver, A., Martinez-Selva, J. M., Garcia-Sanchez, F. A., & Gomez-Amor, J. (1989). Individual differences in psychophysiological and subjective correlates of speech anxiety. *Journal of Psychophysiology, 3*, 75–81.

Rapee, R. M., Sanderson, W. C., & Barlow, D. H. (1988). Social phobia features across the DSM-III-R anxiety disorders. *Journal of Psychopathology and Behavioral Assessment, 10*, 287–299.

Rapp, S., & Leary, M. R. (1994). *Psoriasis and social evaluation.* Unpublished data, Wake Forest University.

Rehm, L. P., & Marston, A. R. (1968). Reduction of social anxiety through modification of self-reinforcement. *Journal of Consulting and Clinical Psychology, 32,* 565–574.

Reis, H. T., Nezlek, J., & Wheeler, L. (1980). Physical attractiveness in social interaction. *Journal of Personality and Social Psychology, 38,* 604–617.

Reis, H. T., Wheeler, L., Spiegel, N., Kernis, M., Nezlek, J., & Perri, M. (1982). Physical attractiveness in social interaction: II. Why does appearance affect social experience? *Journal of Personality and Social Psychology, 43,* 979–996.

Reisenzein, R. (1983). The Schachter theory of emotion: Two decades later. *Psychological Bulletin, 94,* 239–264.

Reznick, J. S. (Ed.) (1989). *Perspectives on behavioral inhibition.* Chicago: University of Chicago Press.

Reznick, J. S., Gibbons, J. L., Johnson, M. O., & McDonough, P. M. (1989). Behavioral inhibition in a normative sample. In J. S. Reznick (Ed.), *Perspectives on behavioral inhibition* (pp. 25–50). Chicago: University of Chicago Press.

Richins, M. L. (1980). Consumer perceptions of costs and benefits associated with complaining. In H. K. Hunt & R. L. Day (Eds.), *Refining concepts and measures of consumer satisfaction and complaining behavior* (pp. 50–53). Bloomington: Indiana University.

Robins, C. J. (1986). Sex-role perceptions and social anxiety in opposite-sex and same-sex situations. *Sex Roles, 14,* 383–395.

Robins, L. N., Helzer, J. E., Weissman, M. M., Orvaschel, H., Gruenberg, E., Burke, J. D. Jr., & Regier, D. A. (1984). Lifetime prevalence of specific psychiatric disorders in three sites. *Archives of General Psychiatry, 41,* 949–958.

Rodin, J., Silberstein, L., & Striegel-Moore, R. (1985). Women and weight: A normative discontent. *Nebraska Symposium on Motivation, 32,* 267–307.

Rosenberg, A., & Kagan, J. (1987). Iris pigmentation and behavioral inhibition. *Developmental Psychobiology, 20,* 377–392.

Rothenberg, A. (1988). Differential diagnosis of anorexia nervosa and depressive illness: A review of 11 studies. *Comprehensive Psychiatry, 29,* 427–432.

Royce, W. S., & Arkowitz, H. (1978). Multimodal evaluation of practice interactions as treatment for social isolation. *Journal of Consulting and Clinical Psychology, 46,* 239–245.

Rubin, K. H., & Both, L. (1989). Iris pigmentation and sociability in childhood: A re-examination. *Developmental Psychobiology, 22,* 717–725.

Russell, D., Cutrona, C. E., & Jones, W. H. (1986). A trait-situational analysis of shyness. In W. H. Jones, J. M. Cheek, & S. R. Briggs (Eds.),

Shyness: Perspectives on research and treatment (pp. 239–249). New York: Plenum Press.

Russell, J. A. (1980). A circumplex model of affect. *Journal of Personality and Social Psychology, 39,* 1161–1178.

Sanderson, W. C., Rapee, R. M., & Barlow, D. H. (1987, November). *The DSM-III-R revised anxiety disorder categories: Descriptions and patterns of comorbidity.* Paper presented at the annual meeting of the Association for Advancement of Behavior Therapy, Boston.

Sansom, C. D., MacInerey, J., Oliver, V., & Wakefield, J. (1975). Differential response recall in a cervical screening program. *British Journal of Preventive and Social Medicine, 29,* 40–47.

Sarason, I. G. (1975). Anxiety and self-preoccupation. In I. G. Sarason & C. Spielberger (Eds.), *Stress and anxiety* (pp. 27–44). New York: Wiley.

Sarason, I. G. (Ed.). (1980). *Test anxiety: Theory, research, and applications.* Hillsdale, NJ: Erlbaum.

Sarason, I. G., & Sarason, B. R. (1986). Anxiety and interfering thoughts: Their effect on social interaction. In W. H. Jones, J. M. Cheek, & S. R. Briggs (Eds.), *Shyness: Perspectives on research and treatment* (pp. 253–264). New York: Plenum Press.

Sarason, I. G., & Sarason, B. R. (1990). Test anxiety. In H. Leitenberg (Ed.), *Handbook of social and evaluation anxiety* (pp. 475–495). New York: Plenum Press.

Sattler, J. M. A. (1965). A theoretical, developmental, and clinical investigation of embarrassment. *Genetic Psychology Monographs, 71,* 19–59.

Scanlan, T. K., & Lewthwaite, R. (1986). Social psychological aspects of competition for male youth sport participants: IV. Predictors of enjoyment. *Journal of Sport Psychology, 8,* 25–35.

Scanlan, T. K., & Passer, M. W. (1978). Factors related to competitive stress among male youth sports participants. *Medicine and Science in Sports, 10,* 103–108.

Scanlan, T. K., & Passer, M. W. (1979). Sources of competitive stress in young female athletes. *Journal of Sport Psychology, 1,* 151–159.

Scarr, S., & Salapatek, P. (1970). Patterns of fear development during infancy. *Merrill-Palmer Quarterly, 16,* 53–90.

Schachter, S. (1959). *The psychology of affiliation.* Stanford: Stanford University Press.

Schachter, S., & Singer, J. E. (1962). Cognitive, social, and physiological determinants of emotional state. *Psychological Review, 69,* 379–399.

Scheier, M. F., & Carver, C. S. (1985). The Self-Consciousness Scale: A revised version for use with general populations. *Journal of Applied Social Psychology, 15,* 687–699.

Schlenker, B. R. (1980). *Impression management: The self-concept, social identity, and interpersonal relations.* Monterey, CA: Brooks/Cole.

Schlenker, B. R., & Darby, B. W. (1981). The use of apologies in social predicaments. *Social Psychology Quarterly, 44,* 271–278.

Schlenker, B. R., & Leary, M. R. (1982). Social anxiety and self-presentation: A conceptualization and model. *Psychological Bulletin, 92,* 641–669.

Schlenker, B. R., & Leary, M. R. (1985). Social anxiety and communication about the self. *Journal of Language and Social Psychology, 45,* 1347–1354.

Schneider, D. (1969). Tactical self-presentation after success and failure. *Journal of Personality and Social Psychology, 13,* 262–268.

Schneider, W., & Shiffrin, R. M. (1977). Controlled and automatic human information processing: I. Detection, search, and attention. *Psychological Review, 84,* 1–66.

Schneier, F. R. (1991). Social phobia. *Psychiatric Annals, 21,* 349–353.

Schneier, F. R., Martin, L. Y., Liebowitz, M. R., Gorman, J. M., & Fyer, A. J. (1989). Alcohol abuse in social phobia. *Journal of Anxiety Disorders, 3,* 15–23.

Scholing, A., & Emmelkamp, P. M. G. (1990). Social phobia: Nature and treatment. In H. Leitenberg (Ed.), *Handbook of social and evaluation anxiety* (pp. 269–324). New York: Plenum Press.

Schwartz, M. F. (1976). *Stuttering solved.* Philadelphia: Lippincott.

Scott, M. B., & Lyman, S. M. (1968). Accounts. *American Sociological Review, 33,* 46–62.

Semin, G. R., & Manstead, A. S. R. (1982). The social implications of embarrassment displays and restitution behavior. *European Journal of Social Psychology, 12,* 367–377.

Sharkey, W. F. (1991). Intentional embarrassment: Goals, tactics, and consequences. In W. R. Cupach & S. Metts (Eds.), *Advances in interpersonal communication research* (pp. 105–128). Normal, IL: Personal Relationships Research Group.

Sharkey, W. F. (1993). Who embarrasses whom? Relational and sex differences in the use of intentional embarrassment. In P. J. Kalbfleisch (Ed.), *Interpersonal communication: Evolving interpersonal relationships* (pp. 147–168). Hillsdale, NJ: Erlbaum.

Sharkey, W. F. (1992). The use of and responses to intentional embarrassment. *Communication Studies, 43,* 257–275.

Sharkey, W. F., & Stafford, L. (1990). Responses to embarrassment. *Human Communication Research, 17,* 315–342.

Sharkey, W. F., & Waldron, V. (1990, November). *The intentional embarrassment of subordinates in the work place.* Paper presented at the meeting of the Speech Communication Association, Chicago.

Sheehan, J., Hadley, R., & Gould, E. (1967). Impact of authority on stuttering. *Journal of Abnormal Psychology, 72,* 290–293.

Shepperd, J. A., & Arkin, R. M. (1990). Shyness and self-presentation. In W. R. Crozier (Ed.), *Shyness and embarrassment: Perspectives from social psychology* (pp. 286–314). Cambridge: Cambridge University Press.

Siegel, G. M., & Haugen, D. (1964). Audience size and variations in stuttering behavior. *Journal of Speech and Hearing Research, 7,* 381–388.

Silver, M., Sabini, J., & Parrott, W. G. (1987). Embarrassment: A dramaturgic approach. *Journal for the Theory of Social Behaviour, 17*, 47–61.

Simmons, R., Rosenberg, R., & Rosenberg, M. (1973). Disturbance in the self-image at adolescence. *American Sociological Review, 38*, 553–568.

Singelis, T. M., & Sharkey, W. F. (in press). Culture, self-construal, and embarrassability. *Journal of Cross-Cultural Psychology.*

Smail, P., Stockwell, T., Canter, S., & Hodgson, R. (1984). Alcohol dependence and phobic anxiety states: I. A prevalance study. *British Journal of Psychiatry, 144*, 53–57.

Smith, C. A. (1991). The self, appraisal, and coping. In C. R. Snyder & D. R. Forsyth (Eds.), *Handbook of social and clinical psychology* (pp. 116–137). New York: Pergamon Press.

Smith, E. N., Allison, R. D., & Crowder, W. E. (1974). Bradycardia in a free ranging American alligator. *Capeia, 3*, 770–772.

Smith, E. N., & Tobey, E. W. (1983). Heart rate response to forced and voluntary diving in swamp rabbits. *Physiological Zoology, 56*, 632–638.

Smith, R. E., & Sarason, I. G. (1975). Social anxiety and the evaluation of negative interpersonal feedback. *Journal of Consulting and Clinical Psychology, 43*, 429.

Smith, R. E., & Smoll, F. L. (1990). Sport performance anxiety. In H. Leitenberg (Ed.), *Handbook of social and evaluation anxiety* (pp. 417–454). New York: Plenum Press.

Smith, R. E., Smoll, F. L., & Curtis, B. (1978). Coach effectiveness training: A cognitive-behavioral approach to enhancing relationship skills in youth sport coaches. *Journal of Sport Psychology, 1*, 59–75.

Smith, R. E., Smoll, F. L., & Schutz, R. W. (1990). Reactions to competition: Measurement and correlates of sport-specific cognitive and somatic trait anxiety: The Sport Anxiety Scale. *Anxiety Research, 2*, 263–280.

Snell, W. E., Jr. (1989). Willingness to self-disclose to female and male friends as a function of social anxiety and gender. *Personality and Social Psychology Bulletin, 15*, 113–125.

Snyder, C. R., & Forsyth, D. R. (Eds.) (1991). *Handbook of social and clinical psychology.* New York: Pergamon Press.

Snyder, C. R., & Smith, T. W. (1986). On being "shy like a fox:" A self-handicapping analysis. In W. H. Jones, J. M. Cheek, & S. R. Briggs (Eds.), *Shyness: Perspectives on research and treatment* (pp. 161–172). New York: Plenum Press.

Snyder, M. L., Kleck, R. E., Strenta, A., & Mentzer, S. J. (1979). Avoidance of the handicapped: An attributional ambiguity analysis. *Journal of Personality and Social Psychology, 37*, 2297–2306.

Spivey, E. (1990). *Social exclusion as a common factor in social anxiety, loneliness, jealousy, and social depression: Testing an integrative model.* Unpublished Master's thesis, Wake Forest University.

Steele, C. M., & Josephs, R. A. (1990). Alcohol myopia: Its prized and dangerous effects. *American Psychologist, 45*, 921–933.

Strahan, R. (1974). Situational dimensions of self-reported nervousness. *Journal of Personality Assessment, 38,* 341–352.

Strickland, B. (1977). Achievement motivation. In T. Blass (Ed.), *Personality variables and social behavior* (pp. 315–356). Hillsdale, NJ: Erlbaum.

Striegel-Moore, R. H., Silberstein, L. R., & Rodin, J. (1993). The social self in bulimia nervosa: Public self-consciousness, social anxiety, and perceived fraudulence. *Journal of Abnormal Psychology, 102,* 297–303.

Strom, J. C., & Buck, R. W. (1979). Staring and participants' sex: Physiological and subjective reactions. *Personality and Social Psychology Bulletin, 5,* 114–117.

Stroufe, L. A. (1977). Wariness of strangers and the study of infant development. *Child Development, 48,* 731–746.

Sullivan, H. S. (1947). *Conceptions of modern psychiatry.* Washington, DC: William Alanson White Psychiatric Foundation.

Sutton-Simon, K., & Goldfried, M. R. (1979). Faulty thinking patterns in two kinds of anxiety. *Cognitive Therapy and Research, 3,* 193–203.

Sweeney, G. A., & Horan, J. J. (1982). Separate and combined effects of cue-controlled relaxation and cognitive restructuring in the treatment of musical performance anxiety. *Journal of Counseling Psychology, 29,* 486–497.

Takahashi, T. (1989). Social phobia syndrome in Japan. *Comprehensive Psychiatry, 30,* 45–52.

Tedeschi, J. T. (1981). *Impression management theory and social psychological research.* New York: Academic Press.

Tedeschi, J. T., & Riess, M. (1981). Predicaments and verbal tactics of impression management. In C. Antaki (Ed.), *Ordinary language explanations of social behaviour.* London: Academic Press.

Tennen, H., & Affleck, G. (1991). Paradox-based treatments. In C. R. Snyder & D. R. Forsyth (Eds.), *Handbook of social and clinical psychology* (pp. 624–643). New York: Pergamon Press.

Thompson, R. A., & Limber, S. P. (1990). "Social anxiety" in infancy: Stranger and separation reactions. In H. Leitenberg (Ed.), *Handbook of social and evaluation anxiety* (pp. 85–137). New York: Plenum Press.

Timms, M. W. H. (1980). Treatment of chronic blushing through paradoxical intention. *Behavioral Psychotherapy, 8,* 59–61.

Torgerson, S. (1983). Genetic factors in anxiety disorders. *Archives of General Psychiatry, 40,* 1085–1089.

Trentham, S., Searcy, S., Jeffcoat, M., Watters, D., & Carpenter, S. (1992). *A comparison of social skills and negative cognitions between shy and non-shy individuals.* Paper presented at the annual meeting of the Southeastern Psychological Association, Knoxville, TN.

Triandis, H. C. (1989). The self and social behavior in differing cultural contexts. *Psychological Review, 96,* 506–520.

Trower, P., & Gilbert, P. (1989). New theoretical conceptions of social anxiety and social phobia. *Clinical Psychology Review, 9,* 19–35.

Trower, P., Gilbert, P., & Sherling, G. (1990). Social anxiety, evolution, and self-presentation. In H. Leitenberg (Ed.), *Handbook of social and evaluation anxiety* (pp. 11–45). New York: Plenum Press.

Trower, P., Yardley, K., Bryant, B., & Shaw, P. (1978). The treatment of social failure: A comparison of anxiety-reduction and skills acquisition procedures on two social problems. *Behavior Modification, 2*, 41–60.

Tunnadine, P. (1980). The role of genital examination in psychosocial medicine. *Clinics in Obstetrics and Gynecology, 7*, 283–291.

Turner, J. C. (1984). Social identification and psychological group formation. In H. Tajfel (Ed.), *The social dimension* (Vol. 2, pp. 518–540). New York: Cambridge University Press.

Turner, R. G. (1977). Self-consciousness and anticipatory belief change. *Personality and Social Psychology Bulletin, 3*, 438–441.

Turner, S. M., & Beidel, D. C. (1989). Social phobia: Clinical syndrome, diagnosis, and comorbidity. *Clinical Psychology Review, 9*, 3–18.

Turner, S. M., Beidel, D. C., Dancu, C. V., & Keys, D. J. (1986). Psychopathology of social phobia and comparison to avoidant personality disorder. *Journal of Abnormal Psychology, 95*, 389–394.

Turner, S. M., Beidel, D. C., Dancu, C. V., & Stanley, M. A. (1989). An empirically derived inventory to measure social fears and anxiety: The Social Phobia and Anxiety Inventory. *Psychological Assessment, 1*, 35–40.

Turner, S. M., Beidel, D. C., & Townsley, R. M. (1990). Social phobia: Relationship to shyness. *Behaviour Research and Therapy, 28*, 497–505.

Twentyman, C. T., & McFall, R. M. (1975). Behavioral training of social skills in shy males. *Journal of Consulting and Clinical Psychology, 43*, 384–395.

Van Hooff, J. (1972). A comparative approach to the phylogeny of laughter and smiling. In R. A. Hinde (Ed.), *Non-verbal communication* (pp. 209–241). Cambridge: Cambridge University Press.

Van Riper, C. G. (1971). *Speech correction: Principles and methods*. Englewood Cliffs, NJ: Prentice-Hall.

Vestre, N. D., & Judge, T. J. (1989). Evaluation of self-administered rational emotive therapy programs for interpersonal anxiety. *Journal of Rational-Emotive and Cognitive-Behavior Therapy, 7*, 141–154.

Videbeck, R. (1960). Self-conceptions and the reactions of others. *Sociometry, 23*, 351–359.

Wagaman, J. R., Miltenberger, R. G., & Arndorfer, R. E. (1993). Analysis of a simplified treatment for stuttering in children. *Journal of Applied Behavior Analysis, 26*, 53–61.

Wainapel, S. F. (1989). Attitudes of visually impaired toward cane use. *Journal of Visual Impairment and Blindness, 83*, 446–448.

Walster, E. (1965). The effect of self-esteem on romantic liking. *Journal of Personality and Social Psychology, 1*, 184–197.

Watson, D., & Friend, R. (1969). Measurement of social-evaluative anxiety. *Journal of Consulting and Clinical Psychology, 33*, 448–457.

Watson, D., & Tellegen, A. (1985). Toward a consensual structure of mood. *Psychological Bulletin, 98*, 219–235.

Weary, G., & Mirels, H. L. (1982). *Integrations of clinical and social psychology.* New York: Oxford University Press.

Wegner, D. M., & Giuliano, T. (1980). Arousal-induced attention to self. *Journal of Personality and Social Psychology, 38*, 719–726.

Wegner, D. M., & Giuliano, T. (1983). On sending artifact in search of artifact: Reply to McDonald, Harris, and Maher. *Journal of Personality and Social Psychology, 44*, 290–293.

Weinberg, M. S. (1968). Embarrassment: Its variable and invariable aspects. *Social Forces, 46*, 382–388.

Weinberg, R. S., & Genuch, M. (1980). Relationship between competitive trait anxiety, state anxiety, and golf performance: A field study. *Journal of Sport Psychology, 2*, 155–160.

Weiner, B. (1989). *Human motivation.* Hillsdale, NJ: Erlbaum.

Weinstein, C. E., Cubberly, W. E., & Richardson, F. C. (1982). The effects of test anxiety on learning at superficial and deep levels of processing. *Contemporary Educational Psychology, 7*, 107–112.

Weinstein, H. M., & Richman, A. (1984). The group treatment of bulimia. *Journal of American College Health, 32*, 208–215.

Wheeless, V. E. (1984). Communication apprehension and trust as predictors of willingness to discuss gynecological health topics. *Communication Research Reports, 1*, 117–121.

Willerman, L. (1979). *The psychology of individual and group differences.* San Francisco: Freeman.

Williams, J. G., Park, L. I., & Cline, J. (1992). Reducing distress associated with pelvic examinations: A stimulus control intervention. *Women and Health, 18*, 41–53.

Wine, J. D. (1971). Test anxiety and direction of attention. *Psychological Bulletin, 76*, 92–104.

Wine, J. (1980). Cognitive-attentional theory of test anxiety. In I. Sarason (Ed.), *Test anxiety: Theory, research, and application* (pp. 349–385). Hillsdale, NJ: Erlbaum.

Wlazlo, Z., Schroeder-Hartwig, K., Hand, I., Kaiser, G., & Munchau, N. (1990). Exposure *in vivo* vs social skills training for social phobia: Long-term outcome and differential effects. *Behaviour Research and Therapy, 28*, 181–193.

Wolpe, J. (1958). *Psychotherapy by reciprocal inhibition.* Stanford: Stanford University Press.

Yoritomo-Tashi (1915). *Timidity: How to overcome it.* New York: Funk & Wagnalls.

Zimbardo, P. G. (1977). *Shyness: What it is and what to do about it.* New York: Jove.

Zimbardo, P. G. (1980, August). *Cognitive and cultural contributions to shyness and loneliness*. Paper presented at the annual meeting of the American Psychological Association, Montreal.

Zimbardo, P. G. (1981). *The shy child*. New York: McGraw-Hill.

Index

Except a man be born
of water and of
spirit, he cannot enter
into the kingdom of God.
(John 3:5)

BORN
of the
SPIRIT

BORN of the SPIRIT

E. Richard Packham

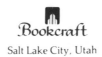

Bookcraft

Salt Lake City, Utah

Library of Congress Catalog Card Number: 79-83680
ISBN 0-88494-361-5

First Printing, 1979

Lithographed in the United States of America
PUBLISHERS PRESS
Salt Lake City, Utah

To those with whom I have shared
the greatest happiness —
my wife and children

Contents

Preface

While I was teaching early morning seminary several years ago, a young lady attended my class every morning for two years. She had an excellent grasp of the principles and doctrines of the Church, could answer almost every question I asked, and received straight A's on all the tests I gave. But in spite of her intellectual knowledge she had great difficulty in applying to her daily life the principles she seemed to understand. Eventually she became inactive in the Church and got caught up in the ways of the world.

Clearly a knowledge of the gospel is not in itself adequate to change the lives of those who embrace it. That requires a spiritual commitment, and it involves the birth of the Spirit. That birth is one of the most tremendous and significant experiences that can come to a mortal being, and indeed is a requirement for exaltation in the kingdom of heaven. Yet one may well ask whether that need is well understood, and whether the transcendent change of heart that the experience involves is sought after as it should be. There are those, for example, who apparently think that the confirmation ordinance in the Church is synonymous with the birth of the Spirit.

Prophets both ancient and modern have made clear the meaning and significance of this birth and the way to obtain it. The deep impression their discussion of this subject has made upon my mind and heart has impelled me to write this book. Its purpose is not to present any new and deep concepts (I have neither the ability nor the desire to do this) but to bring together in one moderately sized volume, as far as words can do this, the essential doctrines and concepts surrounding and supporting this profound spiritual experience and the God-ordained means by which each of us can obtain it.

In doing this I have earnestly sought to be in harmony with the scriptures, the teachings of the Brethren, and the Spirit of the Lord. It is my hope that, given that basis, this book will make a meaningful contribution to the lives of those who read it.

Acknowledgments

I take full responsibility for what is contained in this book. However, there are many to whom I owe much. Without their help and encouragement, this work would still be distributed throughout my files.

Elder Boyd K. Packer's personal counsel to me provided me with the time to organize and write the accumulated thoughts of many years. President Earl Leroy Gunnell contributed significantly in his organizational and editorial help. Joyful hours of discussion with George W. Pace about the doctrine of Christ helped solidify random feelings into hard conclusions. I appreciate the professional typing and final editing of Sister Carolyn Taylor, who prepared the manuscript for the publisher. Finally, without the constant encouragement of my loving wife, Beverly, and her unselfish dedication in typing the rough draft, I would have given up long ago. A most grateful thanks to all.

1
What It Means to Know

In order that the subsequent chapters may be understood with clarity, some definitions are necessary. Let's start with *testimony*. We have frequently heard the statement: "I know that the gospel is true." What does this mean? Why is knowing important? And who can know?

Most of us have heard young children stand and say: "I know the Church is true. I'm thankful for my Mommy and Daddy. I'm thankful for my friends and for my bishop...." Is this a testimony?

Certainly small children have strong feelings in their hearts. But contrast their innocent expression with the words of President David O. McKay, who once said, in effect: "I know that Jesus is the Christ, the Son of the living God. I know with the knowledge of Thomas that He lives...."

Is this a testimony?

Both of the above declarations are testimonies. But are they the same? Certainly not. I think the conclusion is inevitable that there are different kinds or degrees of testimony.

I'm not sure that one can precisely define and exactly categorize this sacred experience of knowing truth. But perhaps we can define some guidelines.

Testimony of Intellect

Because the basic principles and doctrines of the Church are true, they carry an inherent verity within themselves. In fact, the very existence of the church of Jesus Christ is an evidence of truth: it was literally restored by the power of God. The intellectual evidences surrounding the principles, doctrines, and organization are such that a rational intellect is compelled to believe. A person can evaluate the evidences, whether they be scriptural, historical, archaeological, or philosophical, and reach the intellectual conclusion that The Church of Jesus Christ of Latter-day Saints is of divine origin. The entrance of many adult converts into the Church is based upon this intellectual conviction.

Is such a condition a testimony? Yes, an intellectual testimony. Can such a person say, "I know the Church is true"? Yes, just as he can say: "I know that the law of gravity is true. My observations and the observations of others in whom I have confidence show it to be true."

But an intellectual testimony often carries with it a basic weakness: Many people come to an intellectual testimony of the restored Church without ever acting on that knowledge. Their commitment is not such that they will sacrifice for the work of the kingdom.

Perhaps the greatest benefit of this intellectual assent is that it can stimulate one to seek and obtain higher levels of knowledge.

Testimony of Faith

It may seem strange to designate faith as a type of testimony. We generally do not think of it as such. Yet, is not faith a conviction of the heart? As Paul defined, "Faith is the substance of things hoped for, *the evidence of things not seen.*" (Hebrews 11:1; italics added.)

He also states that faith is a gift of God: "For by grace are ye saved through faith; and that not of yourselves: it is the gift of God: Not of works, lest any man should boast." (Ephesians 2:8-9.)

This gift often begins as a barely discernible feeling in the heart. Each individual can nourish and cultivate the particle of faith, or he can reject and kill it. In his great discourse on faith, Alma helps us understand how faith can grow. Faith, he says, is not a perfect knowledge at first. But we can help our faith develop, as he says, "if ye will awake and arouse your faculties, even to an experiment upon my words, and exercise a particle of faith, yea, even if ye can no more than desire to believe, let this desire work in you, even until ye believe in a manner that ye can give place for a portion of my words." (Alma 32:27.)

Then, to help us understand the principle further, Alma compares the words of God to a seed that we plant in our hearts:

> Now, . . . if it be a true seed, or a good seed, if ye do not cast it out by your unbelief, that ye will resist the Spirit of the Lord, behold, it will begin to swell within your breasts; and when you feel these swelling motions, ye will begin to say within yourselves — It must needs be that this is a good seed, or that the word is good, for it beginneth to enlarge my soul; yea, it beginneth to enlighten my understanding, yea, it beginneth to be delicious to me. (Alma 32:28.)

Can you see how faith increases as a person follows Alma's experiment? As Alma goes on to explain, the person doesn't yet have a perfect knowledge — but he knows the seed is good, and he continues to let it grow within him.

Then a marvelous thing happens: the seed begins to bear fruit, "for every seed bringeth forth unto its own likeness." (Alma 32:31.)

At that point the experiment is over. You planted the seed; you let it grow; it bore fruit; and you know without a doubt that the seed is good.

> And now, behold, is your knowledge perfect? Yea, your knowledge is perfect in that thing, and your faith is dormant; and this because ye know, for ye know that the word hath swelled your souls, and ye also know that it hath sprouted up, that your understanding doth begin to be enlightened, and your mind doth begin to expand. (Alma 32:34.)

Nourished faith leads to perfect faith, and, as Alma concluded, perfect faith is indeed knowledge.

We cannot point to the day or the hour that faith comes or begins to be discernible. But if we compare various periods of our life, we can perceive significant changes in the degree of our faith.

Does faith have an impact on our lives and our willingness to sacrifice? Yes, it does — without question. Faith is one of the most powerful and dynamic forces on the earth. Faith can and does change lives.

I had an experience at age ten that illustrates the strength of this type of testimony. It was a hot summer afternoon, and my mother and

I were sitting out on the front lawn in the shade when a neighbor lady came over to visit. During the conversation our neighbor said, "Sometimes I just wonder if the Church is true." I vividly remember the powerful reaction that went through me on hearing that remark. (Fortunately, for the condition of my backside, I didn't vocalize my thoughts, but I still remember them.) I thought: "How can you be so dumb as to make a statement like that. *Of course the Church is true!*" I had attended Primary and Junior Sunday School, but I hadn't read the Book of Mormon or any of the scriptures. In fact, I don't remember even considering before whether or not the Church was true. But even at that early age I apparently had a testimony of faith.

Witness of the Spirit

The growth of the testimony of faith is generally a long and gradual process. Before a person has that testimony he can benefit from a form of testimony that I call the witness of the Spirit.

Moroni's promise, so frequently quoted by missionaries, illustrates how this type of testimony can come:

> And when ye shall receive these things, I would exhort you that ye would ask God, the Eternal Father, in the name of Christ, if these things are not true; and if ye shall ask with a sincere heart, with real intent, having faith in Christ, he will manifest the truth of it unto you, by the power of the Holy Ghost.
>
> And by the power of the Holy Ghost ye may know the truth of all things. (Moroni 10:4-5.)

Moroni promises that, on certain conditions, the Holy Ghost will give one a witness of the truthfulness of the Book of Mormon. It will be a witness so real and spiritually tangible that it will leave the seeker without doubt.

An experience printed in the Great Lakes Mission newsletter, *The Messenger*, in the 1960s, illustrates the witness of the Spirit. Elder Stephen Thompson related the experience as follows:

> About four years ago a member friend and I were talking with a close friend who had just had all six discussions without a baptism result. While we were talking, the [gospel] soon became the topic of our conversation. . . . He said he knew it was true logically and intellectually, but said he just didn't . . . know within his own heart it was true.

His sense of reason said yes, but his heart said no. When questioned about prayer he admitted he had not yet prayed personally. He prayed in the discussions and it was assumed by my companion and me as well as the missionaries that he had prayed personally. We told him what we could about prayer and its importance and gave him the challenge to pray.

Well, the conversation and evening ended with that thought and we went our ways. Late that night, he and my friend and his brother came to my home and told me of a most choice experience. He had gone home and prayed very earnestly for the warm feeling he needed to be baptized. He prayed for about fifteen minutes unsuccessfully. He soon felt an air of discouragement and a bit of disappointment. But the thought of now knowing enabled him to continue on in humble prayer. He was determined to get an answer if it took him all night. He continued on for the next two hours, praying with all the seriousness he could muster. After praying on into the third hour, he was not concerned about the length of prayer and the thought of how tired he was. Thoughts of physical things left his mind. (Was the door locked, and the alarm set, etc.?) He became solely concerned with an answer to his prayers. It was at that instant that his prayers were answered. Not a bolt of lightning, not even a voice, but a personal visitation of the Holy Ghost, a feeling he had he could not describe with words, a feeling that bore witness to the divine calling of the Prophet Joseph Smith. He could not sleep, but was wide awake as it was pushing 2:00 A.M. He felt he had to tell someone about his wonderful experience; that was why he was at my home with my member friend and his younger brother. He was baptized that Saturday night. . . .

This experience is typically what we refer to as a testimony. We can usually point to the day and hour when such a witness comes to us. This gift is available to both members and nonmembers of the Church who desire to

— put Moroni's promise to the test
— know of the divinity of Jesus Christ
— know that Joseph Smith was indeed a prophet
— know the validity of a principle of the gospel
— know of the divine call of existing leaders of the Church, local or general.

It's obvious from the experience just related that a price must be paid before such a sacred gift can be given. Hardened hearts must be softened by fasting and prayer. Obedience to known principles is required. Desire and commitment are the keys. Remember, the Lord desires that his children have every gift he has available to give them. If we haven't received a particular gift we desire, it is because we have yet to pay the complete price.

It may seem strange to some to have to pay a price for a gift. Perhaps I could explain it this way: Suppose you wish to buy an item that costs $100. But all you have is $1. The owner, though, is a generous man. "If you'll give me the $1, to show you really want the item, then I'll give it to you," he says. In effect, you received it as a gift, even though you had to pay a price for it. The difference between your resources and the value of the item is the gift. In the case of a gift of God, this difference is one aspect of the *grace of Christ*.

Like faith, a witness of the Spirit can have great impact in our lives. The preparation of our hearts to be worthy of receiving the witness of the Spirit and the very process of receiving it build commitment and determination toward greater service and sacrifice.

Born of the Spirit

Subsequent chapters will go into greater depth on the birth of the Spirit, so only a brief distinction will be made here. Suffice it to say that receiving the witness of the Spirit does not satisfy the requirement given by Jesus to Nicodemus: "Except a man be born of water and of the spirit, he cannot enter into the kingdom of God." (John 3:5.)

While the purpose of the *witness* of the Spirit is to testify of truth, the function of the *birth* of the Spirit is to create a "mighty change" in our hearts: to purge out the carnality and worldliness in man's nature, to bear witness that a forgiveness of sins has been achieved, to create a new creature of the Holy Ghost — "submissive, meek, humble, patient, full of love, willing to submit to all things which the Lord seeth fit to inflict upon him, even as a child doth submit to his father" (Mosiah 3:19) — in other words, to sanctify the soul of man.

With such a process we literally become part of the household of Christ, his sons and his daughters. President Marion G. Romney states:

> It would appear that membership in the Church and conversion are not necessarily synonymous. Being converted, as we are here using the term, and having a testimony are

not necessarily the same thing either. A testimony comes when the Holy Ghost gives the earnest seeker a witness of the truth. A moving testimony vitalizes faith; that is, it induces repentance and obedience to commandments. Conversion, on the other hand, is the fruit of, or the reward for, repentance and obedience. (*Improvement Era,* Dec. 1963, p. 1066.)

Thus we see the difference between a witness of the Spirit (testimony) and the birth of the Spirit (conversion).

Calling and Election Made Sure

Perhaps the highest level of testimony, if it can be called testimony, is the knowledge by revelation and ordinance that one is sealed up to eternal life. Joseph Smith frequently challenged the Saints to make their calling and election sure. (See *Teachings of the Prophet Joseph Smith,* Salt Lake City: Deseret Book Co., 1972, pp. 298-99, 305.)

One of the greatest messages of a living prophet to the world is that he indeed saw God the Eternal Father and his Son, Jesus Christ. As significant as Joseph's message was, perhaps just as significant is his message to members of the Church that they can know the Savior as he knew Him.

An authoritative discussion on calling and election, the Second Comforter, the more sure word of prophecy, and being sealed by the Holy Spirit of Promise is given in Elder Bruce R. McConkie's *Doctrinal New Testament Commentary*, 3:323-53. (Salt Lake City: Bookcraft, 1973.)

It is clear, then, that not all testimonies or levels of knowledge are the same. A great blessing to members of the Church is that there is always something more to strive for. With such strivings, we grow much closer to our standard of the Christlike life.

2   *Born of Fire*

The scriptures make frequent reference to being born of God, being born of the Spirit, even being baptized with fire and with the Holy Ghost. Just what is that rebirth, and how is it brought about?

Sacrifice and the Birth of the Spirit

King Benjamin taught that the nature of mortal man was alien to God's nature. He also defined, in the same verse, the desired status of a saint: "submissive, meek, humble, patient, full of love, willing to submit to all things which the Lord seeth fit to inflict upon him." (Mosiah 3:19.) A true saint is willing to be completely submissive to God.

Joseph Smith gives a similar definition:

> Let us here observe, that a religion that does not re-quire the sacrifice of all things never has power sufficient to produce the faith necessary unto life and salvation; for, from the first existence of man, the faith necessary unto the enjoyment of life and salvation never could be obtained without the sacrifice of all earthly things. . . .
>
> It is in vain for persons to fancy to themselves that they are heirs with those, or can be heirs with them, who have offered their all in sacrifice, . . . unless they, in like manner,

offer unto him the same sacrifice, and through that offering obtain the knowledge that they are accepted of him. (*Lectures on Faith*, Salt Lake City: N. B. Lundwall, n.d., 6:7-8.)

This chapter defines the process whereby man can be changed to that condition described by Joseph Smith and King Benjamin, where he is willing to sacrifice all things; wherein he indeed becomes "meek, humble, patient, full of love, willing to submit" himself completely to the Lord. The desirability of such a state requires no discussion. It should be the never-ceasing quest of every Latter-day Saint.

Nicodemus went to Jesus by night desiring to know what the requirements were for salvation. Succinctly, Jesus replied, "Except a man be born again, he cannot see the kingdom of God." Not understanding, thinking Jesus was referring to a second mortal birth, Nicodemus asked how such could be. Then the Savior further defined the requirement: "Except a man be born of water and of the Spirit, he cannot enter into the kingdom of God." (John 3:5.)

Thus the requirements were outlined for entrance into God's kingdom. "Born of water" is certainly water baptism. Have we fulfilled this ordinance? For those of us in the Church, the answer is yes.

But have we been "born of the Spirit"? That is not quite so easy to answer. We have received the ordinance of laying on of hands called confirmation, but is that all there is to it? Does everything happen automatically after hands are laid upon our heads by those who have the Melchizedek Priesthood?

Have we been born of the Spirit? Have we been baptized with fire and with the Holy Ghost?

Let Alma ask it in a different way: "And now behold, I ask of you, *my brethren of the church*, have ye spiritually been born of God? Have ye received his image in your countenances? *Have ye experienced this mighty change in your hearts?*" (Alma 5:14; italics added.)

Church members commonly give several different answers to Alma's questions:

"Well, how do I know? Is it something like receiving the gifts of the Spirit?"

"Well, I have had hands laid upon my head and have been given the Holy Ghost."

"I have felt the influence of the Spirit many times in my life. Is that what you mean?"

Of course, there is no simple answer to the question, "Have you been spiritually reborn?" But there is an answer. To understand it, we must first understand the two separate and distinct blessings that can result from the ordinance of confirmation — first, the right of enjoyment of certain gifts of the Spirit, and second, that marvelous change that comes from the baptism of fire and the Holy Ghost.

Gifts of the Spirit

Most members tend to think of the gifts of the Spirit as the only blessing coming from the ordinance of confirmation. The scriptures specify that the gifts of the Spirit are to
— know that Jesus is the Christ
— believe on the words of those that know
— know the differences of administrations
— have the gift of discernment
— have the word of knowledge
— have the gift of wisdom
— have the faith to be healed
— have the faith to heal
— have the opportunity of working miracles
— have the gift of prophecy
— speak in tongues
— have interpretation of tongues.
None of the preceding gifts speak of the mighty change that must be wrought upon the heart of man or of the forgiveness of sins that comes with the birth of the Spirit. Elder Bruce R. McConkie defines the "Gifts of the Spirit" as follows:

> By the grace of God — following devotion, faith, and obedience on man's part — certain special spiritual blessings called *gifts of the Spirit* are bestowed upon man....
>
> Their purpose is to enlighten, encourage, and edify the faithful so that they will inherit peace in this life and be guided toward eternal life in the world to come....
>
> Faithful persons are expected to seek the gifts of the Spirit with all their hearts. They are to "covet earnestly the best gifts."... To some will be given one gift; to others, another.... (*Mormon Doctrine*, 2nd ed., Salt Lake City: Bookcraft, 1966, p. 314.)

Baptism of Fire

Contrast the preceding comments on the gifts of the Spirit with Elder McConkie's definition under "Baptism of Fire":

To gain salvation every accountable person must receive two baptisms. They are baptism of water and of the Spirit. . . . The baptism of the Spirit is called the baptism of fire and of the Holy Ghost. . . . *By the power of the Holy Ghost – who is the sanctifier* (3 Nephi 27:19-21) —*dross, iniquity, carnality, sensuality, and every evil thing is burned out of the human soul as if by fire; the cleansed person becomes literally a new creature of the Holy Ghost.* (Mosiah 27:24-26.) He is born again.

The baptism of fire is not something in addition to the receipt of the Holy Ghost; rather, it is the actual enjoyment of the *gift* which is offered by the laying on of hands at the time of baptism. "Remission of sins," the Lord says, comes "by baptism and by fire, yea, even the Holy Ghost." (D & C 19:31; 2 Nephi 31:17.) *Those who receive the baptism of fire are "filled as if with fire."* (Helaman 5:45.) (*Mormon Doctrine*, 2nd ed., p. 73; italics added.)

He also states under the section "Born Again":

To gain salvation in the celestial kingdom men must be *born again* (Alma 7:14); born of water and of the Spirit (John 3:1-13); born of God, so that they are changed from their "carnal and fallen state, to a state of righteousness," becoming new creatures of the Holy Ghost. (Mosiah 27:24-29.) They must become newborn babes in Christ (1 Peter 2:2); they must be "spiritually begotten" of God, be born of Christ, thus becoming his sons and daughters. (Mosiah 5:7.)

. . . The elements of water, blood, and Spirit are present in both births. (Moses 6:59-60.) The second birth begins when men are baptized in water by a legal administrator; it is completed when they actually receive the companionship of the Holy Ghost, becoming new creatures by the cleansing power of that member of the Godhead. (*Mormon Doctrine*, 2nd ed., p. 101.)

From Elder McConkie's discussion, describing the gifts of the Spirit and birth of the Spirit, it is easy to discern the differences. First, the birth of the Spirit is essential to salvation, while the gifts of the Spirit are available as a great blessing to assist and give comfort to the Saints as they pursue the course of their lives. Second, the birth of the Spirit purges and sanctifies an individual so that as a "new creature of the Holy Ghost" he is capable of a life that approaches the standard necessary for exaltation — he is willing to sacrifice all earthly things.

The ancient prophets made it clear that a baptism of fire is necessary for us to be able to live in God's presence eternally. One good example is Nephi's explanation of what is required to be "in the straight and narrow way":

> Wherefore, my beloved brethren, I know that if ye shall follow the Son, with full purpose of heart, acting no hypocrisy and no deception before God, but with real intent, repenting of your sins, witnessing unto the Father that ye are willing to take upon you the name of Christ, by baptism — yea, by following your Lord and your Savior down into the water, according to his word, behold, then shall ye receive the Holy Ghost; *yea, then cometh the baptism of fire and of the Holy Ghost*; and then can ye speak with the tongue of angels, and shout praises unto the Holy One of Israel. (2 Nephi 31:13; italics added.)

A few verses later Nephi reiterates what we must do to be born again:

> Wherefore, do the things which I have told you I have seen that your Lord and your Redeemer should do; for, for this cause have they been shown unto me, that ye might know the gate by which ye should enter. For the gate by which ye should enter is repentance and baptism by water; *and then cometh a remission of your sins by fire and by the Holy Ghost*. (2 Nephi 31:17; italics added.)

Alma, during his great discourse on priesthood, states:

> Therefore they were called after this holy order, and were sanctified, and their garments were washed white through the blood of the lamb.
>
> *Now they, after being sanctified by the Holy Ghost*, having their garments made white, being pure and spotless before God, could not look upon sin save it were with abhorrence; and there were many, exceeding great many, who were made pure and entered into the rest of the Lord their God. (Alma 13:11-12; italics added.)

Alma also vividly describes his own conversion:

> ... I have repented of my sins, and have been redeemed of the Lord; behold I am born of the Spirit.
>
> And the Lord said unto me: *Marvel not that all mankind, yea, men and women, all nations, kindreds, tongues and people,*

must be born again; yea, born of God, changed from their carnal and fallen state, to a state of righteousness, being redeemed of God, becoming his sons and daughters;

And thus they become new creatures; and unless they do this, they can in no wise inherit the kingdom of God.

I say unto you, unless this be the case, they must be cast off. . . .

Nevertheless, after wandering through much tribulation, repenting nigh unto death, the Lord in mercy hath seen fit to snatch me out of an everlasting burning, and I am born of God. (Mosiah 27:24-28; italics added.)

As the Savior taught the Nephites, he specifically declared their need to be born of the Spirit, saying: "After that ye are baptized with water, behold, *I will baptize you with fire and with the Holy Ghost*; therefore blessed are ye if ye shall believe in me and be baptized, after that ye have seen me and know that I am." (3 Nephi 12:1; italics added.)

The Nephites then prayed that they would receive this great blessing, and " . . . when they were all baptized and had come up out of the water, *the Holy Ghost did fall upon them, and they were filled with the Holy Ghost and with fire.*

"And behold, they were encircled about as if it were by fire; and it came down from heaven, . . . and angels did come down out of heaven and did minister unto them." (3 Nephi 19:13-14; italics added.)

Many other references show the consistency of the prophets with regard to the doctrine of the birth of the Spirit. See, for instance, Mosiah 5:2-5, 7; 15:11-12; Alma 7:14; 22:14-16; Moroni 6:4; 8:24-26; and Moses 6:64-66.

Our modern leaders also have been quite explicit in their explanation of being born of the Spirit. Elder James E. Talmage said: "The power of the Holy Ghost then, is the spirit of prophecy and revelation; His office is that of enlightenment of the mind, quickening of the intellect, *and sanctification of the soul.*" (*Articles of Faith*, 12th ed., London: The Church of Jesus Christ of Latter-day Saints, 1924, p. 163; italics added.)

Next listen to Orson Pratt:

Water baptism is only a preparatory cleansing of the believing penitent; it is only a condition of a cleansing from sin; *whereas, the Baptism of fire and the Holy Ghost cleanses more thoroughly, by renewing the inner man, and by purifying the affections, desires, and thoughts which have long been habituated in the impure ways of sin*. Without the aid of the Holy Ghost, a person who has long been accustomed to love sin, and whose affections and desires have long run with delight in the degraded channel of vice, would have but very little power to change his mind, at once, from its habituated course, and to walk in newness of life. Though his sins may have been cleansed away, yet so great is the force of habit that he would, without being renewed by the Holy Ghost, be easily overcome, and contaminated again by sin. Hence, it is infinitely important that the affections and desires should be, in a measure, changed and renewed, so as to cause him to hate that which he before loved, and to love that which he before hated: *to thus renew the mind of man is the work of the Holy Ghost....*

Every believing penitent who will follow this example of Jesus, by being baptized first with water, is entitled to, and will receive the second baptism of the Holy Ghost and of fire; for the promise is, that Jesus who was himself baptized with the Holy Ghost, should confer this same glorious baptism upon all his children. The two baptisms, therefore, received by the Son of God, are the same that all men *must* receive, in order to become the sons of God....

The Baptism of fire, without doubt, had reference to the purifying qualities of the Holy Ghost, which, like fire, consumes or destroys the unholy affections of those who are made partakers of it. (N. B. Lundwall, comp., *Discourses on the Holy Ghost*, Salt Lake City: Bookcraft, Inc., pp. 33, 35; italics added.)

A beautiful description of the effect of a spiritual rebirth is given by Elder B. H. Roberts:

In addition to this splendid array of powers and gifts of the Holy Ghost, we are told that the result of possessing him "is love, joy, peace, longsuffering, gentleness, goodness, faith, meekness, and temperance." Indeed we may say with the Apostle Parley P. Pratt — though slightly changing his language — the Holy Spirit adapts himself to all the organs and attributes of man. His influence quickens all the intellectual faculties, increases, enlarges, expands and purifies all the natural passions and affections; and adapts them by the gift of wisdom to their lawful use. It inspires, develops, cultivates and matures all the fine-toned sympathies, joys, tastes, kindred feelings and affections of our nature. It inspires virtue, kindness, goodness, tenderness, gentleness and charity. It develops beauty of person, form and feature. It tends to health, vigor, animation and social feeling. It develops and invigorates all the faculties of the physical and intellectual man. It strengthens, invigorates and gives tone to the nerves. In short, it is, as it were, marrow to the bone, joy to the heart, light to the eyes, music to the ears, and life to the whole being. (*Key to Theology*, p. 102) (*The Gospel*, 9th ed., Salt Lake City: Deseret Book Co., 1950, pp. 204-5.)

No Automatic Bestowal

With the preceding powerful statements of ancient and modern prophets fresh in our minds, some may be led to say in their hearts: "I have received the gift of the Holy Ghost by the laying on of hands; why have I not received such an experience?"

The answer to that may well be that indeed they have *not* received the "gift" of the Holy Ghost! The ordinance of laying on of hands only entitles one to the gift when he qualifies for it. Listen to Elder McConkie:

Mere compliance with the formality of the ordinance of baptism does not mean that a person has been born again. No one can be born again without baptism, but the immersion in water and the laying on of hands to confer the Holy Ghost do not of themselves guarantee that a person has been or will be born again. The new birth takes place only for those who actually enjoy the gift or companionship of the Holy Ghost, only for those who are fully converted, who have given themselves without restraint to the Lord. Thus Alma addressed himself to his "brethren of the church," and pointedly asked them if they had "spiritually been born of God," received the Lord's image in their countenances, and had the "mighty change" in their hearts which always attends the birth of the Spirit. (Alma 5:14-31.) (*Mormon Doctrine*, 2nd ed., p. 101.)

Also President Joseph F. Smith states:

Therefore, the presentation or "gift" of the Holy Ghost simply confers upon a man the right to receive at any time, when he is worthy of it and desires it, the power and light of truth of the Holy Ghost, although he may often be left to his own spirit and judgment. (*Gospel Doctrine*, Salt Lake City: Deseret Book Co., 1977, pp. 60-61.)

Again from Elder McConkie:

> Further, the fact that a person has had hands laid on his head and a legal administrator has declared, "Receive the Holy Ghost," does not guarantee that the gift itself has actually been enjoyed.... The Spirit will not dwell in an unclean tabernacle. (1 Cor. 3:16-17; 6:19.) Those who actually enjoy the gift or presentment of the Holy Ghost are the ones who are born again, who have become new creatures of the Holy Ghost. (Mosiah 27:24-26.) (*Mormon Doctrine*, 2nd ed., p. 313.)

It is obvious from the preceding statements that the birth of the Spirit will not come automatically. A person must make a concentrated effort in seeking this great blessing. Sometimes months and years of preparation will be required.

Will we know when we receive the birth of the Spirit? Does it come gradually so that we may have received it already and do not recognize it? There is no question that spiritual preparation to receive this "new birth" could be a long, gradual process. But the distinctive change spoken of by Alma leads me to believe that one cannot receive such an experience without a powerful awareness of it. Like the "witness of the Spirit," we will easily recognize this gift when it comes, and we will know the day and the hour we receive it.

Another reason I believe we will know when the birth of the Spirit comes is that at that point our sins will be cleansed from us — an experience described by such words as "fire" and "burning." Surely such an inward purging will be noticeable.

A modern prophet, President Marion G. Romney, says:

> Conversion is effected by divine forgiveness, which remits sins. The sequence is something like this. An honest seeker hears the message. He asks the Lord in prayer if it is true. The Holy Spirit gives him a witness. This is a testimony. If one's testimony is strong enough, he repents and obeys the commandments. *By such obedience he receives divine forgiveness which remits sin.* Thus he is converted to a newness of life. His spirit is healed. (*Improvement Era*, Dec. 1963, p. 1066; italics added.)

And Nephi says that after we enter the gate of repentance and baptism, "then cometh a remission of your sins by fire and by the Holy Ghost." (2 Nephi 31:17.) We can know that our sins have been forgiven. When the cleansing occurs we will have been filled as if with fire. Thus we will know, as did the people of Zarahemla (Mosiah 4:1-3; 5:1-7), of the "mighty change wrought in our hearts."

Rebirth Experiences

Perhaps if we look at some of those who have experienced the spiritual rebirth we can better identify and relate to the process. A good starting point is the experience of Peter; his spiritual development is clearly delineated in the scriptures. Peter was closely associated with the Savior throughout most of His three-year ministry. Peter saw the healing of the sick, the raising of the dead, the calming of the seas. He saw Christ transfigured with Moses and Elias on the mount and heard the voice of God declare, "This is my beloved Son, in whom I am well pleased." (Matthew 17:5.)

Can we say that Peter had a testimony prior to the Savior's death? Most certainly we can. At one point Jesus asked his disciples, "Whom say ye that I am?" And "Peter answered and said, Thou art the Christ, the Son of the living God.

"And Jesus answered and said unto him, Blessed art thou, Simon Barjona: *for flesh and blood hath not revealed it unto thee, but my Father which is in heaven.*" (Matthew 16:15-17; italics added.) Here Jesus confirmed that Peter did indeed *know*, by revelation, of the divinity of Christ's mission.

But even though Peter had a testimony, he still wasn't converted. A year later Jesus said to him, "*When thou art converted*, strengthen thy brethren." (Luke 22:32; italics added.)

It is interesting to see the remarkable change that took place in Peter when he did become converted. Look at Peter before true conversion, the Peter of the Gospels:

Now Peter sat without in the palace: and a damsel came unto him, saying, Thou also wast with Jesus of Galilee.

But he denied before them all, saying, I know not what thou sayest.

And when he was gone out into the porch, another maid saw him, and said unto them that were there, This fellow was also with Jesus of Nazareth.

And again he denied with an oath, I do not know the man.

And after a while came unto him they that stood by, and said to Peter, Surely thou also art one of them; for thy speech betrayeth thee.

Then began he to curse and to swear, saying, I know not the man. And immediately the cock crew.

And Peter remembered the word of Jesus, which said unto him, Before the cock crow, thou shalt deny me thrice. And he went out, and wept bitterly. (Matthew 26:69-75.)

Contrast the Peter of the preceding events with the powerful Peter in the book of Acts:

Then Peter, filled with the Holy Ghost, said unto them, Ye rulers of the people, and elders of Israel,

Be it known unto you all, and to all the people of Israel, that by the name of Jesus Christ of Nazareth, whom ye crucified, whom God raised from the dead, even by him doth this man stand here before you whole.

And [the council] called them, and commanded them not to speak at all nor teach in the name of Jesus.

But Peter and John answered and said unto them, Whether it be right in the sight of God to hearken unto you more than unto God, judge ye.

For we cannot but speak the things which we have seen and heard.

So when they had further threatened them, they let them go, finding nothing how they might punish them, because of the people: for all men glorified God for that which was done. (Acts 4:8, 10, 18-21.)

The power and strength of Peter in the book of Acts is beyond question. When did Peter receive this "mighty change" in his heart? Keep in mind that Peter's preaching in Acts was directed to the very people who had killed Christ and could do the same to him. The "mighty change" that drove out the fear, intensified the commitment, and gave power to his testimony came forty-nine days after the resurrection of our Savior:

And when the day of Pentecost was fully come, [the apostles] were all with one accord in one place.

And suddenly there came a sound from heaven as of a rushing mighty wind, and it filled all the house where they were sitting.

And there appeared unto them cloven tongues like as of fire, and it sat upon each of them. (Acts 2:1-3.)

Could it be that the Twelve Apostles were "born of fire" at this time? I believe they were. Peter's experience not only verifies the difference between testimony and conversion, but it also dramatically reveals the intensity of the impact which the "mighty change" makes upon the hearts of men.

Another excellent scriptural example of the process of being born again is seen in the experience of the Nephites in King Benjamin's day. After King Benjamin had delivered an address to all his people, they humbled themselves to the earth and cried:

O have mercy, and apply the atoning blood of Christ that we may receive forgiveness of our sins, and our hearts may be purified; for we believe in Jesus Christ, the Son of God, who created heaven and earth, and all things; who shall come down among the children of men.

And it came to pass that after they had spoken these words *the Spirit of the Lord came upon them, and they were filled with joy, having received a remission of their sins, and having peace of conscience*, because of the exceeding faith which they had in Jesus Christ who should come, according to the words which king Benjamin had spoken unto them. (Mosiah 4:2-3; italics added.)

Then Benjamin spoke to them again; and after this second, shorter sermon (Mosiah 4:4-30), the people of Zarahemla responded to him by saying: "We believe all the words which thou hast spoken unto us; and also, we know of their surety and truth, *because of the Spirit of the Lord Omnipotent, which has wrought a mighty change in us, or in our hearts, that we have no more disposition to do evil, but to do good continually.*" (Mosiah 5:2.)

King Benjamin's next words were: "Because of the covenant which ye have made ye shall be called the children of Christ, his sons, and his daughters; for behold, *this day he hath spiritually begotten you*; for ye say that *your hearts are changed* through faith on his name; *therefore, ye are born of him and have become his sons and his daughters.*" (Mosiah 5:7; italics added.)

Note the great joy that came into their hearts with a remission of their sins. Also note that they recognized that a mighty change had occurred in their natures. They no longer had a "disposition to do evil, but to do good continually."

President Marion G. Romney in his October 1963 general conference talk draws the following conclusion:

> Somebody recently asked how he could know when he is *converted*. The answer is simple. He may be assured of it when by the *power of the Holy Spirit his soul is healed*. When this occurs, he will recognize it by the way he feels, *for he will feel as the people of Benjamin felt when they received remission of sins*. The record says, the spirit of the Lord came upon them and they were filled with joy, having received a remission of their sins, and having peace of conscience. (*Improvement Era*, Dec. 1963, p. 1066; italics added.)

Some more modern examples may also help the reader to evaluate his status relative to spiritual rebirth. Note how similar these examples are to the scriptural accounts. Elder Parley P. Pratt recounts the following incident in his autobiography:

> My dear wife had now lived to accomplish her destiny; and when the child was dressed, and she had looked upon it and embraced it, she ceased to live in the flesh. Her death happened about three hours after the birth of this child of promise. A few days previous to her death she had a vision in open day while sitting in her room. *She was overwhelmed or immersed in a pillar of fire, which seemed to fill the whole room, as if it would consume it and all things therein; and the Spirit whispered to her mind, saying: "Thou art baptized with fire and the Holy Ghost."* It also intimated to her that she should have the privilege of departing from this world of sorrow and pain, and of going to the Paradise of rest as soon as she had fulfilled the prophecy in relation to the promised son. This vision was repeated on the next day at the same hour, viz: — twelve o'clock. She was overwhelmed with a joy and peace indescribable, and *seemed changed in her whole nature from that time forth*. (*Autobiography of Parley P. Pratt*, Salt Lake City: Deseret Book Co., 1972, p. 166; italics added.)

President Lorenzo Snow also relates the choice experience of his rebirth:

> Some two or three weeks after I was baptized, one day

while engaged in my studies, I began to reflect upon the fact that I had not obtained a *knowledge* of the truth of the work . . . and I began to feel very uneasy. I laid aside my books, left the house, and wandered around through the fields under the oppressive influence of a gloomy, disconsolate spirit, while an indescribable cloud of darkness seemed to envelope me. I had been accustomed, at the close of the day, to retire for secret prayer, to a grove . . . but at this time I felt no inclination to do so. The spirit of prayer had departed and the heavens seemed like brass over my head. At length, realizing that the usual time had come for secret prayer, I concluded I would not forego my evening service, and, as a matter of formality, knelt as I was in the habit of doing, and in my accustomed retired place, but not feeling as I was wont to feel.

I had no sooner opened my lips in an effort to pray, than I heard a sound, just above my head, like the rustling of silken robes, and immediately the Spirit of God descended upon me, completely enveloping my whole person, filling me, from the crown of my head to the soles of my feet, and O, the joy and happiness I felt! No language can describe the almost instantaneous transition from a dense cloud of mental and spiritual darkness into a refulgence of light and knowledge, as it was at that time imparted to my understanding. . . . *It was a complete baptism – a tangible immersion in the heavenly principle or element, the Holy Ghost; and even more real and physical in its effects upon every part of my system than the immersion by water;* dispelling forever, so long as reason and memory last, all possibility of doubt. . . .

I cannot tell how long I remained in the full flow of the blissful enjoyment and divine enlightenment, but it was several minutes before the celestial element which filled and surrounded me began gradually to withdraw. On arising from my kneeling posture, . . . I *knew* that He had conferred on me what only an omnipotent being can confer — that which is of greater value than all the wealth and honors worlds can bestow. That night, as I retired to rest, the same wonderful manifestations were repeated, and continued to be for several successive nights. The sweet remembrance of those glorious experiences . . . impart[s] an inspiring influence . . . and I trust will to the close of my earthly existence. (*Biography and Family Record of Lorenzo Snow*, comp.

Eliza R. Snow, Salt Lake City: Deseret Book Co., 1884, pp. 7-9; most italics added.)

With these examples fresh in your mind, can you visualize the spiritual impact of such an experience? Can you picture how those who have been reborn can more fully live the law of sacrifice after such a rebirth? Can you see how the ability to live much closer to the standard of a Christlike life would be increased? The desirability of the spiritual rebirth is beyond question.

Have we had that experience? As Alma asked: "Have ye spiritually been born of God? Have ye received his image in your countenances? Have ye experienced this mighty change in your hearts?"

3   *A Signed Contract*

C hurch members who have not been born of the Spirit need to evaluate their position. The Savior told Nicodemus that a person must "be born of water and of the Spirit" in order to enter into the kingdom of God. (John 3:5.) Latter-day Saints past the age of accountability have fulfilled the requirements of water baptism and the laying on of hands, which authorizes them to receive the Holy Ghost. What is the relationship between water baptism, the forgiveness of sin, and actual enjoyment of the *gift* of the Holy Ghost?

Peter declared to the Jews:

> Repent, and be baptized every one of you in the name of Jesus Christ for the remission of sins, and ye shall receive the gift of the Holy Ghost.
>
> For the promise is unto you, and to your children, and to all that are afar off, even as many as the Lord our God shall call. (Acts 2:38-39.)

Apparently sins cannot be remitted without baptism. And since the Holy Ghost will not dwell in impure tabernacles, we cannot enjoy his gift without a remission of sin. Through the great patriarch Enoch, God helps us to further understand the interrelationship between water baptism and the remission of sin — and how the atonement of Christ fits in:

That by reason of transgression cometh the fall, which fall bringeth death, and inasmuch as ye were born into the world by water, and blood, and the spirit, which I have made, and so became of dust a living soul, *even so ye must be born again into the kingdom of heaven, of water, and of the Spirit, and be cleansed by blood,* even the blood of mine Only Begotten; that ye might be sanctified from all sin, and enjoy the words of eternal life in this world, and eternal life in the world to come, even immortal glory;

For by the water ye keep the commandment; by the Spirit ye are justified, and by the blood ye are sanctified. (Moses 6:59-60; italics added.)

The sacrifice of the Savior actually pays the price of sin and cleanses the individual; the Spirit justifies us to the Father, verifying that we have fulfilled all of the requirements; and by the water we keep the commandment. Book of Mormon prophets add their witness to this interrelationship. For instance, Nephi says:

If ye shall follow the Son, with full purpose of heart, acting no hypocrisy and no deception before God, but with real intent, repenting of your sins, witnessing unto the Father that ye are willing to take upon you the name of Christ, by baptism — yea, by following your Lord and your Savior down into the water, according to his word, behold, then shall ye receive the Holy Ghost; yea, then cometh the baptism of fire and of the Holy Ghost. (2 Nephi 31:13.)

In the New Testament, Paul explains that baptism's immersion in water is symbolic of the atonement of Christ:

Shall we continue in sin . . .?

God forbid. How shall we, that are dead to sin, live any longer therein?

Know ye not, that so many of us as were baptized into Jesus Christ were baptized into his death?

Therefore we are buried with him by baptism into death: that like as Christ was raised up from the dead by the glory of the Father, even so we also should walk in newness of life. (Romans 6:1-4.)

These scriptures bring into sharp focus the fact that the sacrifice of Christ is the foundation upon which a new life rests. Literally, a contract is made between the individual and Jesus Christ. The Savior's contractual commitment is that he will pay the price of our sins, cleanse us of sin, and remember our sins no more. Our commitment is that we will love him, remember him, take his name upon us, keep his commandments, and repent of our sins. Water baptism is our signature on the contract; the gift of a spiritual rebirth is his ratification that the contract has been consummated. Thus, Latter-day Saints have fulfilled the ordinance. The contract has been signed. If it has not been ratified, what is yet lacking in the individual's efforts?

4   *A Broken Heart*

W e have submitted to the ordinances and thereby have formally signed the contract committing ourselves to partake of the atonement of Christ. We have a mighty desire to receive a forgiveness of sins and to be reborn, to be changed from our carnal natures. We might be led to plead as did the Lamanite king of the land of Nephi: "What shall I do that I may have this eternal life of which thou hast spoken? Yea, what shall I do that I may be born of God, having this wicked spirit rooted out of my breast, and receive his Spirit, that I may be filled with joy, that I may not be cast off at the last day? Behold," he said, "I will give up all that I possess, yea, I will forsake my kingdom, that I may receive this great joy." (Alma 22:15.)

If such an experience has not come into our lives, what could be lacking ? Aaron answered the king and defined the way: "If thou desirest this thing, if thou wilt bow down before God, yea, if thou wilt repent of all thy sins, and will bow down before God, and call on his name in faith, believing that ye shall receive, then shalt thou receive the hope which thou desirest." (Alma 22:16.)

Both ancient and modern prophets declare that repentance is a key element in the process of conversion. Could inadequate repentance be the reason a rebirth has not come?

"Who me! repent? What are you talking about? I keep the Word of

Wisdom, pay my tithing, attend my meetings. . . . What do I have to repent of?"

Were those your thoughts? Such feelings are not uncommon. But, sadly, that attitude reflects

— the ease with which we justify our sins.
— a lack of understanding of the desperate need we all have to be forgiven and cleansed.
— a lack of understanding of the standard of righteousness required of us.
— a lack of understanding of how sin affects the soul and how we are cleansed from the effect of sin.

Justification of Sin

Perhaps the greatest barrier to true repentance is the ease with which we justify our sins. The subtle whisperings of the adversary help us to excuse our departures from the path of obedience. I'm sure each of us has seen in our own lives how very effectively Satan uses the tool of self-justification. Usually active members concede and rationalize away only the "little sins" without repentance. Sometimes, however, the adversary is sufficiently clever to get us to justify even the major sins.

President Spencer W. Kimball tells of a young couple who did just that:

Across the desk sat a handsome, young nineteen-year-old and a beautiful, shy, but charming, eighteen-year-old. They appeared embarrassed, apprehensive, near-terrified. He was defensive and bordering on belligerency and rebellion. There had been sexual violations throughout the summer and intermittently since school began, and as late as last week. I was not so much surprised. I have had these kinds of visits many times; but what did disturb me was that they seemed little, if any, remorseful. They admitted they had gone contrary to some social standards, but quoted magazines and papers and speakers approving pre-marital sex and emphasizing that sex was a fulfillment of human existence.

Finally, the boy said, "Yes, we yielded to each other, but we do not think it wrong because we *love* each other." I thought I had misunderstood him. Since the world began, there have been countless immoralities, but to hear them justified by Latter-day Saint youth shocked me. He repeated, "No, it is not wrong because we *love* each other."

They had repeated this abominable heresy so often that they had convinced themselves, and a wall of resistance had been built, and behind this wall they stubbornly stood almost defiantly. If there had been blushes of shame at first, such had been neutralized with their logic. ("Love versus Lust," *BYU Speeches of the Year*, Provo, Utah: BYU Extension Publications, January 5, 1965, pp. 4-5.)

I myself had a similar experience as a stake president. An active Church member came to confess what turned out to be a major transgression, one worthy of excommunication. He started the conversation rather lightly by saying, "It isn't so serious, is it?"

Nephi was familiar with this powerful tactic of Satan. "And others will he pacify," Nephi said of Satan, "and lull them away into carnal security, that they will say: All is well in Zion; yea, Zion prospereth, all is well — and thus the devil cheateth their souls, and leadeth them away carefully down to hell." (2 Nephi 28:21.)

Probably it will be the "little sins" that will condemn the majority of us:

— the small "necessary" purchases on the Sabbath.
— tossing a load of washing in the washing machine on Sunday with the excuse that the machine does all the work.
— watching TV ten hours a week, while reading the scriptures a half hour — if at all.
— reading the newspaper an hour a day while spending five minutes a day in personal prayer.
    telling little white lies to keep out of trouble.
— failing to discuss the gospel with our friends.
— failing to set aside the time to do our genealogical or temple work.
— spreading an unpleasant rumor.
— lightly partaking of the sacrament.
— doing ineffective home teaching or visiting teaching.
— and many, many others.

For example, what could be the damage of one cup of coffee? Obviously, one cup would hardly damage the physical body. The major damage would be spiritual. It would come from the attitude that says to Christ: "You asked me not to use coffee, but I don't care what you want me to do; I am going to do what I want to do."

So many of us picture ourselves standing before the judgment bar and appealing to the love of the Savior, saying: "But it is such a small, insignificant thing; surely one cup of coffee won't matter."

I have heard in my heart what the Savior's answer may be: "It was such a small request — surely you must have loved me enough to do *at least* that."

He has given us a standard: "If ye love me, keep my commandments." (John 14:15). If we love little, then there is little tendency to obey. If we love with all our heart, then should we not *"live with all our heart"*?

The Nature of Man

Perhaps the first step toward repentance is to honestly, deeply feel the need to be cleansed and to have forgiveness. Moroni testified that the Lord will help us feel that need by revealing our sins to us: "And if men come unto me I will show unto them their weakness." (Ether 12:27.)

But feeling a need for cleansing does not necessarily come naturally. King David pondered the question: "What is man, that thou art mindful of him?" (Psalm 8:4.) If we add a word, we have a similar question that Latter-day Saints have frequently pondered and debated: "What is man's nature?"

As we first begin to contemplate this in some depth, our thoughts often develop along this line:

1. All men are the direct offspring of God, his sons and daughters.
2. God is perfect and divine.
3. As children of God we must inherit his divine qualities and goodness.
4. Man must then be naturally good.

I have had numerous nonmember friends at different times in my life, and I wouldn't consider any of them to be an evil person. Every one was basically good, trying most of the time to do what he felt was right. But our logic, though seemingly sound, has led us to a conclusion that contradicts the truths taught by the scriptures and modern prophets. What have the prophets said? "The natural man is an enemy to God, and has been from the fall of Adam, and will be, forever and ever, unless he yields to the enticings of the Holy Spirit, and putteth off the natural man and becometh a saint through the atonement of Christ the Lord." (Mosiah 3:19.)

How could this be true of God's children? How could man be an enemy to God?

Abinadi explains that the rift between man and God came about because of the fall of Adam and Eve:

"For they are carnal and devilish, and the devil has power over them; yea, even that old serpent that did beguile our first parents, which was the cause of their fall; *which was the cause of all mankind becoming carnal, sensual, devilish*, knowing evil from good, subjecting themselves to the devil." (Mosiah 16:3; italics added.)

The fall of our first parents caused *all mankind* to become "carnal, sensual, and devilish"? Surely my friends are not like that! But again a prophet speaks: "Because of the fall our natures have become evil continually." (Ether 3:2.)

Of course the modern prophets agree. In a letter to his son David, quoted in the *Instructor*, President David O. McKay discusses the nature of man:

"In the beginning" whenever that was, man found himself shut out from God's eternal presence. He remembered little and in time would have remembered nothing of his associations with eternal beings. "In his humiliation his judgment was taken away." (Acts 8:33.) Earth and earthly things were everything to him. When he became hungry, it was the earth that satisfied him; when he became thirsty, it was an earthly element that quenched his thirst; when he became cold it was the skins of animals that protected him and kept him warm; or it was the great moving luminary in the sky that shed his genial rays on man's chilly limbs.

When he sought comfort in repose, it was from the trees, or from skins of animals, or from vegetation of the earth that gave him a downy bed.

In short, the earth became not only man's "foster mother," she was to him the source of his very existence.

Self-preservation became not only the first law, but I can imagine, *the only law he knew*. As the race increased, and the struggle for existence became more acute, selfishness and strife would manifest themselves. Man would struggle with man for supremacy or for the best things nature could offer for the prolongation of the comforts of life. *Thus would man become "carnal, sensual, and devilish, by nature."* (Alma 42:6-13). ("The Atonement," March 1959, p. 65; some italics added.)

In his great and scholarly treatment of sin, repentance, and forgiveness, *The Miracle of Forgiveness*, President Spencer W. Kimball states:

"The way to eternal life is clear. It is well marked. It is difficult. Evil and good influences will be ever present. One must choose. *Generally the evil way is easier, and since man is carnal that way will triumph* unless there be a conscious and consistently vigorous effort to reject the evil and follow the good." (Salt Lake City: Bookcraft, 1969, p. 15; italics added.)

As I researched this subject, I could find nothing in the standard works that directly stated that man's basic nature after the Fall is good or godlike. The nearest I could find was a statement in the Doctrine and Covenants: "Every spirit of man was innocent in the beginning; and God having redeemed man from the fall, men became again, in their infant state, innocent before God." (D&C 93:38.)

There are also several other scriptures that state in essence, that "little children are alive in Christ." (See Moroni 8:8-22; Mosiah 3:16; D&C 29:47; 74:6-7.) Do such statements contradict those quoted earlier? Obviously the prophets will not contradict themselves; both concepts are harmonious. These scriptures do not define man's nature after arriving at the age of accountability. They tell us merely that when a person is born as a mortal child, he is innocent and free from the bondage of sin. He will not be punished for the disobedience of his parents or the original transgression of Adam and Eve. He is free, when accountable, to choose his course in life, and then he must accept the consequences of that course. But the atonement of Christ freely pays any price, penalty, or debt incurred prior to accountability.

I didn't doubt the words of the prophets about man's nature, but for a while I had difficulty in reconciling their view of man with the basic goodness I saw in society about me. Then as I was reading and pondering the fourth chapter of 2 Nephi I had a sudden burst of insight. The great prophet Nephi relates:

> Behold, my soul delighteth in the things of the Lord; and my heart pondereth continually upon the things which I have seen and heard.
>
> Nevertheless notwithstanding the great goodness of the Lord, in showing me his great and marvelous works, my heart exclaimeth: O wretched man that I am! Yea, my heart sorroweth because of my flesh; my soul grieveth because of mine iniquities.

I am encompassed about, because of the temptations and the sins which do so easily beset me.

And when I desire to rejoice, my heart groaneth because of my sins; nevertheless, I know in whom I have trusted. (2 Nephi 4:16-19.)

Here is a prophet who never faltered, never wavered. Even when Lehi momentarily lost faith on one occasion, Nephi didn't. Even in the most adverse circumstances, Nephi's faith prevailed and persevered. So how could Nephi say such things about himself? Was Nephi a wicked person? No! In fact, in the eyes of society he would have been considered the most righteous of men.

Then the light dawned for me! The prophets, living as close to Christ as they do, have a different standard of measurement than we do! *Their standard is that of a Christlike life:* a life that holds back nothing with respect to time, talent, energy, and means in the service of God; a life reflective of father Abraham's willingness to sacrifice his most precious possession, his son Isaac.

Now, if this is the scriptural standard for good, how many men are good? Indeed are not *all* men enemies to God, unless they "put off the natural man" and become Saints "through the atonement of Christ"? The prophets are not trying to tell us that all men are evil according to *our* standards; they are saying that we have a long way to go with respect to living *Christlike* lives.

In other words, men are selfish. They would rather do what they want, rather than what God wants. Many people go to Church for an hour on Sunday, but how many of our neighbors would be willing to give a tithe of their time — or more — to the Lord? Aren't baseball, movies, TV, boating, skiing more important than keeping the Sabbath Day holy? How many men will give 10 percent, 15 percent, 20 percent, or all they have to the Lord? Or are new cars, lovely homes, summer cottages more important?

How about members of the Church? Are we "carnal, sensual, devilish"? The law of tithing has been strongly taught as a commandment since 1831. Yet what percentage of the Church keeps this commandment? Generally less than 50 percent. Since 1831 the Lord has said that Church members should attend sacrament meeting each week. It requires only 1½ hours a week to do so. But only about 45 percent of all members regularly attend sacrament meeting. More recently the Lord, through his prophet, commanded us to have family home evening once a week, for the preservation of our families. Surely more would respond to such an important need, at such a small price. How many have? Again, perhaps 35 percent at most.

In these cases are not many Church members saying, "What I want to do is more important than what God wants me to do"? And are they not "carnal, sensual, and devilish" to give in to the earthly desires of seeking pleasure, ease, and no responsibility?

I wonder if we could not all be indicted for the bad habits and sins we refuse to give up.

One gets the impression from the scriptures dealing with the nature of man that there are but two levels of righteousness — the "carnal" level and the "Christlike" level. But I don't believe that this conclusion is consistent with sections 76 and 131 of the Doctrine and Covenants. The prophets have not stated that there could not be varying degrees of carnality. To be consistent with section 76, we have to conclude that there are at least terrestrial, telestial, and son of perdition levels of carnality — and certainly there are many levels within each of those.

Of what value is the knowledge of the carnality of man? Is it important to our exaltation?

Without the understanding of our own desperate condition in relation to God's standard of righteousness, we can become very complacent. But knowing our need draws us to the only source of relief — Jesus Christ and his sacrifice. The more we know him, the more we love him and the greater power we have to emulate his life and partake of his cleansing sacrifice.

At the times in my life when I have become complacent — feeling I have it made because I pay my tithes and offerings, live the Word of Wisdom, attend my meetings, render Church service — Nephi's perspective of a Christlike life returns to humble me. If Nephi was concerned about his worthiness, oh, then, how much more does each of us need to be concerned about his own condition! We must not become like the Pharisees of old and feel that because we are good according to the world's standard of measurement we have no further room for improvement. Until we become Christlike through his atonement and consecrate every effort to doing the Father's will — and then endure to the end — we will know we still have much work to do.

The Standard of Righteousness

It is important that we reflect more deeply about the standard of a Christlike life the prophets used as their frame of reference.

Jesus was born of a mortal mother and an immortal Father almost two thousand years ago. He was a spiritual giant beyond compare. Of all who have ever lived or will yet live on this earth, none can match his intellectual genius. Likewise none will ever in mortality reach the level of his unfathomable wisdom, his spiritual strength and powers. No one will ever be closer to the Father in unity, thought, determination, and action. If any man had the ability to determine his own course or to say "I did it my way," it was Christ the Lord, for his combination of intellectual and spiritual capacity would have given him that ability. But notwithstanding his great wisdom and ability —*and here is the key to a Christlike life* — he states: "Verily, verily, I say unto you, The Son can do nothing of himself, but what he seeth the Father do: for what things soever he doeth, these also doeth the Son likewise." (John 5:19.)

"For I came down from heaven, not to do mine own will, but the will of him that sent me." (John 6:38.)

"I speak not of myself: but the Father that dwelleth in me, he doeth the works." (John 14:10.)

Even with the great ability he had, Jesus did nothing of himself. His whole effort was to do the Father's will. All that he did, all that he spoke was given of the Father. If Jesus found it necessary to draw his course of action from God, how much more so do we have a need to be dependent upon the Father to determine the course of our lives in every detail! Those who would follow Christ cannot subscribe to the slogan, "I did it my way."

The Effects of Sin

The soul is like a sponge. It absorbs that to which it is exposed. It is a composite of all our acts, all our thoughts, and all our experiences. If we expose ourselves to the good, the virtuous, the uplifting, they become part of us. In contrast, when we participate in evil acts, see X- or R-rated movies, read filthy novels or magazines, associate with bad companions, think evil thoughts, lie, cheat, or steal, these become a part of us, just as dirty water becomes part of a sponge. Our decisions and actions reflect those things we have absorbed.

When we cease the act of sinning, we merely stop pouring the dirty water over the sponge. Stopping the addition of new stains does not remove the old, however, and we are left with the problems of the past. What is there to eliminate the accumulation of years of stain? What is there in the gospel plan to wring out the sponge of our souls so that we can become clean and pure as Alma describes?

Therefore they were called after his holy order, and were sanctified, and their garments were washed white through the blood of the Lamb.

Now they, after being sanctified by the Holy Ghost, having their garments made white, being pure and spotless before God, could not look upon sin save it were with abhorrence; and there were many, exceeding great many, who were made pure and entered into the rest of the Lord their God. (Alma 13:11-12.)

Preliminary Steps

How many times have you heard the Rs of repentance (the number seems to vary with the speaker), concepts such as recognition, resolve, remorse, and restitution? Did a *knowledge* of these principles bring the miracle of forgiveness into your life? Our ability to recite the Rs of repentance does not necessarily bring the blessing that we desire. There is a "grand key" that unlocks the door to a forgiveness of sin. However, there is much that we must do before the grand key will unlock the door. Let's discuss some of those preliminary requirements; then we'll examine the key to repentance.

Cessation of sin. We cannot continue to add dirty water and hope to clean the sponge. Before the Savior allows us to partake of his sacrifice and receive his sanctifying influence, we must demonstrate our love and sincerity of purpose by obedience to his will. "If ye love me, keep my commandments" (John 14:15). To do otherwise would be hypocritical and insincere. We cannot say we love him and appreciate his efforts on our behalf, then mock him by deliberate disobedience to his will. The saving influence of his grace is limited to those who are willing to pay the price of obedience. President Spencer W. Kimball clearly outlines the need to make a concentrated effort to be worthy in all areas before forgiveness can come:

In connection with repentance, the scriptures use the phrase, "with all his heart" (see D&C 42:25). Obviously this rules out any reservations. Repentance must involve an all-out, total surrender to the program of the Lord. That transgressor is not fully repentant who neglects his tithing, misses his meetings, breaks the Sabbath, fails in his family prayers, does not sustain the authorities of the Church, breaks the Word of Wisdom, does not love the Lord nor his fellowmen. A reforming adulterer who drinks or curses is not repentant. The repenting burglar who has sex play is not ready for forgiveness. God cannot forgive unless the transgressor shows a true repentance which spreads to all areas of his life.

The Lord knows, as does the individual concerned, the degree of contrition exhibited, and the reward will be received accordingly, for God is just. He knows the heart. He knows whether or not one is making but a show of repentance. Feigning repentance or bluffing is futile, for both the transgressor and the Lord know the degree of sincerity. (*The Miracle of Forgiveness*, Salt Lake City: Bookcraft, 1969, pp. 203-4.)

Forgiveness of others. In the Sermon on the Mount, Jesus outlines one of the fundamental prerequisites to forgiveness:

"For if ye forgive men their trespasses, your heavenly Father will also forgive you:

"But if ye forgive not men their trespasses, neither will your Father forgive your trespasses." (Matthew 6:14-15.)

The Lord confirms this in modern revelation: "Wherefore, I say unto you, that ye ought to forgive one another; for he that forgiveth not his brother his trespasses standeth condemned before the Lord; for there remaineth in him the greater sin." (D&C 64:9.)

A clear and unbending rule thus is established: before we can be forgiven, we must forgive *all* who trespass against us.

Confession of Sin. With the more serious sins — those where a member's status in the Church may be in question — the transgressor will not be forgiven without confession to a bishop or stake president. The purpose of confession is not for the Church authority to grant forgiveness, for it is not within his authority to do so except as it pertains to Church court action. His function is to share the burden, outline a course required for repentance, and give loving follow-through to see that the individual does not give up hope and discontinue the quest for forgiveness. President Spencer W. Kimball clearly outlines the need for confession:

"Especially grave errors such as sexual sins shall be confessed to the bishop as well as to the Lord. There are two remissions which one might wish to have. First, the forgiveness from the Lord, and second, the forgiveness of the Lord's Church through its leaders." ("Be Ye Clean," *BYU Speeches of the Year*, Provo, Utah: BYU Extension Division, May 4, 1954, p. 10.)

The Grand Key

Once the preceding requirements have been complied with, the grand key to repentance can unlock the door. That key is given to us by the Savior in these words: *"Ye shall offer for a sacrifice unto me a broken heart and a contrite spirit.* And whoso cometh unto me with a broken heart and a contrite spirit, him will I baptize with fire and with the Holy Ghost." (3 Nephi 9:20; italics added.)

The Savior gave this commandment in the context that it replaced another law, the law of animal sacrifice. This former law was one of the significant higher laws of the gospel and not merely a part of the lesser law given through Moses. This is not to suggest that righteous men and women in ancient times did not also offer the sacrifice of a broken heart and a contrite spirit, but now the Savior was putting an added emphasis on this law: "Ye shall offer for a sacrifice unto me a broken heart and a contrite spirit." And whoever would do this, he said, "Him will I baptize with fire and with the Holy Ghost."

Thus the Savior himself confirms that the key to being born of the Spirit, the key to total repentance, is to offer as a sacrifice a broken heart! If you have not received "a mighty change in your heart," could it be that you have not yet experienced a broken heart? Father Lehi also affirms the need of a broken heart:

> Wherefore, redemption cometh in and through the Holy Messiah; for he is full of grace and truth.
>
> Behold, he offereth himself a sacrifice for sin, to answer the ends of the law, unto all those who have a broken heart and a contrite spirit; and unto none else can the ends of the law be answered. (2 Nephi 2:6-7.)

It is a broken heart that will complete our repentance; then the Lord will wring out the sponge of our souls, purging and cleansing us. But what is there in the gospel to break our hearts? Webster's dictionary says that those who have "broken hearts" have been "crushed" spiritually. Have you ever been crushed spiritually? Have you ever experienced a broken heart?

How *can* we be crushed or broken? Everything in the doctrines of the Church brings joy. Think about it — from eternal marriage to the universal resurrection to our knowledge that God is our Father, everything in the gospel brings joy.

So what is there that can crush us spiritually? Some have felt that they have suffered a broken heart when a sweetheart has broken off a relationship. Others, at the death of loved ones or friends, feel their hearts have been broken. But while we can feel deep sorrow through experiences like these, they are not what the Savior says will cleanse and purify us.

We can probably best understand the broken heart — and its causes — by looking at the experience of someone who has gone through it. Lynn A. McKinlay of the BYU faculty shares with us his very personal witness:

> Such laboring in the spirit I have never known before. My wife and children were away for an hour or so, visiting her mother, and I was in the house alone. I felt the old familiar earthborn loneliness but was entirely unprepared for that which came. I knelt down beside the couch, began to pray to draw the Spirit to my breast for comfort and relief. But soon I felt an overwhelming power fill my being — not a power of light and exaltation which I wanted and expected, that I'd tasted measurably before at times, but a power that seemed almost to bruise my flesh and crush my spirit with the awful knowledge of my earthly guilt. The shameful vivid memories of sins I had committed tore my heart apart as they passed before my eyes and settled in my bosom. I could almost feel the anguish that the Master bore for me there in Gethsemane; the aching sorrow that I felt, to know with burning knowledge every sin I had committed or — God help me — I might yet commit, had of necessity to be absolved by bitter pain within his own pure, perfect, patient body. How the sobs tore through my throat. My spirit groaned with grief. With all the strength in me I bared my soul, confessed as deeply as my consciousness could stretch and still beyond, and pled forgiveness at the feet of him, my Savior and my King. I offered him my life, whatever it was worth to him. He bought it with his blood, the blood that oozed from every pore. (*The Spirit Giveth Life*, Salt Lake City: Deseret Book Co., 1955, pp. 52-53.)

This, as I understand it, is the only way we will come to the point where we feel our spirits have been crushed and our hearts broken. We come to love the Savior with all our hearts and then know with burning knowledge that we literally and personally contributed to his suffering in Gethsemane and on the cross by the individual acts of disobedience in our lives. If we have not received the experience of a broken heart, we have not yet turned the key that unlocks the door to a forgiveness of sin and a birth of the spirit. To receive it we need to truly understand the sacrifice that Christ made for us.

The Suffering Redeemer

President Joseph Fielding Smith relates the following with regard to the suffering of Christ.

> A great many people have an idea that when he was on the cross, and nails were driven into his hands and feet, that was his great suffering. His great suffering was before he ever was placed upon the cross. It was in the Garden of Gethsemane that the blood oozed from the pores of his body: "Which suffering caused myself, even God, the greatest of all, to tremble because of pain, and to bleed at every pore, and to suffer both body and spirit — and would that I might not drink the bitter cup, and shrink."
>
> That was not when he was on the cross; that was in the garden. That is where he bled from every pore in his body.
>
> Now I cannot comprehend that pain. I have suffered pain, you have suffered pain, and sometimes it has been quite severe; but I cannot comprehend pain, which is *mental anguish more than physical*, that would cause the blood, like sweat, to come out upon the body. It was something terrible, something terrific; so we can understand why he would cry unto his Father:
>
> "If it be possible, let this cup pass from me: nevertheless not as I will, but as thou wilt." (*Doctrines of Salvation*, Salt Lake City: Bookcraft, 1954, 1:130.)

The Book of Mormon prophets bore powerful testimony of Christ's suffering. (For example, see 2 Nephi 9:20-21; Mosiah 14:1-12; 15:7-12; Alma 7:11-14; 34:8-16; 42:13-15; 3 Nephi 27:13-15, 20-21.) Hear, for instance, the words of King Benjamin:

> And the things which I shall tell you are made known unto me by an angel from God. And he said unto me: . . .
>
> For behold, the time cometh, and is not far distant, that with power, the Lord Omnipotent who reigneth, who was, and is from all eternity to all eternity, shall come down from heaven among the children of men, and shall dwell in a tabernacle of clay, and shall go forth amongst men, working mighty miracles, such as healing the sick, raising the dead,

causing the lame to walk, the blind to receive their sight, and the deaf to hear, and curing all manner of diseases.

And lo, he shall suffer temptations, and pain of body, hunger, thirst, and fatigue, even more than man can suffer, except it be unto death; for behold, blood cometh from every pore, so great shall be his anguish for the wickedness and the abominations of his people. (Mosiah 3:2, 5, 7; italics added.)

The Savior revealed to Joseph Smith the depth of his suffering:

For behold, I, God, have suffered these things for all, that they might not suffer if they would repent;

But if they would not repent they must suffer even as I;

Which suffering caused myself, even God, the greatest of all, to tremble because of pain, and to bleed at every pore, and to suffer both body and spirit – and would that I might not drink the bitter cup, and shrink —

Nevertheless, glory be to the Father, and I partook and finished my preparations unto the children of men. (D&C 19:16-19; italics added.)

Elder James E. Talmage discussed the suffering of Christ in his profound work, *Jesus the Christ*:

Christ's agony in the garden is unfathomable by the finite mind, both as to intensity and cause. The thought that He suffered through fear of death is untenable. Death to Him was preliminary to resurrection and triumphal return to the Father from whom He had come, and to a state of glory even beyond what He had before possessed; and, moreover, it was within His power to lay down His life voluntarily. He struggled and groaned under a burden such as no other being who has lived on earth might even conceive as possible. It was not physical pain, nor mental anguish alone, that caused Him to suffer such torture as to produce an extrusion of blood from every pore; but a spiritual agony of soul such as only God was capable of experiencing. No other man, however great his powers of physical or mental endurance, could have suffered so; for his human organism would have succumbed, and synocope would have produced unconsciousness and welcome oblivion. In that hour of anguish Christ met and overcame all the horrors that Satan, "the prince of this world" could inflict. The frightful struggle incident to the temptations immediately following the Lord's baptism was surpassed and overshadowed by this supreme contest with the powers of evil. . . .

At the ninth hour, or about three in the afternoon, a loud voice, surpassing the most anguished cry of physical suffering issued from the central cross, rending the dreadful darkness. It was the voice of the Christ: *"Eloi, Eloi, lama sabachthani? which is, being interpreted, My God, my God, why hast thou forsaken me?"* What mind of man can fathom the significance of that awful cry? It seems, that in addition to the fearful suffering incident to crucifixion, the agony of Gethsemane had recurred, intensified beyond human power to endure. In that bitterest hour the dying Christ was alone, alone in most terrible reality. That the supreme sacrifice of the Son might be consummated in all its fulness, the Father seems to have withdrawn the support of His immediate Presence, leaving to the Savior of men the glory of complete victory over the forces of sin and death. . . .

If the soldier's spear was thrust into the left side of the Lord's body and actually penetrated the heart, the outrush of "blood and water" observed by John is further evidence of a cardiac rupture; for it is known that in the rare instances of death resulting from a breaking of any part of the wall of the heart, blood accumulates within the pericardium, and there undergoes a change by which the corpuscles separate as a partially clotted mass from the almost colorless, watery serum. . . .

The present writer believes that the Lord Jesus died of a broken heart. The psalmist sang in dolorous measure according to his inspired prevision of the Lord's passion: "Reproach hath broken my heart; and I am full of heaviness: and I looked for some to take pity, but there was none; and for comforters, but I found none. . . ." (Salt Lake City: Deseret Book Co., 1977, pp. 613, 660-61, 668-69.)

It is significant that the prophets spend as much time as they do relating the suffering of our Savior and Redeemer. We can only surmise that it is important for us to understand and know of it.

Many have wondered that an all-powerful God would require the suffering of his most beloved Son as the method of redeeming his children. As we read the prophets, we see that there are two significant reasons. First, the eternal law of justice requires suffering as payment for sin. (Alma 42:15, D&C 19:16-19.) Second, a more subtle but equally important reason is that through his sacrifice and suffering Christ would be able to draw all men to him, he would be able to enter into their hearts and "wring out" their souls. In no other way could the hearts of men be broken and their lives so changed that the Holy Ghost could come upon them.

"And my Father sent me that I might be lifted up upon the cross; and after that I had been lifted up upon the cross; that I might draw all men unto me." (3 Nephi 27:14.)

If there had been an easier way, I'm sure the Father would have chosen it to save his Son the agony he endured. But there was no other way.

Punishment, Justice, and Mercy

If men do not partake of the atonement of Christ, they must literally suffer for their sins in payment of the demands of justice. As already related, the Lord has explained that he suffered "for all, that they might not suffer if they would repent; but if they would not repent they must suffer even as I." (D&C 19:16-17.)

Alma tells us why this must be.

> Now, repentance could not come unto men except there were a punishment, which also was eternal as the life of the soul should be, affixed opposite to the plan of happiness, which was as eternal also as the life of the soul.
>
> Now, how could a man repent except he should sin? How could he sin if there was no law? How could there be a law save there was a punishment?
>
> Now, there was a punishment affixed, and a just law given, which brought remorse of conscience unto man.
>
> Now, if there was no law given — if a man murdered he should die — would he be afraid he would die if he should murder?
>
> And also, if there was no law given against sin men would not be afraid to sin.
>
> And if there was no law given, if men sinned what could justice do, or mercy either, for they would have no claim upon the creature?
>
> But there is a law given, and a punishment affixed, and a repentance granted; which repentance mercy claimeth;

otherwise, justice claimeth the creature and executeth the law, and the law inflicteth the punishment; if not so, the works of justice would be destroyed, and God would cease to be God.

But God ceaseth not to be God, and mercy claimeth the penitent, and mercy cometh because of the atonement; and the atonement bringeth to pass the resurrection of the dead; and the resurrection of the dead bringeth back men into the presence of God; and thus they are restored into his presence, to be judged according to their works, according to the law and justice.

For behold, justice exerciseth all his demands, and also mercy claimeth all which is her own; and thus, none but the truly penitent are saved. (Alma 42:16-24.)

Why does justice require the payment of suffering? Is God vindictive? No! God could not be vindictive and continue to be God. President Joseph Fielding Smith said: "The Lord does not delight in punishment, however there is the demand of justice which must be met, and therefore the wicked are forced to suffer, and this suffering helps to cleanse them from their sins." (*Answers to Gospel Questions*, Melchizedek Priesthood Course of Study, 1972-73, p. 91.) However, the cleansing that comes from suffering for one's own sins is not comparable to the cleansing that can come from Christ, which leaves a person without spot or blemish and worthy to dwell in the presence of God. It does, however, cleanse one enough to allow him a measure of salvation and the ability to live with himself in some degree of happiness throughout the eternities.

A Broken Heart

A knowledge of Christ's suffering is literally the key to a person's being able to offer the sacrifice of a broken heart. This is why the prophets spend a significant amount of time discussing his infinite sacrifice. Through deep and fervent prayer, and through a searching scriptural study of Jesus Christ, we come to know him. One cannot walk where he walked, experience vicariously what he experienced, without knowing him. And to know him is to love him.

Elder Melvin J. Ballard, a late member of the Council of the Twelve, once related a great experience that demonstrates how knowing Christ is loving him:

Two years ago, about this time, I had been on the Fort Peck Reservation for several days with the brethren, solving the problems connected with our work among the Lamanites. Many questions arose that we had to settle. There was no precedent for us to follow, and we just had to go to the Lord and tell Him our troubles, and get inspiration and help from Him. On this occasion I had sought the Lord, under such circumstances, and that night I received a wonderful manifestation and impression which has never left me. I was carried to this place — into this room. I saw myself here with you. I was told there was another privilege that was to be mine; and I was led into a room where I was informed I was to meet someone. As I entered the room I saw, seated on a raised platform, the most glorious being I have ever conceived of, and was taken forward to be introduced to Him. As I approached He smiled, called my name, and stretched out His hands toward me. If I live to be a million years old I shall never forget that smile. He put His arms around me and kissed me, as He took me into His bosom, and He blessed me until my whole being was thrilled. As He finished I fell at His feet, and there saw the marks of the nails; and as I kissed them, with deep joy swelling through my whole being, I felt that I was in heaven indeed. The feeling that came to my heart then was: Oh! if I could live worthy, though it would require four-score years, so that in the end when I have finished I could go into His presence and receive the feeling that I *then* had in His presence, I would give everything that I am and ever hope to be! (*Melvin J. Ballard, Crusader for Righteousness*, Salt Lake City: Bookcraft, 1966, p. 66.)

To love Christ, to know of his suffering, and then to realize that through our disobedience we personally, literally contributed to his suffering — this produces a broken heart and a contrite spirit.

I would like to relate a story in which you are the chief character. I am indebted to a great friend and teacher, George W. Pace of the Brigham Young University faculty, for this excellent illustration on how one can personally bring the power of Christ's atonement into his life and truly come to the point of offering a broken heart. Picture in your mind the following:

As a result of your study of the scriptures you are left with a lively desire to bring the power of the atonement into your life, to receive his image in your countenance, to receive a remission of your sins and to be born of fire and the Holy Ghost. Night after night you wrestle with the Lord, pleading for the gift of repentance and forgiveness to come into your life. Over a period of days, months, or maybe even years, you try to improve your life so that you are worthy of this gift.

One evening, as you kneel in an attitude of fasting and mighty prayer, you notice the room growing lighter. Soon you see a person standing before you and recognize him as your Savior. He smiles as he softly speaks your name. You fall at his feet in worship as did Elder Ballard. He raises you to your feet and asks if you truly desire to be forgiven of your sins.

Your heart leaps with joy; perhaps he has come to forgive you! You answer, "Yes."

"But we have one thing yet to do before I can grant you that great blessing."

You reply, "Anything, anything you ask!"

"Will you take me by the hand and walk back through the corridors of your life as we review the events of your life together." Now you are not so sure of your desire for forgiveness. There are events you would rather not have the Savior see, especially while you are in his presence.

With his gentle urging you pull your courage together, cast aside the cover of false pride, throw your shoulders back, and agree to proceed. You take the Savior by the hand and begin to journey back through your life. Things go well for a while; then suddenly you see ahead an incident you're not proud of. You slow down, but with gentle encouragement you proceed. There it is!

Shame and embarrassment fill your being. You can't look at the Savior! But then you notice that he is no longer standing at your side. You look more closely. There, kneeling, is your Savior and Redeemer. No longer is he smiling; you see sorrow and agony written on his face. You see blood coming from the pores of his body. You see the Son of God suffering for your disobedience. Embarrassment and shame leave, and your heart fills with remorse. He whom you love as you love no one else is suffering as you have never seen anyone suffer before, and he is suffering because of you.

The same thing happens as one by one you review other events of your life of which you are ashamed. Finally your heart breaks; you are crushed spiritually! You offer everything to him, for you recognize that he has bought you with his blood!

One need not literally behold the Savior to experience a broken heart. However, we do have to deeply realize his suffering on our behalf. When we have offered broken hearts, we can then be forgiven of our sins. We can then be worthy of the baptism of fire and of the Holy Ghost. We are then new creatures born of the Holy Ghost. We are the begotten sons and daughters of Christ, with his image in our countenances. We have then received "this mighty change in our hearts."

Forgiveness

It is important that we understand that a knowledge of forgiveness comes with true and complete repentance. Young Alma is an excellent example of this. Though he had been instrumental in diverting many souls from the teachings of Christ, the magnitude of his angelic encounter softened his hard heart and rebellious nature, enabling him to acknowledge and accept responsibility for his guilt. Consider the words of his confession as he pleaded for mercy, for release from the bonds of iniquity:

> But I was racked with eternal torment, for my soul was harrowed up to the greatest degree and racked with all my sins.
>
> Yea, I did remember all my sins and iniquities, for which I was tormented with the pains of hell; yea, I saw that I had rebelled against my God, and that I had not kept his holy commandments.
>
> Yea, and I had murdered many of his children, or rather led them away into destruction; yea, and in fine so great had been my iniquities, that the very thought of coming into the presence of my God did rack my soul with inexpressible horror. (Alma 36:12-14.)

But when, in anguish, he cried out to Jesus for mercy, he "could remember [his] pains no more." "And oh, what joy," he says, "and what marvelous light I did behold; yea, my soul was filled with joy as exceeding as was my pain!" (Alma 36:19-20.)

We have examined many incidents of repentance in the Book of Mormon, and in every one those involved knew of their forgiveness and understood that they had become clean and pure before the Lord. (See Enos 2-5; Mosiah 4:2-3, 11-12; 27:23-28.) The common thread running through all of these accounts is the fact that a knowledge of the remission of sins came when the people were sufficiently humbled and offered a broken heart.

President Spencer W. Kimball pleaded with the youth of the Church to seek a knowledge of the forgiveness of their sins:

> As soon as one has an inner conviction of his sins, he should go to the Lord in "mighty prayer" as did Enos, and never cease his supplications until he shall, like Enos, receive the assurance that his sins have been forgiven by the Lord. It is unthinkable that God absolves serious sins upon a few requests. He is likely to wait until there has been long sustained repentance as evidenced by a willingness to comply with all His other requirements. ("Be Ye Clean," p. 9.)

I remember giving a talk in a BYU student ward on a Sunday when President Marion G. Romney made a surprise visit to our ward. I spoke of the experience of Enos and the need that we all have to know that we have been forgiven. During the course of my remarks I stressed several times that we didn't have to hear a voice as Enos did, but that we would know by the power of the Spirit when we had been forgiven. At the conclusion of the meeting President Romney was asked to speak to the congregation. I remember vividly how emphatically he testified, "I want you to know that you *can* hear a voice!"

President Harold B. Lee gave us some valuable instruction on receiving forgiveness of sins. He said: "If the time comes when you have done all that you can to repent of your sins, whoever you are, wherever you are, and have made amends and restitution to the best of your ability; if it be something that will affect your standing in the Church and you have gone to the proper authorities, then you will want that confirming answer as to whether or not the Lord has accepted of you. In your soul-searching, *if you seek for and you find that peace of conscience, by that token you may know that the Lord has accepted of your repentance.*" ("Stand Ye in Holy Places," *Ensign*, July 1973, p. 122; italics added.)

Cleansed by Christ

Sometimes we are taught that we cannot be completely cleansed from our sins; we can "pull the nails out but the holes are still there in the board." Such a philosophy seems to me to question the Savior's ability to cleanse. The vision that came to Peter preparing him to receive the gentile, Cornelius, could possibly apply here. In the vision

Peter was presented with foods that were forbidden by the Mosaic law and was commanded to eat. "But Peter said, Not so, Lord; for I have never eaten any thing that is common or unclean." Then the voice spoke to Peter again, saying, "What God hath cleansed, that call not thou common." (Acts 10:14-15.)

Isaiah also confirmed that what Christ cleanses is clean when he recorded: "Come now, and let us reason together, saith the Lord: though your sins be as scarlet, they shall be as white as snow; though they be red like crimson, they shall be as wool." (Isaiah 1:18.)

Alma's testimony of the power of the atonement of Christ supports the idea of a total cleansing:

> Therefore they were called after this holy order, and were sanctified, and their garments were washed white through the blood of the Lamb.
>
> Now they, after being sanctified by the Holy Ghost, having their garments made white, being pure and spotless before God, could not look upon sin save it were with abhorrence; and there were many, exceeding great many, who were made pure and entered into the rest of the Lord their God. (Alma 13:11-12.)

Perhaps the most comforting of all the Savior's statements about repentance is that when we have fully partaken of the sacrifice of Christ through repentance the Lord forgets our sins: "Behold, he who has repented of his sins, the same is forgiven, and I, the Lord, remember them no more." (D&C 58:42.)

If the Lord forgets our sins after he has forgiven us, then we likewise can forget them, and, as long as we remain repentant, we will never be confronted with them again. Thus it seems that the old allegory of the nail holes left in the board does not square with the scriptures. Now, I fear some may say, "If the atonement of Christ can cleanse and purify and make one as though he had not sinned, why not enjoy life: 'eat, drink, and be merry,' and in our later lives we can repent and be as though we had not sinned." To them I offer the following, for theirs is the logic of Satan and it has crucial flaws:

— when we knowingly disobey, we, by our own choice, separate ourselves from Christ and the Spirit of God. We set up a momentum toward evil that we may never be able to reverse.

— in the circumstance described, we place ourselves in subjection to the power of Satan, and once having gained power over us he can create great barriers that will make it difficult for the Spirit of God to provide the motivation to change our course.

— the difficulty of repentance increases with the seriousness of our sins. At best it is not an easy process. (See Alma 36.)

— sin brings unhappiness and the loss of the Spirit of the Lord. We lose the "peace that passeth all understanding" and the joy of a righteous life. These lost years and the good that we could have achieved can never be returned. If there are holes left in the board after repentance, they would represent such loss.

— if we want to live where God lives, we must develop the character attributes he has. This takes time. The years we may spend in sinful living rob us of time.

An excellent summarizing testimony to this section is provided by President Joseph F. Smith:

> Men cannot forgive their own sins; they cannot cleanse themselves from the consequences of their sins. Men can stop sinning and can do right in the future, and so far their acts are acceptable before the Lord and worthy of consideration. But who shall repair the wrongs they have done to themselves and to others, which it seems impossible for them to repair themselves? By the atonement of Jesus Christ the sins of the repentant shall be washed away; though they be crimson they shall be made white as wool. This is the promise given to you. (*Gospel Doctrine,* Salt Lake City: Deseret Book, 1977, pp. 98-99.)

5   *The First Principle*

W hen asked, "What is the first principle of the gospel?" many
people will immediately respond, "Faith." Faith is not the
whole answer. According to Joseph Smith, the first principle of the
gospel is "Faith in the Lord Jesus Christ." The difference is real. While
it is important to have faith in Joseph Smith, faith that the Book of
Mormon is true, faith in the Church, faith in the present-day prophet,
faith in these areas is not the first principle.

The previous chapter related the ability to truly repent to a person's ability to love Christ. In fact, while a person could cease sinning
without knowing the Savior, it is impossible to repent unto forgiveness
without a knowledge of him. Repentance is totally related to the depth
of love, conviction, or faith that one has for Jesus Christ.

Just as repentance is dependent upon faith in Christ, being born
of the Spirit is dependent upon repentance and on having completed
the ordinances of baptism and confirmation. Mormon ties these concepts together:

> The first fruits of repentance is baptism; and baptism com-
> eth by faith unto the fulfilling the commandments; and the
> fulfilling the commandments bringeth remission of sins;
>
> And the remission of sins bringeth meekness, and
> lowliness of heart; and because of meekness and lowliness

of heart cometh the visitation of the Holy Ghost, which Comforter filleth with hope and perfect love, which love endureth by diligence unto prayer, until the end shall come, when all the saints shall dwell with God. (Moroni 8:25-26.)

Joseph Smith with just a little different wording said the same thing:

We believe that through the Atonement of Christ, all mankind may be saved, by obedience to the laws and ordinances of the Gospel.

We believe that the first principles and ordinances of the Gospel are: first, Faith in the Lord Jesus Christ; second, Repentance; third, Baptism by immersion for the remission of sins; fourth, Laying on of hands for the gift of the Holy Ghost. (Articles of Faith 3 and 4.)

This entire book really deals with nothing more than faith in the Lord Jesus Christ, repentance, baptism by immersion for the remission of sin, and receiving the Holy Ghost by the laying on of hands. When Joseph Smith taught, "Teach nothing but faith and repentance," he saw these as the fundamental elements that would bring everything else into focus.

To Love Christ

One of the most popular songs in the blasphemous rock opera *Jesus Christ Superstar* is "I Don't Know How to Love Him." The beauty of the melody is in total contrast to the blasphemy of the lyrics. However, the title may reflect the deep concern of many Latter-day Saints. Indeed, how do we develop a love for Christ? What kind of love do we have for him? Is it deep and moving or is it academic and remote?

Think of the experience of Elder Melvin J. Ballard, reported in the previous chapter. The love expressed by Elder Ballard is so poignant that the written words bring tears to the eyes and chills to the spine. But Elder Ballard's love didn't begin with this experience, although it may have been intensified by it. His powerful and motivating love for the Savior was evident from his sermons prior to this particular event. In fact, this experience came because he had such a deep love for Christ, not because the Lord wanted to give him that love. In any case, his experience gives us a frame of reference by which we can measure the status of our own condition. However, the key question may remain: "I don't know how to love him."

To Know Christ

Abraham was given the privilege of viewing the premortal existence, and as he beheld the "noble and great ones" there was only one that was "like unto God." (See Abraham 3:22-24.) Many of God's children are "noble and great," but Jesus Christ is the greatest of them all.

The power of Christ is partially evident as we look up into the heavens on a starry night and realize that our sun is merely one of approximately 100 billion other suns in our Milky Way galaxy. Our galaxy is about 100,000 light years across — too far to even comprehend in terms of miles.

The power of Christ becomes more evident from the great vision of Moses, wherein God said to him: "Worlds without number have I created; . . . *and by the son I created them,* which is mine Only Begotten." (Moses 1:33; italics added.)

Christ had the power and the knowledge to create "worlds without number," and yet he willingly offered himself as a sacrifice to suffer as no man can comprehend. How can one doubt his love for us?

The Savior is indeed the foundation of our religion. As Joseph Smith declared: "The fundamental principles of our religion are the testimony of the Apostles and Prophets, concerning Jesus Christ, that He died, was buried, and rose again the third day, and ascended into heaven; and all other things which pertain to our religion are only appendages to it." (*Teachings of the Prophet Joseph Smith*, Salt Lake City: Deseret Book Co., 1972, p. 121.)

It is easier to see how central Jesus is to our religion if we look at it as if he had never atoned for our sins. Without that atonement
— obedience would lose its value, since without him we still could not be cleansed. The smallest infraction would condemn us.
— the ordinances would lose their value. All of them — baptism, confirmation, the sacrament, the endowment — center in him.
— the priesthood would lose its value. Its power rests in Christ.
— the Church would no longer hold any value. Without Christ there would be no hope in this life or hereafter.
Elder James E. Talmage writes: "However incomplete may be our

comprehension of the scheme of redemption through Christ's vicarious sacrifice in all its parts, we cannot reject it without becoming infidel; for it stands as the fundamental doctrine of all scripture, the very essence of the spirit of prophecy and revelation, the most prominent of all the declarations of God unto man." (*Articles of Faith*, Salt Lake City: Deseret Book Co., 1977, p. 77.)

We need to ponder in our hearts the great testimonies of Christ given in the scriptures. We need to fast with the specific purpose that we might come to know the Savior more completely. We need to pray and wrestle with the Lord to help us to be worthy to know our Redeemer. Of all the requirements that will bring the knowledge of Christ into our hearts, mighty prayer will bring the greatest success; but all areas working together will pave the way.

A Modern Witness

I now relate one final account that outlines in a beautiful way the entire process of being born again. I cannot document this account or personally vouch for its authenticity; I received a copy of it second or third hand, and it contained no note of authorship. But it certainly rings true and in every detail fits my understanding of the sequence of events that brings us to the spiritual rebirth. The sister relating this account may have desired to remain anonymous so that it wouldn't appear that she was boasting of her spiritual experience.

All my life I have had a love of the scriptures. I have enjoyed reading all the standard works, and have known the thrill of excitement of discussing the different points of doctrine and finding some new piece of knowledge which I had not known before.

However, I have never understood the Atonement. I knew that there was something that I must learn about it, but I had never had a teacher who could explain it to me — at least to the extent that I could comprehend it. For several years as I have taken of the sacrament I have prayed that I could understand the Atonement, but no understanding came to me. . . .

As I sat in class that night, the subject of the Atonement came up and I seized the opportunity to ask my teacher, "Do you understand the Atonement?"

"Yes, I believe I do," came the answer. . . .

"Then tell me about it," I said. And I was hardly able to contain my excitement because I thought that at last perhaps my prayers would be answered.

He led me with scripture. First, one in the Doctrine and Covenants, then one in the Bible, then back to the Book of Mormon. Then to the Pearl of Great Price. I cannot remember the chapters or the verses where these things were found because I was so intent in my concentration on the matter itself that I paid no attention. But I was conscious of the excitement growing within me, for I was beginning to understand things which I had read before but never understood. It was as though a light were beginning to flash on in my mind. (I had been aware of this light flashing on before, during my study and conversations and during some especially spiritual sacrament meetings, but before I could fully grasp it, the light would be gone again. I could not recognize it for what it was.) Several hours and many, many scriptures went by, but I was not conscious of time. I struggled within myself to understand. It took all of my powers of concentration.

Occasionally my teacher would stop and say, "Now does that light stay on for you?"

I would answer, "No, but keep talking." I was afraid that any interruption might break my chain of thought and the light would go off completely, never to flash on again. Several times during the evening the thought left me completely, and I was left in a void of darkness; at these times I prayed with all my soul that I could understand. For I now realized that I was on the threshold of a most tremendous thing. I did not want to take the chance of losing it.

One of the main things that had me stumped was — if God is all-powerful (as I had always believed that he was), why must there be an atonement made? Being all-powerful, could he not simply say — "You are redeemed from the fall," and we would be redeemed? The answer was beautifully pointed out for me in the forty-second chapter of Alma.

I realized also that man was naturally carnal and sensual because of the fall, and in this condition he could never dwell in the presence of a perfect being, but I could not comprehend how the Savior could cleanse us. Would we simply say to Jesus, "Here, take my sins!" and then we would be clean?

My teacher began to rehearse for me the great suffering of our Lord, the terrible suffering of both the body and spirit to the extent that it caused him, even God, to bleed at every pore! It was a suffering which he willingly took upon himself, and he paid the penalty for each sin committed, even from the fall of Adam to the end of the Millennium. It was a suffering both physical and spiritual, which was so terrible that it caused his great heart to break. And to think that all the time he could have withdrawn! At any time he could have said, "Be gone," and all his accusers would have withered as a dried reed. He had the power over death, and could have, at the slightest wish, saved himself — but he would not! He even refused the narcotic vinegar that was pressed to his lips that his suffering might be somewhat relieved: and this he did because of his love for us!

To realize that my own sins were amongst those which gave him pain brought me down into the depths of sorrow. I wept because of my sins — my angry thoughts, my unholy thoughts, my backbiting, the hate and anger and greed which I had felt within me and allowed to canker my soul. I wept because of them, not only because I was sorry that I had had them (for I had always been sorry before), but because I knew that I had added to my Savior's suffering. . . . My heart was borne down into the dust with this new realization, and I cried. I found myself wishing that some suffering might come upon me that I could in some way pay the penalty for my own transgressions and thus rid my conscience of the guilt of the blood of him who died. I had been evil — happy to do wrong. Yes, I'd even gloried in it at times. Then afterwards I would perhaps feel a little twinge of conscience and vow that I would do better. But I did not realize that by my wicked ways I added to the incomprehensible suffering of him on that dreadful day!

Thus in my sorrow I wished for some suffering to come upon myself so that I could pay, not him! But I have known no suffering. No great sorrow has come into my life. No sorrow has come to me because of my transgressions. I have gone my merry way, basking in his love and kindness, sinned and was flippant, sorry, and then sinned again. And at none of these times did I realize that I, in even my slightest evils, was causing some of the suffering of my Lord.

Suddenly there stood before me a bright picture of all my sins. Not that I was evil with regard to our civil or moral laws, for I knew that in these things I had not erred, but in the light of this new thing I was painfully aware of all my carelessness — yes, of even blasphemy! For I now realized how irreverent I had been in remembering the emblems of his death!

How many times I had looked at his picture, and said, under my breath, "Yes, Lord, I do love thee!" Then I had tossed his holy sacrament into my mouth and immediately begun wishing for a dress like the one the woman in front of me was wearing!

How many times had I prayed during the sacrament (for ever since I was a little girl I had been taught to pray during the sacrament) and said, "Dear Lord, I thank thee for all that I have, and now please give me this, and give me that." And never once did I thank him for his gift to me — or ask his forgiveness for my sins!

Or how many times had I come to the sacrament table and asked forgiveness for my own transgressions, and still held a grudge against those who had transgressed against me!

All these things and many, many others stood bright and clear before me, and I was weak and sick with shame!

How he must despise me for my hypocrisy! How he must despise me, for I was even worse than those at Calvary! They at least had not protested their love then turned their faces! But even in my darkest moment I knew that he did not despise me. For even then — in fact, then more than ever — I could feel the warmth and peace of his love.

Then, suddenly, that light flashed on bright and perfect and as clear as crystal. "This is it!" I exulted. This is the love of God!

My heart leaped with joy! My heart leaped up, and I wept again, but this time not with sorrow and shame, but with joy, for I had tasted of his love and forgiveness, and now I knew what it was! It was this same thing which I had felt on many occasions before, a feeling of love and warmth

— but I had not recognized it and thus had "denied the Spirit!" . . .

I had indeed been "born again," and this time not of the water, but of the Spirit. My first reaction beyond my pangs of joy was of astonishment. Even though it was late at night, I wanted to run out and pound on the doors of the houses and shout, "I know about these things, I know about it — do you know about it?" I restrained myself, however, and instead of running and shouting, I sat and meditated. But I still could not, and cannot to this day, get over my surprise, for I had been in the Church all my life, and had loved the gospel, and had not dreamed that there was so much more to be had.

The first thing which came to my mind during my meditation was that I had never before known the real meaning of our fourth Article of Faith. Faith in the Lord Jesus Christ and repentance now means: a knowledge (and I do not say belief because I had always believed) of our Savior and his atonement to the extent that we are brought down into the depths of repentance, thus to plead for his mercy upon us; for this is the only way we can enter again into the presence of the perfect God.

And I know that he can purify us, for I have felt his cleansing power. How can I be filled with hate or envy or malice when I know that his Spirit is upon me and I am conscious of his love?

Then there flooded into my mind verse after verse of scripture — scripture which I had known since childhood, scripture which I had loved and often repeated. And to my surprise they had a new meaning. In the light of the new knowledge which I received, these scriptures had taken on a new significance. It was as though I was seeing them for the first time. I thought of the words of Paul: "Now we see through a glass, darkly, but then face to face: now I know in part; but then shall I know even as also I am known."

I cannot begin to enumerate the scriptures which coursed through my mind, but they were many. There were so many that I could not even fathom that I had known so many, and they all had bearing on this one thing — the Atonement.

I had felt this power and witnessed this presence, and for the first time I understood *how* we are cleansed by the refiner's fire, how the gift of tongues comes, how Joseph Smith could prophesy in the name of the Lord, how the lame are made to walk, the blind to see, the dead raised. I even understood how the brother of Jared could remove the veil so that he could see Jesus. And all these things I could see, because at last I had been able to exercise my faith as a "grain of mustard seed."

As the full realization of this surged upon me, I said to my teacher, "I am afraid of this thing," for I knew that Joseph Smith and Sidney Rigdon had seen a vision in which they saw how Satan makes war on the Saints who have been made partakers of this power. And he and his hosts encompass them and try to lead them away.

I knew that I had received a witness of my Savior. And I knew that I could not sin again without doing so with a full knowledge that I was heaping agony on him who was lifted up, and thus helping to crucify him to myself. And should Satan lead me so far away as to deny this, I would be denying the Holy Ghost which bore witness of it.

I fear and tremble to think of this, and know that I must cleave to the word of God with all my soul, for I know that I am weak — quick to pride!

I do not say these things to boast, because I know that this witness had come to a great many other people at a much younger age than I am, and I know that it is because of my pride and my inability to humble myself that it could not come to me before.

The next day as I began my day's work, I could not resist the urge to sit down and read the scriptures, and to my astonishment the true meaning of these things flooded into my understanding. I suddenly knew what all these things meant — and I knew that I knew! I saw for the first time what all these prophets were trying to say. And they were all trying to say one thing — that Jesus died that we might live!

Now I know what it is that the writers would say again and again: "And it is marvelous before our eyes — and we were astonished and the eyes of our understanding were opened and it is the faith which we have had that has brought us to this great knowledge, whereby we do rejoice with exceeding great joy."

As I went about my day's duties, my heart swelled up in an unsurpassable love for those about me, even the strangers whom I passed on the street. My heart went out in love to them, and I couldn't help looking at them and wondering if they knew what I knew.

To my surprise not only had my spirit been quickened, but all of my senses also. I found a new enjoyment in the landscape about me. I saw beauty in all the commonplace things which had meant nothing to me before. The same old songs now seemed new and beautiful. And even colors seemed brighter and more vibrant because my senses were quickened so that I could enjoy them more!

I thought to myself, "This is the means by which all things come — not by man's own knowledge but by the Holy Ghost which bears record of Him!"

And I must sing like Job of old — "I know that my redeemer liveth, and that he shall stand at the latter day upon the earth"; and if I am true and faithful and endure to the end, "though after my skin worms destroy this body, yet in my flesh shall I see God."

6

A Great Work of Love

M uch confusion exists in the religious world on the doctrines of salvation, grace, justification, and obedience to moral law. A lack of understanding even seems to persist within the membership of The Church of Jesus Christ of Latter-day Saints. The important questions are:

Are we saved by the grace of Christ?

Does obedience to law cleanse from sin?

Do we merit or deserve Christ's sacrifice?

What is the interrelationship between the grace of Christ and obedience to law?

Some Latter-day Saints go so far as to say that Christ's grace applies only to the resurrection of our physical bodies; while our good works alone qualify us for exaltation in the celestial kingdom of our Heavenly Father. I have in my library a book written for LDS missionaries stating that the grace of Christ relates to the resurrection only. On the other extreme there are sectarian ministers who say that keeping God's commandments is not vital to salvation. In other words, they say you do not have to obey God's laws or commandments to be acceptable to him. To illustrate, let me quote from a sermon given in the 1970s by a minister of a large Michigan congregation.

But, people, when you live by the law, God is always

predictable. This is why we like the law. We think we know what God is going to be like and what He thinks and what He wants us to do. We can corral God then because we've got him locked up in His own law. He has said this is the way it's going to be and that's the way it's going to be, friend, but it's a lie! It's not the truth. God will be himself and He will choose to do what He will choose to do. And He would choose to love whom He would love. And we don't like it that way. You have to understand how insidiously this thing works. We are given over to self-delusions when we choose to live by the law rather than by grace. A man living by the law has a measurable device against which to measure his life; the law says so. His life is like such. And he looks at the two and he says, "Ha! Ha! I'm not quite what I ought to be, so I will change myself. I will be something other than I am. I'm going to be what the law tells me to be." And so he starts living that way. And that device is a good thing. It's measurable; it's predictable. It's understandable — no surprises, no gimmicks, nothing. . . . And so we begin to accelerate in our righteousness and our achievements at that point. And we become closer and closer to living to the law and we become less and less a human being. And you know why? Because we live by *imitation*, and success comes to us by imitation. By being something other than what we really are, we think we are going to merit the love of God and we're going to find happiness. People, it's false to live by imitation. You can't be something you are not. God doesn't call you to the law. He doesn't call you to such *phoniness*. He comes to you in His grace and says, "I love you the way you are. Why can't you learn to love yourself? I accept you as you are. Why can't you accept yourself?" And we don't want it that way. We cast the grace, and with it the truth, aside and we insist on being phonies — living by imitation, living to be someone else or something other than what we are. . . . Thus, the person who lives by grace becomes himself. . . .

This point of view is usually justified by two significant scriptures — first, the incident of the thief on the cross in which Jesus said, "To day shalt thou be with me in paradise" (Luke 23:43), and second, Paul's statement, "For by grace are ye saved through faith; and that not of yourselves; it is the gift of God: not of works, lest any man should boast" (Ephesians 2:8-9).

These scriptures certainly express the truth — but a doctrine must be established in the full light of all that God has revealed, not just from a couple of isolated scriptures.

Is Obedience to Law Required?

Does our Father require obedience to the law? In answering that, we must first define sin. John, the beloved apostle, states:

> Whosoever committeth sin transgresseth also the law: *for sin is the transgression of the law*.

> He that committeth sin is of the devil; for the devil sinneth from the beginning. For this purpose the Son of God was manifested, that he might destroy the works of the devil.

> *Whosoever is born of God doth not commit sin [transgress the law]*; for his seed remaineth in him: and he cannot sin, because he is born of God. (1 John 3:4; 8-9; italics added.)

Since sin is transgression of the law, the real question is: Can we be saved while being disobedient to law? In the preceding scripture, John clearly answered this question. The scriptures are replete with statements that man cannot be saved in sin. The Savior himself repeatedly states the necessity of obedience to the commandments.

> And he said unto [the rich young man], . . . *if thou wilt enter into life, keep the commandments*.

> He saith unto him, Which? Jesus said, Thou shalt do no murder, Thou shalt not commit adultery, Thou shalt not steal, Thou shalt not bear false witness,

> Honour thy father and thy mother: and, Thou shalt love thy neighbour as thyself.

> The young man saith unto him, All these things have I kept from my youth up: what lack I yet?

> Jesus said unto him, If thou wilt be perfect, go and sell that thou hast, and give to the poor, and thou shalt have treasure in heaven: and come and follow me. (Matthew 19:17-21; italics added.)

> Not everyone that saith unto me, Lord, Lord, shall enter into the kingdom of heaven; but he that doeth the will of my Father which is in heaven. (Matthew 7:21.)

Does this sound as if the Lord accepts everyone as they are? To be approved of him we not only have to accept Christ but we have to keep his commandments. In fact, Christ not only required that his followers live the commandments, but he took the Ten Commandments and added a standard to them that would bring his followers up to a new level of righteousness. The commandment against murder was no longer enough — the Lord commanded his disciples against even anger. (Matthew 5:21-22.) No longer was it sufficient to avoid adultery — the Lord commanded against lust as well. (Matthew 5:27-28.) No longer was it sufficient just to love one's neighbor. Now the Saint would be expected to love his enemy. (Matthew 5:43-44.)

And so it was with many aspects of the Mosaic law. The Lord reaffirmed the commandment — and then gave additional requirements. At the end of that section of the Sermon on the Mount he said: "Be ye therefore perfect, even as your Father which is in heaven is perfect." (Matthew 5:48.)

Do these things confirm that God accepts us as we are; or does he expect us to repent and accept a Christlike life? The basic message of the gospel preached by Jesus and the apostles was that of repentance. (See Luke 24:46-47.) Repentance implies a changed life.

Does Obedience Cleanse from Sin?

Why does God require obedience to his law? Does our obedience today cleanse from previous transgressions of the law? Many Latter-day Saints feel that that is the case. They feel that when we begin keeping the commandments we are automatically cleansed from our previous sins and thus become able to return to God's presence. But the prophets clearly say that such is a false understanding. Listen to Lehi: "And men are instructed sufficiently that they know good from evil. And the law is given unto men. *And by the law no flesh is justified* [*made acceptable*]; *or, by the law men are cut off.* Yea, by the temporal law they were cut off; and also, by the spiritual law they perish from that which is good, and become miserable forever." (2 Nephi 2:5; italics added.)

Hear also the martyr Abinadi: "*Salvation doth not come by the law alone;* and were it not for the atonement, which God himself shall make for the sins and iniquities of his people, that they must unavoidably perish, notwithstanding the law of Moses." (Mosiah 13:28; italics added.)

Thus we find the Book of Mormon prophets upholding Paul's position, in which he stated: "For all have sinned, and come short of the glory of God. Where is boasting then? It is excluded. By what law? of works? Nay: but by the law of faith. Therefore we conclude that a man is *justified by faith without the deeds of the law*." (Romans 3:23, 27-28; italics added.)

If obedience to law does not cleanse, why then obey the law? There are four profound reasons why. First, character development comes by obedience to eternal law. This is how we develop the godlike character attributes associated with each law. The Prophet Joseph taught that. "God himself, finding he was in the midst of spirits and glory, because he was more intelligent, saw proper to institute laws whereby the rest could have a privilege to advance like himself. . . . He has power to institute laws to instruct the weaker intelligences, that they may be exalted with himself." (*Teachings of the Prophet Joseph Smith*, Salt Lake City: Deseret Book, 1972, p. 354.)

Second, all of God's commandments will produce maximum happiness in this life for all of his children who will obey them. The prophets have said, "Wickedness never was happiness." (See Alma 41:10.) Thus obedience to the basic commandments produces the environment that brings joy to the soul. But anger, jealousy, greed, dishonesty, and immorality canker the soul and bring unhappiness and sorrow.

Third, but equally important, once having been cleansed from sin, obedience to law keeps us from further uncleanliness. In fact, had a person lived a perfect life without an infraction of a single law, as did Christ our Savior, he would not fall under the condemnation of law and the atonement of Christ would be unnecessary on his behalf (except to redeem him from physical death). But, unfortunately, as Paul states: "As it is written, There is none righteous, no, not one. For all have sinned, and come short of the glory of God." (Romans 3:10, 23.)

Thus, a *single* infraction brings us under the condemnation of law, unclean and unworthy of the presence of God. As James said, "For whosoever shall keep the whole law, and yet offend in one point, he is guilty of all." (James 2:10.)

A person cannot be cleansed by the process of repentance and forgiveness and then return to disobedience without nullifying the cleansing previously received. As the Lord said to some of the Saints in Joseph Smith's day: "I, the Lord, will not lay any sin to your charge; go your ways and sin no more; but unto that soul who sinneth shall the former sins return, saith the Lord your God." (D&C 82:7.)

Briefly, the fourth reason for keeping the commandments relates to the statement of Jesus, "If ye love me, keep my commandments." (John 14:15.) Before the Savior allows us to partake of his sacrifice and receive of his sanctifying influence, we must demonstrate our love and sincerity of purpose by obeying his will. We cannot say we love Christ and appreciate his efforts on our behalf, then deliberately mock him by disobedience. The saving influence of his grace is limited to those willing to pay the price of obedience. It should be kept in mind, however, that there are differing degrees of unworthiness or filthiness, depending upon the degree of our disobedience. The more unworthy we become, the more effort we need to expend to become clean in the sight of God.

What Cleanses from Sin

Remember, though, that our own efforts will only take us so far. Something more is needed.

Nephi explains: "For we labor diligently to write, to persuade our children, and also our brethren, to believe in Christ, and to be reconciled to God: *for we know that it is by grace that we are saved, after all we can do.*" (2 Nephi 25:23; italics added.)

And from Abinadi we leard that *"salvation doth not come by the law alone; and were it not for the atonement,* which God himself shall make for the sins and iniquities of his people, that *they must unavoidably perish,* notwithstanding the law of Moses." (Mosiah 13:28; italics added.)

By some profound, inexplicable process, Christ's infinite suffering in Gethsemane and on the cross somehow mediates the demands justice makes that disobedience must be compensated for by suffering. All sin and transgression of law, *past, present,* and *future,* have been paid by him. Thus, those who are obedient and thereby qualify for his grace are cleansed and able to enter the presence of God without spot or blemish. But it is his sacrifice, not our obedience, that cleanses from sin.

Since all have sinned and fallen under condemnation of law, none of us merit (or deserve) this cleansing power. It is a gift. As Aaron explained: "Since man had fallen *he could not merit anything of himself;* but the sufferings and death of Christ atone for their sins, through faith and repentance." (Alma 22:14; italics added.)

And Paul said, "By grace are ye saved through faith; and that not of yourselves: it is the gift of God: Not of works lest any man should boast." (Ephesians 2:8-9.)

Since we cannot merit the cleansing that can come from Christ, we can truly say we are saved by the grace of Christ. As Nephi declares: "Brethren, reconcile yourselves to the will of God, and not to the will of the devil and the flesh; and remember, after ye are reconciled unto God, that it is only in and through the grace of God that ye are saved." (2 Nephi 10:24.)

Without Christ's infinite sacrifice for the sins of man, could justice ever be satisfied? It could not. All who are under the bondage of sin are in debt to justice and are in no position to pay the price. But the Savior's love for us caused him to be willing to make the payment that purchased us from both death and hell. Truly we are "bought with a price." Truly we are "saved by grace," as the prophets have declared.

On what condition will he grant this great gift? We have already discussed the requirements. We gain access to the grace of Jesus Christ, first, by believing, accepting, and having great faith in Christ; second, by repenting with all our hearts — meaning that we have *broken hearts* and *contrite spirits* — and by walking in a newness of life, keeping the commandments of Christ. Third, baptism by water signs and seals the contract between Christ and the individual. Fourth, the gift of the Holy Ghost brings the process of conversion, which purges our souls, sanctifies, and brings a spiritual rebirth.

The Key to the Gospel

By what process can the power of the gospel be brought into our lives? There is one simple key — to know Jesus Christ, or to desire to know him, so that by study, fasting, and prayer Christ can be revealed to us. As we begin to know the Son of Man and begin to comprehend the love he had for us, then (and only then) will our hearts respond with a similar love, a love that produces a desire to obey.

"If ye love me, keep my commandments." (John 14:15.) As we begin to realize the pain and suffering we personally brought upon his pure, perfect body and soul, our love will cause our own hearts to break and reach a degree of contrition possible in no other way. We will then offer him our lives to do with as he will. Then a sure knowledge of our forgiveness will come into our hearts and produce "joy as exceeding as was [our] pain" (Alma 36:20), which forgiveness and joy come as a result of the grace and love of Christ.

7

A Perspective
of Life

Much of what we have discussed to this point has seemed to depreciate the importance of man, particularly as the carnal nature of man was outlined in chapter 4. Some may have felt that the position of man was diminished as we learned that people are naturally evil and as we read how Nephi cried, "O wretched man that I am!" It is important in this concluding chapter that we understand clearly man's position in the scheme of things, the importance of this mortal experience, and how the whole of it fits together.

Who Are You?

God leaves no doubt as to his view of man: "For behold, this is my work and my glory — to bring to pass the immortality and eternal life of man." (Moses 1:39.) God's whole purpose relates to the eternal position of man. We are his children, and if we will partake of the atonement of Christ he will help us to become like him. He would not have offered his Only Begotten Son for us if we were unimportant to him.

However, we cannot become puffed up in the knowledge of our relationship to God. Only as we totally submit our own will to God's will can he mold us, as clay, to become as he is. We must consider ourselves and our selfish desires as "less than the dust of the earth" as did the people of Zarahemla. (Mosiah 4:2.) Man is quick to pride and quick to selfishness.

The importance of mortal life is diminished by the nature of mortality itself. Who do you know best in all the world of mortality? Yourself, of course. Likewise, I know myself better than anyone else. Yet, even here, I wonder if our knowledge isn't dimmed by "seeing through the glass darkly".

Let me use myself for an example. My name is Richard Packham; I am forty-five years old. I remember well my mother and father. I can remember parts of my early childhood. But what about prior to my mortality? Who am I really? What or where was I fifty years ago? Ever so dimly my spirit pierces the curtain of memory and whispers that I was something, that I was somewhere.

> Our birth is but a sleep and a forgetting;
> The soul that rises with us, our life's star,
> Hath had elsewhere its setting,
> And cometh from afar;
> Not in entire forgetfulness,
> And not in utter nakedness,
> But trailing clouds of glory do we come
> From God, who is our home. . . .
>
> The homely nurse [Earth] doth all she can
> To make her foster-child, her inmate man,
> Forget the glories he hath known,
> And that imperial palace whence he came.

(William Wordsworth, "Ode: Intimations of Immortality," ll. 59-66, 82-85, in *Major British Writers*, New York: Harcourt, Brace & World, 1959, 2:99.)

I appreciate the poet, but more especially the prophets, through whom the veils are parted just a little more. Through them I can see dimly into the glory and splendor of my premortal existence.

But I don't want to speak of me. What about you? Where were you a hundred years ago? A thousand? Who were you? What was your name? What did you look like? What events did you experience? What associations did you form? Of course, the veil is not sufficiently parted to give complete answers to the questions raised. But we do know enough to place our life here in proper perspective.

What the Prophets Have Said

I can't tell you your name, nor do we know your age as a spirit child of Heavenly Parents, but I can tell you that you did live. The Lord said to Jeremiah: "Before I formed thee in the belly I knew thee; and before thou camest forth out of the womb I sanctified thee, and I ordained thee a prophet unto the nations." (Jeremiah 1:5.)

Likewise, the Lord implied to Job that the sons and daughters of God shouted for joy and sang together as the foundations of the earth were laid. (Job 38:3-7.)

We can tell you what you looked like in your premortal state. Jesus showed himself to man many times prior to his birth in Jerusalem almost two thousand years ago. One of the best accounts of such an appearance is recorded in Ether. The brother of Jared had such great faith that he saw the finger of the Lord. Then, because the brother of Jared's faith was so strong, the Lord revealed himself to him and said: "This body, which ye now behold, is the body of my spirit; and man have I created after the body of my spirit; and even as I appear unto thee to be in the spirit will I appear unto my people in the flesh." (Ether 3:16.)

This incident occurred more than two thousand years prior to the birth of Christ's mortal body. Notice that the Savior stated that his spirit had the same visual appearance as his physical body would have. In the same way, your spirit body looks like you, without the imperfections of mortality. The Lord confirmed this in a revelation to Joseph Smith: "That which is spiritual [is] in the likeness of that which is temporal," he said. "And that which is temporal [is] in the likeness of that which is spiritual; the spirit of man in the likeness of his person, as also the spirit of the beast, and every other creature which God has created." (D&C 77:2.)

We have also been given some insight into how old we are. "Man was also in the beginning with God," the Lord says. "Intelligence, or the light of truth, was not created or made, neither indeed can be." (D&C 93:29.)

The intelligence of man is eternal; he never had a beginning, nor will he have an end. Joseph Smith gave an eloquent discourse on the eternal nature of man in his King Follett funeral sermon, in which he elaborated on this scripture and declared that we were coeternal with our Heavenly Father as conscious, intelligent, active entities. (See *Teachings of the Prophet Joseph Smith*, Salt Lake City: Deseret Book Co., 1972, pp. 342-62.)

The Perspective

Now you may be saying, "Okay, so what does this have to do

with me and my perspective of life?" You will have to help me now by letting me use your imagination. Imaginations are wonderful things. When I mention the word *elephant* you can close your eyes and actually picture an elephant in your mind.

But I don't want you to picture an elephant; I want you to picture yourself in this premortal world we have been speaking of. Go back even before your spirit birth. I don't believe that it is inconsistent with the eternal law of free agency to believe that you were able to see into the far distant future to that goal of becoming an exalted being. There were challenges to meet, hurdles and tests to overcome in order for you to move forward. For countless thousands of years, perhaps, you overcame each obstacle, and while there may have been some setbacks, by exerting great effort you moved forward. You followed the path; you kept the laws that allowed you to move forward to the next stage of your eternal journey.

Is it possible to imagine the joy that welled up in your heart when Heavenly Parents finally gave you a spirit body to house the intelligent "ego" of your previous existence? Can you slightly comprehend the love that grew and filled your being for those pure, perfect Parents who nurtured you to spiritual maturity? However, even there in the presence of your Heavenly Father it wasn't easy to do everything right. Free agency again allowed you to choose the path you would follow. There were laws to obey, tasks to be performed, and lessons to learn.

We have no way of knowing just how long we were involved in this process of progression as spirit children of Heavenly Parents, but the indications are that, judged by our earthly standards of time, it was an immense period. Our Father had in mind for us a much shorter span of life in mortality. The scriptures indicate that one day after the manner of the Lord's reckoning is equal to a thousand years of earthly time. (Abraham 3:4.) On a proportionate basis that would mean that a mortal span of, say, eighty years would correspond to about two hours of the Lord's time. This is of course rather a crude comparison, but it has considerable validity for our present purpose.

We can imagine the great excitement that swept through Father's family when it was heard that a great council was being called. Perhaps we were ready to gain bodies — and to have our faithfulness tested. Maybe the time had come! You were thrilled with our Father's words, which may have sounded something like this:

"Children, the time has come for you to receive one final test — perhaps the hardest test of all. We will make an earth for you to dwell on. There you will no longer be in my presence. And we will prove you thereby to see if you will do everything I command you to do.

"But you will have to keep my commandments based only upon faith and the inspiration of the Holy Spirit that I will send to help guide you. By meeting and overcoming opposition, conflict, pain, hardship, and suffering, you will develop humility, long-suffering, patience, control over the physical appetites, and the other qualities of character that will help you to become like me."

I'm sure you were astonished when Lucifer stood in opposition to the Father's plan. But Jehovah, our beloved Elder Brother, the first-born of the Father, stood in support of the Father and volunteered to go upon the earth, suffer for the sins of his brothers and sisters, and redeem those that would stray from the path. Many followed Lucifer because his plan was easy and safe. But you followed Jehovah.

Satan and his followers then rebelled and were subsequently cast out. After this great contest, Father had Jehovah lay the foundation of the earth. You were among the sons of God who shouted for joy and the daughters of our God who sang together on that occasion. The test was soon at hand. It would be difficult, but you knew you would be faithful, *for it was only going to last two hours of God's time. You could endure anything for two hours*.

Just prior to your coming, Father probably warned you of the great power that Satan and his angels would have in the earth. He warned that Satan would use glamorous enticements to try to distract you from the way. Your answer may have been; "But, Father, it is for such a short time. Surely I won't fall in just two hours of being tested. I would be willing to endure anything for two hours just to have the privilege of becoming like you. Anything — blindness, disease, loss of loved ones, pain, suffering, anything. I know that my love for you will carry me through."

And so here you are. The very fact that you are here tells me that for an eternity of years before this you have walked the strait and narrow path; you have climbed upward step by step, not looking backward; for countless ages you have added success to success, faithfulness to faithfulness. *Here you are at the last test; the final examination*. Most college final exams are two hours long, aren't they? What you do here and now determines everything that follows. Your efforts, strivings, and successes over the countless thousands of years gone on before hangs in the balance. What will you do with this test?

Now do you see why the Brethren feel as they do? Some years

back, in an early morning seminary instructors' manual, President Spencer W. Kimball counseled the youth of the Church in this way:

> Do you see why the spiritual should not be made second to temporal, why sacrament meeting, Sunday School, seminary and priesthood assignments should not be placed second to scholastic achievement? Why working to build the Kingdom should not be second to professional success, material wealth, or social prominence? Why temple marriage takes absolute priority over civil marriage? Why doing what the crowd does is of much less importance than doing what is right? Why necking, petting, vulgarity, profanity, and fornication are to be avoided at all costs? Why we should accept and not refuse the calls of the priesthood to go on missions and to other areas of service within the Kingdom?

These words of the prophet to the youth of the Church need little change to be applied to adults. Perhaps a few additional words may be substituted, like home teaching, family home evening, genealogy, willingness to sacrifice in all things.

And so here we are looking through the glass darkly. Somehow we don't seem to remember the love we had for our Father and our Elder Brother. Somehow it doesn't seem quite so important to follow in every detail the counsel of our leaders. We find it easy to justify what we want to do rather than what God has asked us to do. In fact, the final exam is just a little harder than we thought it would be.

But do you see that everything you have worked for throughout an eternity hangs in the balance? It is the final test. It is so short. And it is worth every effort.

Index

on spiritual rebirth, 12
McKay, David O.
  on nature of man, 33
  testimony of, 1
McKinlay, Lynn A., on broken heart, 41
Mercy, justice, and punishment, 45-46
Mormon, on spiritual rebirth, 53-54
Moroni
  on sin, 32
  on testimony, 4
Mosaic law, 66

-N-

Nature of man, 32-36
  Abinadi on, 33
  David O. McKay on, 33
  Spencer W. Kimball on, 34
Nephi
  on baptism of fire, 13, 26
  on grace, 68
  on remission of sins by fire, 13, 17-18
  on sin, 31
  and spiritual rebirth, 13
  and worthiness, 34-35
Nicodemus, and salvation, 10

-O-

Obedience, 38, 65-68
  and witness of the Spirit, 6

-P-

Pace, George W., 47
Paul
  on baptism, 26
  on faith, 2
  on sin, 66-67
Peter
  and cleansing power of Christ, 51
  on gift of the Holy Ghost, 25
  and spiritual rebirth, 18-20
Pratt, Orson, on baptism of fire, 14-15
Pratt, Parley P., on spiritual rebirth, 21
Premortal existence, 72-75
Punishment, justice, and mercy, 45-46

-R-

Rebirth, spiritual. See Birth of the Spirit
Repentance, 29-51, 66
  and forgetting of sins, 51
  grand key to, 40
  preliminary requirements to, 38-39
  Spencer W. Kimball on, 38-39
Roberts, B. H., on spiritual rebirth, 15-16
Romney, Marion G., 50
  on birth of the Spirit, 6-7
  on conversion, 17
  on spiritual rebirth, 21

-S-

Sacrifice
  and faith, 3
  Joseph Smith on, 9-10
  as key to repentance, 40
Salvation, Abinadi on, 66, 68
Sanctification
  Alma on, 13, 38
  Enoch on, 25-26
Satan, 75
Savior. See Jesus Christ
Selfishness, 35
Self-justification, 30-32
Sin
  cleansing from, 68-69
  definition of, 65
  effects of, 37
Smith, Joseph, 54
  on law, 67
  and making calling and election sure, 7
  revelation to, on spirit of man, 73
  on sacrifice, 9
  and suffering of Christ, 43
Smith, Joseph F.
  on forgiveness, 52
  and gift of the Holy Ghost, 16-17
Smith, Joseph Fielding
  on justice, 46
  on suffering of Christ, 42
Snow, Lorenzo, on spiritual rebirth, 21-22
Spirit, birth of. See Birth of the Spirit
Spirit, gifts of. See Gifts of the Spirit
Spiritual rebirth. See Birth of the Spirit
Spirit, witness of. See Witness of the Spirit

Standard of righteousness, 35, 36-37

-T-

Talmage, James E.
  on power of the Holy Ghost, 14
  on redemption, 55-56
  on suffering of Christ, 43-44
Testimony
  definition of, 1

of faith, 2-4
  intellectual, 2
  Moroni on, 4
Thompson, Stephen, and witness of the
  Spirit, 4-5
Tithing, 35

-W-

Witness of the Spirit, 4-6

Book designed by Bailey-Montague and Associates
Composed by Column Type
in Palatino with display lines in Palatino Italic
Printed by Publishers Press
on 70# Publishers Smooth Offset
Bound by Mountain States Bindery
in Kivar 5, Midnight Blue, Skiver